Clinical Immunology

Catherine Sheehan, MS, CLS, SI

Associate Professor
Department of Medical Laboratory Science
College of Arts and Sciences
Southeastern Massachusetts University
North Dartmouth, Massachusetts

Clinical Immunology
Principles and Laboratory Diagnosis

With 9 Contributors

J. B. Lippincott Company

Philadelphia

Grand Rapids
New York   London
St. Louis   Sydney
San Francisco   Tokyo

Project Editor: Melissa B. McElroy
Indexer: Katherine Pitcoff
Design Coordinator: Ellen C. Dawson
Cover and Interior Designer: Liz Doles
Production Manager: Carol A. Florence
Production Coordinator: Caren Erlichman
Compositor: Tapsco, Inc.
Printer/Binder: R. R. Donnelley & Sons Company

6   4   2   1   3   5

Library of Congress Cataloging in Publication Data
Clinical immunology.

  Includes bibliographical references.
    1. Immunodiagnosis.   2. Immunology.   I. Sheehan,
Catherine.   [DNLM: 1. Diagnosis, Laboratory.   2. Immune
System.   3. Immunity.   4. Immunologic Diseases.
QW 504 C6418]
RB46.5.C546   1990   616.07′56   89-12882
ISBN 0-397-54809-5

Any procedure or practice described in this book should be applied by
the health-care practitioner under appropriate supervision in accordance with professional standards of care used with regard to the
unique circumstances that apply in each practice situation. Care has
been taken to confirm the accuracy of information presented and to
describe generally accepted practices. However, the authors, editors,
and publisher cannot accept any responsibility for errors or omissions
or for any consequences from application of the information in this book
and make no warranty, express or implied, with respect to the contents
of the book.

Every effort has been made to ensure drug selections and dosages are
in accordance with current recommendations and practice. Because of
ongoing research, changes in government regulations and the constant
flow of information on drug therapy, reactions, and interactions, the
reader is cautioned to check the package insert for each drug for
indications, dosages, warnings, and precautions, particularly if the
drug is new or infrequently used.

Dedication

To my family and friends for their support and encouragement.

Preface

Clinical Immunology: Principles and Laboratory Diagnosis was developed for students and practitioners in health-related programs who are interested in basic concepts of human immunology and its application to diagnostic testing. Although this book assumes little or no previous exposure to immunologic concepts, it does assume some understanding of related sciences, such as genetics, anatomy, physiology, microbiology, and chemistry. Experimental aspects of immunology are minimized, and immunologic principles of laboratory diagnosis in human disease are emphasized. The book is intended for clinical laboratory science students in 2- or 4-year programs and in hospital- or college-based programs, practicing laboratorians who wish to update their knowledge of immunology and serology, and other health professionals.

The text is divided into three sections. The first is a discussion of immune reactions by the human host in response to a challenge. It addresses fundamental mechanisms of the immune system, such as antigen recognition, self versus nonself, expected specific and nonspecific reactions, tumor surveillance, and hypersensitivity. The second section is an in-depth discussion of antigens and antibodies and their interaction in serologic testing. It addresses the principles of *in vitro* serologic reactions and the sources of error and quality control in testing; however, it is not designed to be a procedure manual. It is intended that the concepts of serologic methods can be applied to specific serologic tests used to diagnose or monitor immunologically mediated diseases. The final section is a discussion of immunologic diseases in which measurement of an immune product or reaction is a significant tool for diagnosing or monitoring the disease.

Though immunology is a rapidly changing field, all attempts have been made to ensure that the information presented is current.

I wish to thank the reviewers who made critical suggestions for improvements in the text: Hendrik Bogaars, Richard Goldschmidt, and Eva Quinley. Special thanks to Shirley Haley for her expert manuscript review, and to Elizabeth Lecour for her assistance in creating the glossary. My sincere appreciation to Jim Feeley, Diane Abeloff, and Marion Poisson for preparing the illustrations in this book. Finally, through their suggestions and by expressing their needs, clinical laboratory science students have encouraged the writing of this book.

Catherine Sheehan, MS, CLS, SI

Contributors

Ann C. Albers, PhD
  Chairman and Associate Professor
  Department of Medical Technology
  School of Health Related Professions
  University of Pittsburgh
  Pittsburgh, Pennsylvania

Alice K. Chen, PhD
  Associate Professor
  Department of Medical Technology
  School of Health Related Professions
  University of Pittsburgh
  Pittsburgh, Pennsylvania

Suio-Ling Chen, PhD
  Surgery Research
  Cleveland Metro-General Hospital
  Cleveland, Ohio

Therese B. Datiles, MA
  Supervisor
  Diagnostic Immunology Laboratory
  Department of Laboratory Medicine
  The Johns Hopkins Hospital
  Baltimore, Maryland

Dorothy J. Fike, MS, MT (ASCP), SBB
  Assistant Professor
  Department of Medical Technology
  School of Allied Health Professions
  Medical College of Virginia Campus
  Virginia Commonwealth University
  Richmond, Virginia

Richard L. Humphrey, MD
  Departments of Medicine and
    Laboratory Medicine
  The Johns Hopkins Oncology Center
  The Johns Hopkins Hospital
  Baltimore, Maryland

Karen James, PhD, MT (ASCP)
  Associate Director of Laboratories
  Central DuPage Hospital
  Winfield, Illinois
  Immunology Consultant
  Loyola University Medical Center
  Maywood, Illinois

Rosemarie Matuscak, PhD, MT (ASCP)
  Assistant Professor
  Department of Medical Technology
  School of Health Related Professions
  University of Pittsburgh
  Pittsburgh, Pennsylvania

Ann Marie McNamara, ScD, MT
    (ASCP)
  Formerly:
  Post-Doctoral Resident in Medical
    and Public Health Microbiology
    Laboratory
  Centers for Disease Control
  Atlanta, Georgia
  Currently:
  Associate Director for Scientific
    Affairs
  Biotechnology Services Division
  Microbiological Associates, Inc.
  Rockville, Maryland

Contents

Clinical Immunology

CHAPTER 1

The Scope of Immunology

Catherine Sheehan

Definition of Immunology

Immunology is the study of the mechanisms that protect an individual from injury. The immunologic response constitutes a broad range of defense mechanisms from preventing and combatting infection from microorganisms to surveillance to identify and eliminate aberrant host cells that may develop into neoplasms. Any challenge to the integrity of the individual, such as irritating substances, toxins, infectious agents, and neoplastic cells, activates appropriate immunologic mechanisms, including inflammation, phagocytosis, antibody synthesis, or T-lymphocyte activation, to eliminate these challenges.

Two types of immunity, innate and adaptive, comprise the immunologic response by the host (Table 1-1). Innate immunity is present from birth in all individuals and is activated in the same manner each time the individual is exposed to a challenge. For each exposure, regardless of the challenge encountered, the mechanisms are the same. On the other hand, adaptive immunity is acquired or learned by an individual *only* when challenges are encountered. The resulting adaptive immunity is specific for the stimulating challenge and is remembered during subsequent challenges.

Innate immunity is the first defense against challenging organisms from the environment. The mechanisms are nonspecific and are ready to be used any time, without delay. The physical barrier of the skin and mucous membranes, for instance, provides the first line of defense from invading organisms by preventing their entry.

Physiologic innate immunity prevents the likelihood of infection by providing an unfavorable environment for the infective organism: the high acidity of the stomach destroys most ingested organisms; the tearing action of the eye flushes foreign material from the eye; the flow of urine prevents bacterial infection of the lower urinary tract; and cilia and mucus of the respiratory tract remove particulate matter that enters from the air.

Table 1-1: Types of Immunity

Innate immunity

Adaptive immunity

Humoral immunity

Cell-mediated immunity

Age and nutritional status also influence immunity; children and older people are more susceptible to certain infections, such as *Escherichia coli* sepsis in the newborn and *Streptococcus pneumoniae* pneumonia in older people. Poor nutrition may adversely influence the immune system to respond to a challenge.

Chemicals secreted by cells also contribute to innate immunity. Lysozyme, an enzyme found in secretions, disrupts the cell wall of bacteria, thus killing the organism. Skin secretions, such as lactic acid and saturated fatty acids, provide resistance to some bacteria and fungi. Mucoprotein in secretions prevents attachment of some viruses to cells; thus, the virus cannot enter the cell. Interferon prevents viral replication.

Should innate immunity fail to protect the individual from the challenge, adaptive mechanisms are stimulated (Table 1-2). These mechanisms are dormant until challenged; therefore, an initial response is delayed until cells are activated and produce immune products.

Table 1-2: Routes of Adaptive Immunity

Active immunity—the host cells produce immune products to generate protection

Passive immunity—preformed immune products are administered to provide protection

Adoptive immunity—immunocompetent cells are administered to reconstitute the immune system

mune products. The adaptive immune response is specific for the challenge, and memory is generated for the stimulus, resulting in a more intense and faster immune response on reexposure to the challenge. Sometimes products of the microorganisms, such as toxins or enzymes, stimulate the adaptive response, thus expanding the diversity of response to a single organism.

Humoral immunity is the form of adaptive immunity in which B lymphocytes and plasma cells produce specific antibodies that recognize and react to a challenge. Antibody is particularly effective in eliminating bacteria.

Cell-mediated immunity is the second form of adaptive immunity where T lymphocytes recognize aberrant host cells, transplanted cells, and foreign organisms and initiate a cellular response through chemical mediators called lymphokines. The cell-mediated response is especially effective in eliminating viruses, fungi, mycobacteria, and tumor cells and in rejecting tissue grafts.

Adaptive immunity may be acquired in three ways. *Active immunity* is generated when an immunocompetent individual is exposed to a foreign challenge and initiates an immune response. *Passive immunity* is acquired when preformed immune products, such as antibodies, sensitized lymphocytes, and lymphokines, are administered to the individual. In *adoptive immunity*, immunocompetent cells are transferred to an immunoincompetent individual who is unable to generate immune products.

Active adaptive immunity requires that the cells of the immune system interact with the stimulating agent. The result is the production of antibodies, sensitized lymphocytes, and lymphokines. These immune products eliminate the stimulating agent and usually provide lifelong immunity. Active immunity requires competent lymphocytes to generate immune products that are specific for the challenge. Exposure to the stimulating agent occurs from natural infection or from immunization. Ideally, if an individual is infected with the live rubella virus or is immunized with the live attenuated rubella virus, the result should be the same—the stimulation of humoral and cellular adaptive mechanisms to generate protection.

Passive immunity occurs when immune products, most often antibody preparations known as immune globulin, are administered to an individual. In this way, immediate protection is provided; active immunity may take weeks to develop. For example, when an individual has been exposed to the hepatitis B virus, hepatitis B immune globulin is administered immediately to prevent hepatitis B infection.

Adoptive immunity is reserved for immunodeficient individuals. When immunocompetent cells or tissue are transplanted into an immunoincompetent individual, the cells or tissue may reconstitute the immune system. This allows the individual to respond to future challenges by initiating an active immune response.

Scope of Immunology

Currently, immunology is divided into 11 main areas of study, some of which overlap; they will be covered in the remainder of the book.[1]

Allergy and hypersensitivity refer to the deleterious effects when the immune responses are exaggerated (Chapters 6 and 27). Autoimmunity is the failure of the immune system to tolerate "self," and immune reactions directed against "self" (Chapter 29). Cancer immunology is the study of tumor antigens and the immunologic response to tumors (Chapter 7). Cellular immunology investigates lymphocytes and lymphoid organs involved in the immune response (Chapters 3, 4, 5, 17, 26, and 28). Immunochemistry studies immunoassays and antigen–antibody interactions (Chapters 10, 11, 12, 13, 14, 15, 16, and 17). Immunogenetics is primarily concerned with the genetic control of immune responses (Chapter 2). Immunohematology is the study of blood groups. Immunopathology is the study of organ damage by immune products or processes. Microbial immunology studies the antigens of bacteria, viruses, and other parasites and the development of vaccines (Chapter 18, 19, 20, 21, 22, 23, and 24). Molecular immunology analyzes the structure of antigens, antibodies, and complement (Chapters 5, 8, 9, and 25). Transplantation investigates tissue typing, graft rejection, and immunologic tolerance (Chapter 2).

References

1. Nicholas R, Nicholas D: Immunology: An information profile. Mansell Publishing, London, 1985, p 11.

CHAPTER 2

Major Histocompatibility Complex

Dorothy J. Fike

The major histocompatibility complex (MHC) is one of the most genetically diverse regions in the human genome. Differences were first recognized in the 1950s, when leukocyte agglutinating antibodies were found in some multiply transfused individuals and multiparous women. Because the antigens were expressed on leukocytes, they were called human leukocyte antigens (HLA). The MHC has been found to be important in transplantation, disease associations, and more recently, the regulation of the immune response during antigen presentation.[1] Since 1968 the HLA Nomenclature Committee of the World Health Organization has met every few years to revise and update the definition of antigens included in the MHC.

MHC Antigens

The MHC region in humans is located on the short arm of chromosome 6 (Fig. 2-1).[2] There are 10 distinct genetic areas located in the MHC: HLA-A, -B, -C, -E, -D/DR, -DQ, -DP, -DN, -DO, and [C2, C4, and Bf]. Each gene yields a specific product. The gene complex yields three classes of antigen products. Class I antigens are cellular proteins and include the HLA-A, -B, and -C antigens. Class II antigens are also cellular proteins and are named HLA-D/DR, -DQ, and -DP. Class III antigens, considered minor MHC antigens, are proteins principally secreted by cells and are complement components, C2, C4, and Factor B.

The class I antigen is a single glycoprotein chain composed of 338 amino acids with a molecular weight of 44,000 d. Most of this protein is on the outer surface of the cell membrane (281 amino acids), but a small portion passes through the cell membrane (25 amino acids) and into the interior of the cell (32 amino acids) (Fig. 2-2). A second protein, β_2 microglobulin, is loosely associated with class I antigens.

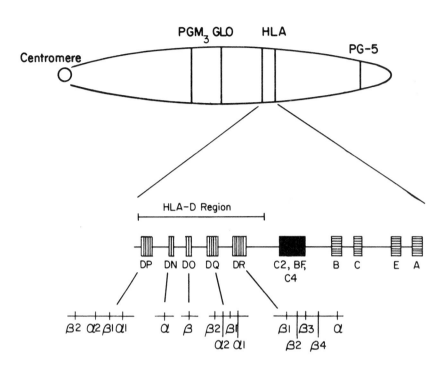

FIGURE 2-1. The major histocompability complex (MHC) is located on the short arm of chromosome 6 between glyoxylase (GLO) and urinary pepsinogen (PG 5) genes. The gene for phosphoglucomutase 3 (PGM 3) is located near the GLO gene. There are three classes of genes located in the MHC. The HLA-A, -B, -C, and -E loci are class I genes (▤). Class II genes (▥) are the HLA-D, -DR, -DP, -DQ, -DN, and -DO loci. In the HLA-DR, -DP, and -DQ loci there are genes for both α and β polypeptide chains necessary for the protein. The class III genes (■) code for complement proteins (C2, C4, and Factor B). Though HLA-E, -DN, and -DO have been described, little is known about them.

Class I antigens are found on almost all nucleated cells and are recognized in graft rejection.[1] Some class I remnants have been found on red cells,[3] though these remnants are not usually involved with transfusion reactions.

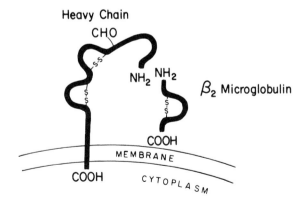

FIGURE 2-2. The class I antigens are transmembrane proteins with the majority of the amino acids on the exterior of the membrane. β_2 microglobulin is associated with the class I molecule.

The class II antigen is composed of two glycoprotein chains, α and β, both of which contain a transmembrane region. The α chain has a molecular weight of 34,000 d and the β chain, one of 29,000 d. (Fig. 2-3).[1] The α and β chains are not covalently bound to each other but are located next to each other on the cell membrane. Since both the chains are transmembrane, they can function together. Each glycoprotein chain is encoded in the MHC locus; multiple alleles exist for different α and β chains for each class II antigen. The DR subregion is composed of four genes: One gene codes for the α chain and three different genes code for β chains. All HLA-DR molecules share the same α chain, which can combine with any β chain. The DP and DQ subregions have two α- and two β-chain genes. It appears that the α chain of one subregion can only combine with the β chain of the same subregion.

The class II antigens, unlike class I antigens, are not found on all nucleated cells. Class II antigens are restricted to immunocompetent cells, particularly B

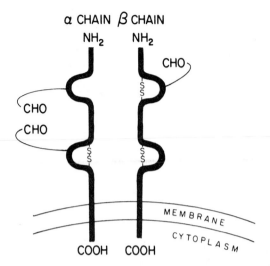

FIGURE 2-3. The class II antigens are two transmembrane proteins. Each antigen has an α and β chain. As with the class I antigens, the majority of the protein is on the cell exterior.

cells and macrophages. These antigens are important for antigen presentation and interactions between immunocompetent cells.

Class III antigens are serum complement components (see Chapter 5) that activate complement factor 3 (C3) by either the classical or alternative pathway.[4] Factor B activates C3 in the alternative pathway, and C2 with C4 activate C3 in the classical pathway. The polymorphism of these antigens is less than that of the class I and class II antigens.

Each of the class I and class II gene complexes has several alleles (gene variants), a partial listing may be seen in Table 2-1. Those antigens (alleles) with a "w" designation are antigens that have not been completely confirmed as a single specific antigen by the World Health Organization's HLA Nomenclature Committee.[5] Early detection of HLA-A and -B antigens used serum from multiply transfused individuals or multiparous women. These sera were not "pure" antibodies, but a mixture of different HLA antibodies. What was originally thought to be one antigen recognized by a specific antiserum

may now be known to be more than one. These antigens are known as "splits"; the original designation is listed in brackets in Table 2-1. HLA-D antigens may not be a unique set of antigens but may be a designation based on the testing procedure. Further studies are being conducted to better define the HLA-D antigens.

HLA Antigen Detection

The HLA antigens are detected by three distinct methods. HLA-A, -B, and -C antigens are serologically defined antigens and may be detected using the lymphocyte cytotoxicity procedure. This procedure uses lymphocytes and known antisera in the presence of complement. If the antigen is present on the lymphocyte, the cells will be lysed, allowing a dye to enter the cell.[1] This procedure, developed by Terasaki, is more completely described in Chapter 17. HLA-DR and -DQ antigens are detected by the modified lymphocyte cytotoxicity procedure in which purified B lymphocytes are used instead of a mixture of lymphocytes used to detect HLA-A, -B, and -C antigens.[6]

The HLA-D antigens are determined by the one-way mixed-lymphocyte culture (MLC). Since serologic reagents are unavailable, this procedure requires cellular typing reagents. Homozygous typing cells have a single known HLA-D antigen expressed on their surface and serve as the source of HLA-D antigen. These stimulator cells are irradiated or treated with mitomycin to prevent them from responding in the assay. The patient lymphocytes express HLA-D antigens to be detected and are the responder cells in the assay. After incubating these two cell populations, the responder cell will react to the stimulator cell if the responder cell does not express the HLA-D antigen found on the stimulator cell. The responder cell becomes activated and undergoes cell division. A radiolabeled nucleic acid precursor, tritiated thymidine, included in the media, is

Table 2-1: Partial Listing of HLA Specificities as of November, 1987

HLA-A	HLA-B	HLA-C	HLA-D	HLA-DR	HLA-DP	HLA-DQ
A1	Bw4	Cw1	Dw1	DR1	DPw1	DQw1
A2	B5	Cw2	Dw2	DR2	DPw2	DQw2
A3	Bw6	Cw3	Dw3	DR3	DPw3	DQw3
A9	B7	Cw4	Dw4	DR4	DPw4	DQw4
A10	B8	Cw5	Dw5	DR5	DPw5	DQw5 [w1]
A11	B12	Cw6	Dw6	DRw6	DPw6	DQw6 [w1]
A23 [9]	B13	Cw7	Dw7	DRw11 [5]		DQw7 [w3]
A24 [9]	B14	Cw8	Dw8	DRw12 [5]		DQw8 [w3]
A25 [10]	B15	Cw9 [w3]	Dw9	DRw13 [w6]		DQw9 [w3]
A26 [10]	B16	Cw10 [w3]	Dw18 [w6]	DRw14 [w6]		
A28	B27	Cw11	Dw19 [w6]	DRw15 [2]		
Aw34 [10]	B38 [16]		Dw20	DRw16 [2]		
Aw36	B39 [16]		Dw21	DRw17 [3]		
Aw66 [10]	Bw41		Dw22	DRw18 [3]		
Aw69 [28]	Bw44 [12]		Dw23	DRw52		
Aw74	Bw45 [12]		Dw24	DRw53		
Minimum of 24 antigens	Bw73		Dw25	Minimum of 20 antigens		
	Bw75		Dw26			
	Bw76		Minimum of 26 antigens			
	Bw77					
	Minimum of 52 antigens					

There are seven HLA antigens with many alleles at each locus. HLA-A and -B antigens were the first to be discovered and are numbered consecutively between the two. HLA-C, -D, -DR, -DP, and -DQ antigens are numbered consecutively for each antigen. w indicates a workshop antigen that is provisionally accepted, though not yet completely characterized. A number in brackets refers to the original broad designation of the antigen; with further study the broad designation was divided into separate antigens, called splits.

incorporated into the actively dividing cells and can be measured. In many instances, HLA-D antigen detection leads to better organ matching and improved graft survival.[7] More details about the MLC are found in Chapter 17, "Cellular Assays."

The HLA-DP antigens are detected using the primed lymphocyte typing. Cells matched for other HLA antigens are allowed to react in a mixed lymphocyte reaction with stimulator cells. These primed cells are allowed to react in a second MLC with irradiated unknown cells to determine if the unknown cells will cause a response.[1,6]

Inheritance of HLA

The genetic information in the HLA region is closely linked, so that it is inherited as a unit, the haplotype. An individual inherits two HLA haplotypes, each containing an allele for each HLA gene. One haplotype is inherited from the mother; the other is inherited from the father. HLA genes are codominant so that both alleles are expressed. The gene product is the class I or class II antigen that is expressed on the surface of the cell. When antigen typing is performed on an individual, it is impossible to determine which genes are inherited as a haplotype, since each antigen is detected individually. For example, the antigens detected could be HLA-A2 and 10, and HLA-B5 and 12. The possible haplotypes would be HLA-A2 associated with HLA-B5 and HLA-A10 with HLA-B12; or HLA-A2 could be linked with HLA-B12, and HLA-A10 with HLA-B5 (Fig. 2-4). In some cases when an individual is typed, only one antigen at a particular locus will be detected (i.e., HLA-A1 or HLA-B8) instead of the expected two.

ANTIGENS TYPED

HLA-A2, 10   HLA-B5, 12

Possibility 1

HAPLOTYPE 1   HLA-A2, -B5
HAPLOTYPE 2   HLA-A10, -B12

Possibility 2

HAPLOTYPE 1   HLA-A2, -B12
HAPLOTYPE 2   HLA-A10, -B5

FIGURE 2-4. In HLA typing the presence of the HLA-A and -B antigens is determined. On each chromosome there is only one HLA-A and one HLA-B gene. Family studies are necessary to determine the actual haplotype.

This lack of expression at a locus is known as a blank. It could be that the individual has inherited the same gene from both parents or that there is an additional antigen present at the locus that cannot be detected by currently available methods.

To determine the antigens of a particular haplotype, family studies must be done. Ideally, at least two generations would be typed to aid in differentiating a blank from duplicate alleles or methodology failure. The following example shows results obtained from a family that had been typed for the HLA-A and HLA-B antigens:

Father	HLA-A2,10; HLA-B5,12
Mother	HLA-A9,10; HLA-B8,16
First child	HLA-A2,9; HLA-B5,16
Second child	HLA-A2,10; HLA-B5,8
Third child	HLA-A10; HLA-B8,12

Looking at the results for the first child and the parents, the first child must have inherited HLA-A2 and HLA-B5 from the father, since the mother does not have these genes. Therefore, one of the haplotypes of the first child is HLA-A2,-B5. The other haplotype of the first child must be HLA-A9,-B16, which must be inherited from the mother (Fig. 2-5). Since one haplotype of the father is HLA-A2,-B5, the second haplotype must be HLA-A10,-B12. The mother's haplotypes are HLA-A9,-B16 and HLA-A10,-B8. The second child inherited haplotype HLA-A2,-B5 from the father and HLA-A10,-B8 from the mother. The third child inherited a blank in the HLA-A locus, since only one HLA-A antigen was detected. Since both parents have the HLA-A10 antigen, this child has two HLA-A10 genes. This child's haplotypes are HLA-A10,-B12 from the father and HLA-A10,-B8 from the mother.

Sometimes the inheritance pattern in a family may not exhibit the expected haplotypes. This may be due to chiasmata, or crossing over, of genetic material (genes coding for the antigen) from one chromosome to the sister chromosome. The process of crossing over occurs during cell division (either

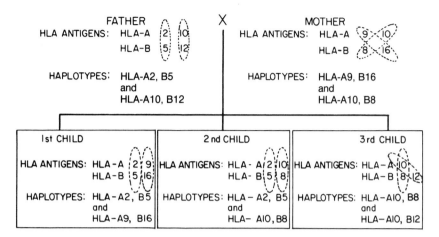

FIGURE 2-5. The HLA antigens have been determined in this family. Since one HLA-A antigen and one HLA-B antigen is inherited from each parent, the haplotypes of each may be determined. Child 1 received HLA-A2, -B5 from the father and HLA-A9, -B16 from the mother. Child 3 has only one HLA-A antigen that was inherited from both parents. Since there is only one HLA-A and one HLA-B antigen inherited on a single chromosome, the haplotypes of the parents may be determined by the combination of HLA-A and -B antigens inherited by the children. The dotted lines around the antigens indicate which antigens are inherited together.

mitosis or meiosis), when the chromosomes line up on the spindle fiber. In the previous example, if the second child had typed as HLA-A2,10 and HLA-B8,12 instead of HLA-A2,10 and HLA-B5,8, the haplotype from the father would be HLA-A2,-B12 instead of HLA-A2,-B8 (Fig. 2-6). Since the haplotype from the father using the results of the first child is HLA-A2,-B5 and HLA-A2,-B12 and the results from the second child are HLA-A2,-B8 and HLA-A2,-B12, this suggests crossing over. What are the haplotypes of the father? The haplotypes could be HLA-A2,-B5 and HLA-A10,-B12 or HLA-A2,-B12 and HLA-A10,-B5. Since the third child inherited HLA-A10,-B12 from the father, it might be assumed that the crossing over occurred in the second child. This might be an error; the crossing over might have occurred in both the first and third children. To determine the father's true haplotypes, one must HLA-type his parents or siblings. Crossing over can

occur between the haplotypes of the mother or father, or it can occur in both parents.

HLA typing has been used to determine the parentage of an individual. Since the HLA loci are highly polymorphic, a greater number of parental exclusions can be made.[8] In parentage testing, a person can only be excluded from being the parent; it can never be said that a person is definitely the parent. Parentage testing may be done to determine paternity, to identify kidnapped children, to use in immigration, and to resolve questions of inheritance. In cases of paternity, the putative (accused or alleged) father, mother, and child are typed. Analyzing the results of the child and comparing them with those of the alleged father and with the mother can result in the evidence to exclude the man as the true biologic father. For example, the putative father typed as HLA-A3,11 and HLA-B5,7, the mother typed as HLA-A2,28 and HLA-B12,14, and the child typed as

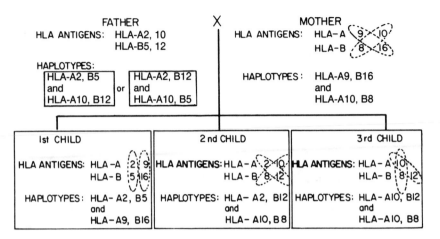

FIGURE 2-6. In some cases the haplotype of a parent may not be determined, since crossing over (chiasmata) has occurred. The same HLA-A and -B antigens are not paired together in the children. The antigens of the parents and children 1 and 3 are the same as those found in Fig. 2-5. In this figure child 2 has inherited the HLA-A2 and -A10 antigens and the HLA-B8 and -B12 antigens. The haplotypes may be determined as HLA-A2, -B12 from the father and HLA-A10, -B8 from the mother. Comparing child 1 and child 2, the HLA-A2 antigen is inherited with both the HLA-B5 and -B12 antigens.

HLA-A2,3 and HLA-B13,14. In this case the putative father may be excluded from paternity, since the child has the HLA-B13 antigen and the mother does not. The antigen must be inherited from the biologic father (Fig. 2-7). Since the putative father does not express HLA-B13, he can be excluded as the father. If the child had typed as HLA-A2,3 and HLA-B5,14, the putative father could not be excluded on the basis of HLA typing. HLA is one of many inherited phenotypic expressions used to determine parentage.[9]

A. EXCLUSION

"Putative Father"	HLA-A3, 11; HLA-B5, 7
Mother	HLA-A2, 28; HLA-B12, 14
Child	HLA-A2, 3; HLA-**B13**, 14

B. NONEXCLUSION

"Putative Father"	HLA-A3, 11; HLA-B5, 7
Mother	HLA-A2, 28; HLA-B12, 14
Child	HLA-A2, 3; HLA-B5, 14

FIGURE 2-7. The HLA antigens may be used to determine parentage. The child in example A has the HLA-B13 antigen that neither parent has. The "putative father" may be excluded in this example. In example B the child's HLA-B5 antigen may have been inherited from the "putative father," so he may not be excluded from paternity.

Transplantation

Almost all organs and tissues in the body may be successfully transplanted from one individual to another (Table 2-2).[10] If the individuals are from the same species but genetically different, the type of transplant is an allograft. This is the most common type of transplant performed in humans. Other types of transplants are xenograft (a graft between individuals of different species), autograft (tissue grafted back to the original donor), and isograft (a graft between genetically identical individuals) (Table 2-3). An example of a xenograft is a graft between a baboon and a human, performed recently

Table 2-2: Organs/Tissues Transplanted

Organ/Tissue	Reason	HLA Antigens Typed
Kidney	End stage renal disease	Yes (HLA-A, -B, -C, -DR, -DQ)
Heart (Heart–lung)	End stage cardiac impairment refractory to medical management	None (due to time constraints)
Liver	Hepatic dysfunction in both synthetic and regulatory ability	None ("privileged" site)
Pancreas	Improve quality of life for diabetics and prevent vascular changes associated with diabetes mellitis	Yes
Skin	Burns	None (usually an autograft)
Bone	To promote healing of un-united fractures, to restore structural integrity and to facilitate cosmetic repair	None (some are autografts; allografts use frozen bones whenever possible to reduce immunogenicity)
Cornea	Diseased corneas	None ("privileged" site)
Bone marrow	Advanced leukemia, severe combined immunodeficiency disease, and aplastic anemia	Yes (HLA-A, -B, -C, -DR, -DQ)
Fetal adrenal tissue	Tic LaRue	None (antigens not developed)

Several organs and tissues may be transplanted. Organ transplantation is performed in individuals with diseases that destroy or damage the tissue/organ and render it nonfunctional. The type of tissue or organ determines which, if any, of the HLA antigens that are typed.

when Baby Fay received a baboon heart. An example of an autograft is the use of skin from one area of an individual to replace burned skin. An example of an isograft would be an identical twin receiving an organ or tissue from the other twin.[11]

Isografts and autografts are usually accepted by the recipient and do not result in rejection because all donor tissue antigens are the same as the recipient and no antigens are recognized as different. Allograft transplantation requires ABO and HLA typing. In most cases, the HLA typing to be performed is for the HLA-A, -B, -C, -DR, and -DQ antigens.[10] The organ to be transplanted dictates the HLA antigens to be tested. Organs vary in the quantity of HLA antigen expressed on the cell surface. In some cases,

the organ must be transplanted before HLA typing can be performed. In these cases, the organ must at least be ABO compatible.

The ABO antigens are found on red cells and other tissues. Individuals usually have antibodies to those antigens not expressed on their tissues and blood cells (Table 2-4). These antibodies will cause an acute rejection of the transplanted tissue. For example, if a donor were blood group B and the recipient were blood group A, the group A recipient would have anti-B antibody, which will recognize the B antigen on the transplanted tissue. The graft would be rejected. Since group O donors do not express A or B antigens, tissue from this blood group may be used for any other blood group. The recipient

Table 2-3: Types of Grafts

Graft	Definition
Xenograft	Tissue transplanted between individuals of two different species
Allograft	Tissue transplanted between individuals of the same species; genetically different
Isograft	Tissue transplanted between individuals who are genetically identical
Autograft	Tissue transplanted back to the original donor

Tissues or organs may be transplanted between individuals of the same or different species.

antibodies of other blood groups will not react to the transplant, since it lacks the A and B antigens. Group O recipients must receive a transplant from a group O donor because group O recipients have anti-A and anti-B antibodies.

In an allograft if the four HLA-A and HLA-B antigens of the donor and the recipient are the same,

this is a four match. If three antigens are shared by the donor and recipient, it is a three match. If two antigens are the same and two are different, it is a two match (Table 2-5). Referring to example 1 in Fig. 2-5, evaluate the match of each child with each parent. The father and mother would both be a two match with each child. Consider the match between siblings. The first child would be a two match with the second child and a zero match with the third child. The second child would be a two match with both the first and third children. The third child would be a zero match with the first child and a two match with the second child. The father and mother would be one matches to each other (Table 2-6).

Kidney transplantation may be done with a cadaver kidney or a kidney from a living related donor. The extent of testing depends on the source of the kidney. In either situation, the donor kidney must be ABO compatible with the patient (Table 2-4). If a living related donor kidney is to be used, the HLA-A, -B, -C, -DR, and -DQ antigens should be identified for the recipient and all potential donors. The best match between the recipient and donor is the kidney of choice, since the survival rate improves as the number of shared antigens increases. If more than

Table 2-4: ABO Antigens and Antibodies

Group	Antigen Present	Antibodies Present	Able to Receive Transplant From
O	None	Anti-A Anti-B	Group O
A	A	Anti-B	Group O Group A
B	B	Anti-A	Group O Group B
AB	A and B	None	All blood groups

ABO blood groups are important in transplantation. Group O organs may be given to individuals of any blood group, but group O individuals may only receive group O organs, because the antibodies that are present will reject organs of any other blood group.

Table 2-5: HLA Antigens Shared
in Transplantation

Match	Antigens Shared
4 match	2A and 2B antigens
3 match	2A and 1B antigens or 1A and 2B antigens
2 match	1A and 1B antigen
1 match	1A or 1B antigen
0 match	No HLA antigens in common

Transplantation of organs may be matched by the number of HLA-A and
-B antigens that are shared between donor and recipient.

one donor is available, a mixed lymphocyte culture between the recipient and each donor may be performed to determine the potential for the recipient to respond to mismatched HLA-DR and -DQ antigens.[12]

If a cadaver kidney is to be transplanted, the organ must be transplanted within 48 hours. Time does not allow the mixed lymphocyte culture to be performed. The HLA-A, -B, and -C antigens of the donor are determined, and all HLA antigens in the recipient are detected, as is done for the living related donor recipient. There is a central registry for all individuals waiting for an organ transplant.[12]

When liver and hearts are transplanted, the organ must be placed in the recipient within four hours

Table 2-6: HLA Antigens Matched in a Family

Transplant		Match	Antigens Shared
DONOR	**RECIPIENT**		
Father	Mother	One match	HLA-A10
Father	Child 1	Two match	HLA-A2, -B5
Mother	Child 1	Two match	HLA-A9, -B16
Father	Child 2	Two match	HLA-A2, -B5
Mother	Child 2	Two match	HLA-A10, -B8
Father	Child 3	Two match	HLA-A10, -B12
Mother	Child 3	Two match	HLA-A10, -B8
Child 1	Child 2	Two match	HLA-A2, -B5
Child 1	Child 3	Zero match	None
Child 2	Child 1	Two match	HLA-A2, -B5
Child 2	Child 3	Two match	HLA-A10, -B8
Child 3	Child 1	Zero match	None
Child 3	Child 2	Two match	HLA-A10, -B8

These are examples of the number of HLA antigens that would be shared by family members if an organ was
transplanted between two family members found in Figure 2-5.

after removal from the donor. HLA typing is performed on the donor for heart transplants, but the recipient may not be of the same HLA type because of the availability of the recipient. HLA typing is not performed on the donor in liver transplants.[12]

Following transplantation, several drugs may be administered to prevent transplant rejection. Drugs used include corticosteroids and, depending on the allograft and tissue match, cyclosporin, cyclophosphamide, azathioprine, antilymphocyte globulin, antithymocyte globulin, and monoclonal antibodies against specific T-cell subsets. Cyclosporin is a fungal product that reduces the interleukin-2 lymphocyte activation. The use of cyclosporin has increased the survival rates of transplanted organs, particularly those found in liver transplants. Azathioprine is an antimetabolite that inhibits DNA proliferation. In graft rejection the cells of the immune system are actively dividing, and the azathioprine prevents cell division. Antilymphocyte globulin contains antibodies that inhibit lymphocytes.

Lymphoplasmapheresis has been used to remove the lymphocytes and immunoglobulin in the recipient. By removing the recipient's lymphocytes, the immunocompetent cells are not present in sufficient numbers to react with the foreign tissue. If the recipient has preformed antibodies, the antibodies are removed by lymphoplasmapheresis, thus preventing an immediate antigen–antibody reaction with the transplanted organ. This procedure allows better organ survival in the recipient.[10]

Host versus graft rejection can be classified as acute, hyperacute, and chronic. Antigens present on the donor organ are recognized as nonself by immunocompetent cells in the recipient, and an immune response occurs. All organs may be rejected by this mechanism except bone marrow. Classic signs of rejection include swelling and tenderness of the graft, increased temperature, malaise, and generalized myalgia. A decrease in the function of the organ is also seen.

Acute rejection occurs within days of the transplant. The blood-borne cells in the graft (antigen-presenting cells) provide the primary stimulus for rejection. Class II antigens on the antigen-presenting cells allow host lymphocytes to recognize self or nonself. The blood-borne cells also provide a second messenger by releasing interleukin-1 (IL-1), which triggers lymphocyte activation. This signal activates CD4 cells, B cells, and CD8 cells. The exact mechanism for the rejection of the grafted tissue is still under study. Most of the early cells found in the graft are recipient lymphocytes; four to seven days later, many cells appear, including monocytes–macrophages and neutrophils. High doses of corticosteroids are often used to prevent acute rejection.

Hyperacute rejection is due to the presence of preformed ABO or HLA class I antibodies. These antibodies are present in sufficient concentration to bind to its specific antigen located on the vascular endothelium of the graft. The complement pathway is activated by the antigen–antibody reaction; complement components activate the coagulation cascade. Microemboli may form that block the vessels and, in the case of the kidney, the glomerular capillary loops and arterioles. There is no effective way of treating hyperacute rejection. Care must be taken to assess the ABO group of the donor and recipient and to detect the presence of anti–class I antibodies in the recipient. The presence of the class I antibodies may be detected during the cross match procedure. This procedure reacts the recipient's serum with the donor's lymphocytes. If the recipient has an antibody to an HLA-A, -B, or -C antigen of the donor, hyperacute rejection will occur, and the organ will not be transplanted.

Chronic rejection occurs months to years after transplantation of the donor organ. The actual control mechanisms for this type of rejection are unknown. In kidney transplantation, the arterial lumen of the graft narrows because of endothelial cell proliferation and ultimately results in loss of renal function. There is no known treatment for this type of rejection.

A second type of rejection is graft versus host disease (GVHD). This occurs when immunocompetent cells in the graft attack the immunoincompetent host. A bone marrow transplant may result in this type of rejection phenomenon.[12,13]

Bone marrow transplantation is unique, compared with other organ transplantation. A bone marrow recipient, in many cases, has functional immunocompetent cells that must be eliminated prior to transplantation. Total body irradiation of the recipient and chemotherapy eliminate functional cells. The donor has 200 to 300 mL of bone marrow removed from his or her iliac crest using repeated bone marrow punctures until sufficient bone marrow has been obtained. The amount taken will not harm the donor immunologically. Once the bone marrow is infused intravenously, it will completely repopulate the recipient's bone marrow within six to eight weeks. Since the immunocompetent cells from the donor circulate throughout the recipient, it is critical to have the best HLA match possible between donor and recipient.

The clinical symptoms of graft versus host disease include skin rash, diarrhea, and jaundice. Competent T cells can be seen in the skin, intestine, and liver. If these symptoms occur 10 to 28 days after transplantation, it is known as acute graft versus host disease. If the symptoms of graft versus host disease occur 30 to 70 days after transplant, this is chronic graft versus host disease. Chronic graft versus host disease resembles many autoimmune or collagen vascular disorders. GVHD can be prevented by using methotrexate, cyclosporin, or cyclophosphamide given for 3 to 12 months posttransplantation.

Another complication of bone marrow transplantation is infection. It takes eight weeks for the bone marrow to become repopulated, during which time the recipient is almost totally immunoincompetent. There are no circulating leukocytes for the first two to four weeks. Bone marrow recipients are kept in a sterile environment until they become immunocompetent again.

HLA and Disease

There has been some correlation between HLA phenotype and specific diseases. In general, these diseases have an unknown cause, have a heritable pattern of distribution, and are associated with immunologic abnormalities. Not all individuals with a particular HLA antigen have the disease, but individuals with the disease have a higher frequency of expressing that particular antigen than is found in the general population.

The first disease associated with an HLA antigen was ankylosing spondylitis. Ninety percent of those individuals with ankylosing spondylitis express the HLA-B27 antigen, compared with 9% of the general population. This yields a relative risk of 91. (Relative risk is the chance that an individual with the antigen will develop the disease, compared with an individual who lacks the antigen.) The frequency of HLA antigens in normal populations varies with race; therefore, the relative risk also varies with race. HLA-B27-positive blacks have a relative risk of 37 of developing ankylosing spondylitis.[1] Other forms of arthritis are associated with HLA-B27. Many autoimmune diseases are associated with an increased frequency of class II antigens.[11] HLA antigens and the disease associations are listed in Table 2-7.

Role of the MHC in Regulating the Immune Response

The major histocompatibility complex has a role in regulating the immune response, as evidenced by MHC restriction. In humans, MHC restriction occurs

Table 2-7: Some Diseases Associated With HLA Antigens

Disease	Antigen	Relative Risk
CLASS I		
Ankylosing spondylitis	B27	87.4
Reiter's disease	B27	37
Post *Shigella, Salmonella, Yersinia,* and gonococcal arthritis	B27	14–30
Subacute thyroiditis	Bw35	13.7
Psoriasis	A1	2.1
	B13	8.7
	Cw6	13
Myasthenia gravis	B8	4
Active chronic hepatitis	B8	9.2
CLASS II		
Goodpasture's syndrome	DR2	13
Multiple sclerosis	DR2	5
Systemic lupus erythematosus	DR3	5.8
Grave's disease	DR3	6
Active chronic hepatitis	DR3	5
Addison's disease	DR3	6
Myasthenia gravis	DR3	3.4
Rheumatoid arthritis	DR4	4
Hashimoto's disease	DR5	3.2

Some HLA antigens are found in a higher frequency in certain diseases when compared with the general population. The relative risk is different for each disease. Some antigens, HLA-B27, -B8, -DR2, and -DR3, may be associated with more than one disease. In some cases more than one HLA antigen is associated with a disease. In psoriasis, all the HLA antigens are in the same class (class I), whereas in chronic active hepatitis and myasthenia gravis, the antigens are found in both class I and class II.

when a lymphocyte population can only be activated in the presence of an antigen and an MHC molecule. If the viral antigen is associated with a class I MHC antigen on a virally infected cell, CD8-positive cells (cytotoxic T cells) will respond. The viral antigen plus the class I antigen on the target cell are recognized by the CD3 and CD8 receptors, respectively, on the surface of cytotoxic T cells. The virus alone or

A Virally Infected Cell and Class I Antigen

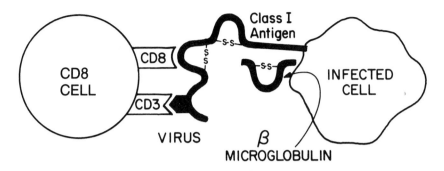

B Virally Infected Cell and Class II Antigen

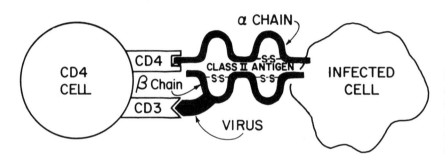

FIGURE 2-8. The MHC is responsible for immune regulation. The virally infected cell may attach to a class I antigen (A) or a class II antigen (B) and stimulate lymphocytes.

class I antigen alone on a virally infected cell will not cause a response.

If the viral antigen is associated with a class II MHC antigen, a CD4-positive cell (helper T cell) can respond. Again, the viral antigen plus the class II antigen together are recognized by the CD3 and CD4 receptors on the helper T cell (Fig. 2-8). It is theorized that with the CD3 molecule interaction there is a signal that activates the lymphocyte.[11]

Summary

The major histocompatibility complex has three classes of antigens. The class I antigens (HLA-A, -B, and -C) are composed of a single transmembrane protein chain. β_2 microglobulin is loosely associated with the class I chain on the exterior portion of the molecule. Class II antigens (HLA-D, -DR, -DP, and -DQ) have two transmembrane protein chains, α and β chains. Class III antigens are minor histocompatibility antigens and in humans are associated with components of the complement system.

Detection of the HLA antigens may be useful in parentage testing, since multiple alleles occur at each locus. In parentage testing, the father or mother may be excluded, but may not be conclusively proved to be the parent. Some HLA antigens have been associated with diseases. All individuals with a particular antigen do not have the disease, but individuals with a particular disease are more likely to have a particular antigen.

HLA antigen detection is also used in organ transplantation. In some cases, matching antigens of a donor with a recipient is important for acceptance of the graft. Rejection may be due to the host rejecting the grafted tissue, as in kidney, heart, and liver transplants, or due to the graft rejecting the host, as in bone marrow transplants.

References

1. Schwartz BD: The human major histocompatibility HLA complex. In Stites DP, Stobo JD, Wells JV (eds): Basic and Clinical Immunology, 6th ed, p 50. Norwalk, Appleton and Lange, 1987

2. Carroll MC, Katzman P, Alicol EM, et al: Linkage map of the human major histocompatibility complex including the tumor necrosis factor genes. Proc Natl Acad Sci USA 84:8535, 1987

3. Issitt PD: Antigens defined by antibodies that may lack clinical significance. In: Applied Blood Serology, 3rd ed, p 422. Miami, Montgomery Scientific Publishing, 1985

4. Fike DJ: unpublished data

5. HLA Nomenclature Committee: Nomenclature for factors of the HLA system, 1987. Vox Sang 55:119, 1988

6. Hartzman RJ, Sheehy MJ: Identification of class II antigens by primed lymphocyte typing and T lymphocyte clones. In Rose NR, Friedman H, Fahey J (eds): Manual of Clinical Laboratory Immunology, 3rd ed, p 849. Washington, DC, American Society for Microbiology, 1986

7. Dubey DP, Yunis I, Yunis EJ: Cellular typing: mixed lymphocyte response and cell mediated lympholysis. In Rose NR, Friedman H, Fahey J (eds): Manual of Clinical Laboratory Immunology, 3rd ed, p 847. Washington, DC, American Society for Microbiology, 1986

8. Duquesnoy RJ, Tranetzki J: Determination of exclusion by HLA system cases of disputed parentage. In Walker, RH (ed): Inclusion Probabilities in Parentage Testing, p 305. Arlington, American Association of Blood Banks, 1983

9. Bias WB, Zachary AA: Basic principles of paternity determination. In Rose NR, Friedman H, Fahey J (eds): Manual of Clinical Laboratory Immunology, 3rd ed, p 902. Washington, DC, American Society for Microbiology, 1986

10. Garovoy MR, Melzer JS, Gibbs VC, et al: Clinical transplantation. In Stites DP, Stobo JD, Wells JV (eds): Basic and Clinical Immunology, 6th ed. Norwalk, Appleton and Lange, 1987

11. Roitt I: Essential immunology, 6th ed, p 215. Oxford, Blackwell Scientific Publications, 1988

12. Garovoy MR, Carpenter CB: Immunological monitoring of renal allograft rejection. In Rose NR, Friedman H, Fahey J (eds): Manual of Clinical Laboratory Immunology, 3rd ed, p 886. Washington, DC, American Society for Microbiology, 1986

13. Hansen JA, Mickelson EM, Beatty PG, et al: Clinical bone marrow transplantation: Donor selection and recipient monitoring. In Rose NR, Friedman H, Fahey J (eds): Manual of Clinical Laboratory Immunology, 3rd ed, p 892. Washington, DC, American Society for Microbiology, 1986

CHAPTER 3

Cells and Tissues of the Immune System

Suio-Ling Chen

Cells of the Immune System

All the cells involved in the immune response arise from pluripotent stem cells in the bone marrow. There are two main lines of cellular differentiation: The lymphoid lineage, which produces lymphocytes; and the myeloid lineage, which produces monocytes, neutrophils, eosinophils, and basophils. The features of these cells are discussed in the following sections.

Lymphocytes

Lymphocytes are produced in the primary lymphoid organs such as bone marrow and thymus. Approximately 20% to 30% of circulating nucleated cells are lymphocytes, and most of these are long lived. These lymphocytes can be classified into two categories based on their size. Small lymphocytes have a diameter of 8 to 10 μm, have a high nuclear to cytoplasm (N/C) ratio, and lack cytoplasmic granules (Fig. 3-1). These small lymphocytes are further divided into two major classes, T and B lymphocytes, based on their functions. Large granular lymphocytes (LGL) may have a diameter up to 16 μm, have a smaller N/C ratio than small lymphocytes, and contain cytoplasmic granules.[1]

B Lymphocytes

B lymphocytes make up approximately 5% to 15% of circulating lymphocytes. As shown in Figure 3-2, they are classically identified by their cell surface immunoglobulin (SIg). The SIg is endogenously synthesized by the B cells and serves as the antigen receptor. The majority of human peripheral blood B cells express both IgM and IgD; however, some B cells express IgG, IgA, or IgE. In mucosal associated lymphoid tissues, the majority of B cells express IgA

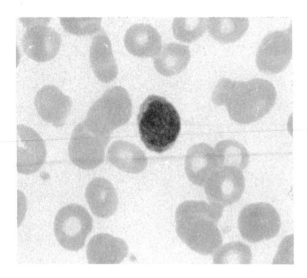

FIGURE 3-1. A mature lymphocyte (×1000). (Courtesy of Dr. JJ Marty.)

as their SIg. Other B-cell markers are Fc receptors for the IgG heavy chain, receptor for complement components (C3b and C3d), MHC class II molecules, and receptors for the Epstein-Barr virus. Recently, a series of monoclonal antibodies has been developed

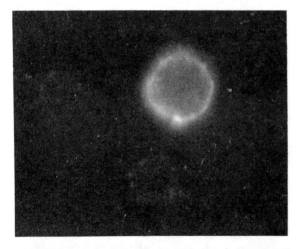

FIGURE 3-2. A surface immunoglobulin positive B cell (×1000).

that identifies the lymphocyte surface glycoproteins known as CD (cluster of differentiation) (Table 3-1). The CD markers that are frequently used to identify B cells are CD19, CD20, and CD21.

B-Lymphocyte Differentiation. Mature B lymphocytes are the products of lymphoid stem cells that undergo a sequence of differentiation under the influence of a special microenvironment. In birds this microenvironment is the Bursa of Fabricius, a discrete lymphoepithelial organ originating from hindgut endoderm.[2] In mammals the differentiation occurs first in the fetal liver and subsequently in the bone marrow.[3] The B-cell development can be divided into two stages, antigen dependent and antigen independent (Fig. 3-3). The stem B cells lacking immunoglobulin products go through a series of events, including cell divisions and immunoglobulin gene rearrangement, to become pre-B cells. A pre-B cell is a large lymphoblast containing IgM heavy chains in the cytoplasm but lacking light chain. It also expresses MHC class II molecules and complement receptors on the cell surface. The pre-B cells differentiate into mature B cells by losing their cytoplasmic IgM heavy chains and acquiring surface IgM and IgD.[4] The B-cell differentiation up to this point is independent of antigenic stimulation. Upon encountering an antigen, the mature B cells are driven to undergo cell activation, proliferation, and differentiation, giving rise to plasma cells that synthesize and secrete immunoglobulins. Although it contains immunoglobulin, a plasma cell lacks SIg and other B-cell markers, such as Fc receptors, complement receptors, MHC class II molecules, and monoclonal antibody–defined CD glycoproteins. It is also a terminally differentiated B cell (Fig. 3-4).

T Lymphocytes

Approximately 80% of the circulating lymphocytes are T cells. The T lymphocytes are associated with two types of immunologic functions, effector and regulatory. The effector functions include activities such as cytolysis of virally infected cells and tumor

Table 3-1: T and B Lymphocyte Markers*

CD Designation	Molecular Weight	Cellular Distribution	Comment	Antibody Clone
CD1	49Kd	Thymocytes	Also expressed on Langerhan cells in skin	Leu-6 OKT6 T6
CD2	45, 50Kd	T-cells	SRBC-receptor associated	Leu-5b OKT11 T11
CD3	19, 25Kd	T-cells	Associated with T-antigen receptor	Leu-4 OKT3 T3
CD4	55, 64Kd	T-helper/inducer cells	Receptor for MHC class II molecule	Leu-3a OKT4 T4
CD8	33, 43Kd	T-suppressor/cytotoxic cells	Receptor for MHC class I molecule	Leu-2 OKT8 T8
CD19	40, 80Kd	B-cells		Leu-12 B4
CD20	35Kd	B-cells		Leu-16 B1
CD21	145Kd	Mature B cells	C3d receptor	B2

* The antibody clones are representative of those commercially available and are not intended to be comprehensive.

targets and lymphokine production. The regulatory functions are represented by their ability to amplify or suppress other effector lymphocytes, including B and T cells. The classical T-cell surface marker is sheep red blood cell (SRBC) receptors. When the T cells are incubated with SRBC, SRBC bind to T cells to form rosettes. Most circulating T cells express three of the following CD markers:

CD2: SRBC Receptor
CD3: Part of T-cell antigen receptor complex
CD4: Receptor for MHC class II molecule
CD8: Receptor for MHC class I molecule

Two subpopulations of T cells are identified in the circulation. In general, the T lymphocytes with CD2, CD3, CD4 phenotype are associated with helper–inducer activity, and the lymphocytes with CD2, CD3, CD8 phenotype are associated with cytotoxic or suppressor activity. However, the functional association with these two markers (CD4 and CD8) appears not to be as simplistic as was once thought.

T-Lymphocyte Differentiation. Like B cells, T cells require a specialized microenvironment for differentiation and maturation. The stem cells or pre-T cells arise in the bone marrow or fetal liver and mi-

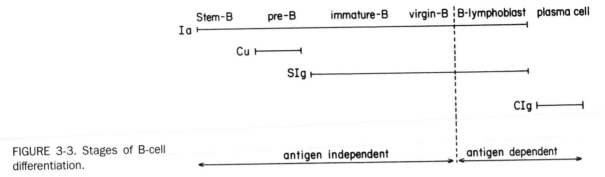

FIGURE 3-3. Stages of B-cell differentiation.

grate into the thymus. The thymus is derived from the third and fourth pairs of embryonic pharyngeal pouches and is thus of endodermal origin. It is in this microenvironment that T cells acquire developmental maturation (Fig. 3-5). The bone marrow T stem cells contain an enzyme, terminal deoxynucleotidyl transferase (TdT) but do not express surface CD glycoprotein. The earliest differentiation event is acquisition of CD2 and CD3, which occurs in the thymic cortex. Further differentiation in the cortex is the expression of both CD4 and CD8. Two major events

occur as the T cells move through the thymic medulla: (1) development of two distinct T-cell populations, helper–inducer T cells (CD4 positive), and suppressor–cytotoxic T cells (CD8 positive); and (2) loss of TdT enzyme. It is interesting to note that approximately 90% of T cells die intrathymically and never enter the peripheral circulation. The most significant outcome of this intrathymic differentiation is that the T cells learn to recognize self-MHC gene products, which is essential for cellular interaction in the immune responses.[5,6]

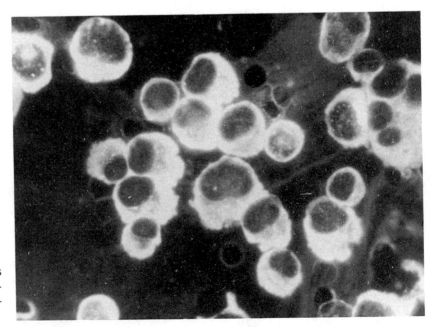

FIGURE 3-4. Plasma cells showing cytoplasmic immunoglobulin by direct immunofluorescence (×1000).

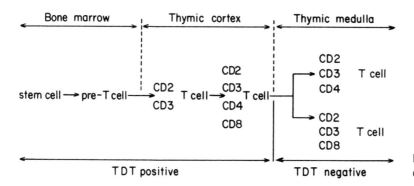

FIGURE 3-5. T-cell maturation sequence.

Large Granular Lymphocytes

Large granular lymphocytes (LGL) are sometimes referred to as the third population of lymphocytes, or natural killer cells (NK cells). They are slightly larger than a resting T or B cell and have cytotoxic granules, but do not consistently express T- or B-cell markers. However, they have surface IgG Fc receptors. NK cells are able to lyse virally infected cells and tumor cells without prior immunization. Unlike cytotoxic T cells, the cytolytic activity of NK cells is not MHC restricted. They also play an important role in antibody-dependent cell-mediated cytolysis (ADCC).[6]

Monocytes and Macrophages

Monocytes represent approximately 4% to 10% of circulating nucleated cells. It has a diameter of 12 to 16 μm. The nucleus is horseshoe shaped, and the cytoplasm contains neutrophilic granules (Fig. 3-6). Circulating monocytes are able to migrate into various tissues and become tissue macrophages. They assume two main functions, removal of particulate antigens and presentation of antigens to the lymphocytes. The surface markers of monocytes and macrophages are IgG Fc receptor, complement receptor, and MHC class II molecule.[6,7]

Polymorphonuclear Granulocytes

Polymorphonuclear granulocytes are a heterogeneous group of cells, including neutrophils, eosinophils, and basophils. The mature form has a diameter of 10 to 15 μm and usually contains a multilobed nucleus and many cytoplasmic granules. They are able to adhere and penetrate the endothelial cell lining of blood vessels and migrate into surrounding tissues. They play an important role in acute inflammation.

Neutrophils

Neutrophils represent about 70% of circulating nucleated cells (Fig. 3-7). The cytoplasm contains azurophilic granules that contain enzymes, including

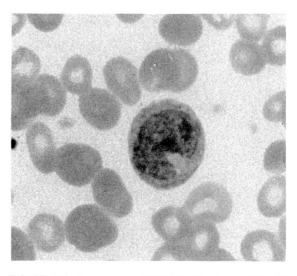

FIGURE 3-6. A monocyte ($\times$1000). (Courtesy of Dr. JJ Marty.)

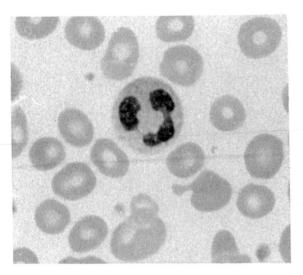

FIGURE 3-7. A neutrophil (×1000). (Courtesy of Dr. JJ Marty.)

hydrolase, myeloperoxidase, and muraminidase. Their major function is phagocytosis. Since Fc and complement receptors are expressed on the cell surface, their phagocytic activities are enhanced when particles or antigens are coated with antibody and/or complement (opsonization). Thus, with the aid of antibody and complement, neutrophils play an important role in protection against extracellular microorganism infection.[6,7]

Eosinophils

In a healthy, nonallergic individual, eosinophils comprise approximately 2% to 5% of circulating nucleated cells. The cytoplasm of an eosinophil contains yellowish-red granules. Its major function is probably to kill the invading organism by releasing the granular contents to the extracellular space. For example, it is thought that eosinophils play an important role in protection against helminth infection.

In the site of allergic response, eosinophils are triggered to release histaminase and aryl sulfatase, which inactivate the allergic mediators, such as histamine and slow-reacting substances of anaphylaxis, therefore, dampening the allergic response.[6,7]

Basophils and Mast Cells

Basophils and mast cells are indistinguishable from each other in a number of properties. They are characterized by deep violet blue cytoplasmic granules that contain histamine and other vasoactive amines. Unlike B cells, monocytes, macrophages, and neutrophils, which express Fc receptors for IgG, basophils and mast cells express Fc receptors for IgE heavy chain. Thus, IgE antibodies bind to these cells and remain stable (*i.e.*, not catabolized) for a long period of time. Cross-linking of the cell surface IgE by an allergen triggers the cell to release granular contents, which initiates allergic reaction.

Regardless of functional similarity, basophils and mast cells are distinct cell populations: (1) Basophils are probably derived from cells resembling a myeloblast, whereas tissue mast cells are connective tissue cells of mesenchymal origin; (2) basophils circulate in peripheral blood, whereas mast cells are widely distributed in the tissues, including thymus, spleen, lung, gastrointestinal tract, and bone marrow; and (3) mast cell membrane is less regular than that of a basophil and it contains more granules that are finer than basophil granules.[8]

Organs and Tissues of the Immune System

For the physical well-being of a host it must have a filtering system that will eliminate the foreign substances. This is accomplished by passing the blood or lymph through a loose meshwork of fibers or reticula to which phagocytes adhere. The entire filtration system is known as reticuloendothelial system and includes lymphoid organs, liver, and lungs.

Based on the primary function, the organs and tissues of the immune system are divided into two main categories: primary (central) and secondary (peripheral) lymphoid organs. In humans the primary lymphoid organ is composed of bone marrow, fetal liver, and thymus. The cells of the immune system are produced and mature in these primary lymphoid organs. Subsequently, these functional cells are released into the circulation and populate the secondary lymphoid organs or tissues. Included in the secondary lymphoid organs are lymph nodes, spleen, and mucosal-associated lymphoid tissues (MALT). The lymph nodes and spleen are encapsulated organs, whereas MALT are lymphoid cell aggregates occurring along the gastrointestinal, respiratory, and urogenital tracts. These secondary lymphoid organs and tissues are located in strategic sites throughout the body to carry out their functions: trapping the antigens, providing the specialized niche for lymphocyte–antigen interactions, and exporting the immune response products (effector T cells and antibodies) to the systemic circulation.

Primary Lymphoid Organs

Bone Marrow

All the cells of the blood, including lymphocytes, are produced in the bone marrow throughout adult life. Whereas T-cell development requires the thymic microenvironment, the bone marrow gives rise to func-tional B cells directly. In addition, adult bone marrow appears to be an important secondary lymphoid organ because it contains many mature T cells and plasma cells.[1]

Thymus

The thymus gland develops from the third and fourth pairs of embryonic pharyngeal pouches. It begins as an outpouching of the endodermal epithelium into which lymphocytes of mesodermal origin migrate. The thymus is bilobed and located in the anterior mediastinum. It reaches its maximal size at puberty; thereafter, it atrophies and is replaced by fatty tissue. This age-related process resulting in partial loss of thymic function is known as thymic involution. The thymus is exceedingly sensitive to corticosteroids; the steroid treatment accelerates involution. "Stress involution" of the thymus is believed to be triggered by stimulating the adrenal gland to release corticosteroid as a result of stress or disease.[9]

The thymus gland is organized into lobules that are separated by connective tissue septa (Fig. 3-8). Microscopically, each lobule is further divided into two distinct areas: outer cortex and inner medulla. The lymphocytes (pre-T cells) migrate from bone

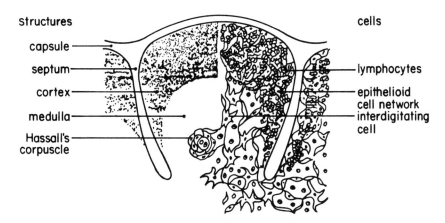

FIGURE 3-8. The structure of a thymus lobule. (From Roitt IM, Brostoff J, Male DK. Immunology. London, Gower Medical Publishing, 1985.)

marrow into the cortex, and then into inner medulla. The T cells mature during this journey. Thus, the T lymphocytes found in the outer cortex are immature, with high mitotic activity, and the inner medulla contains mature T cells that are ready to be exported to the systemic circulation. The network of epithelial cells and interdigitating cells is thought to be important in the lymphocytes' learning processes for self–nonself recognition. Hassall's corpuscles are found in the thymic medulla; the function of these cells is not well understood.[2]

The thymus produces a number of soluble mediators that maintain the cell-mediated immunity. These mediators most likely act on T cells at different stages of development. Thymosin (molecular weight 3100 to 5250 d) is one of the best characterized thymic factors or hormones; it restores T-cell deficiencies in thymectomized mice. Thymopoietin (molecular weight 5500 d) induces T-cell maturation. Serum thymic factor (molecular weight 847 d) induces the T-cell markers. Although most of the thymic factors are probably produced by thymic epithelial cells, thymic macrophages are also known to secrete a mitogenic factor that acts on developing T cells.[9]

Secondary Lymphoid Organs

The immune responses are initiated in the secondary lymphoid organs or tissues. Several common structural characteristics are observed among the secondary lymphoid organs. They have (1) specialized ports of entrance for the lymphocytes, (2) discrete areas to which T and B cells home, and (3) elaborate architectural organization that maximizes the trapping of antigens and lymphocyte–antigen interactions.

Lymph Node[10]

A typical lymph node is 1 to 25 mm in diameter and is round or bean shaped. The entire organ is encapsulated with subcapsular sinuses that surround the lymphoid tissue. The lymphoid tissue is organized into an outer cortex and an inner medulla (Fig. 3-9). The cortex is further divided into two domains: follicles and diffuse paracortex. Mature T and B cells released from primary lymphoid organs inherently home to the paracortex and follicles, respectively. This characteristic homing ability has been elegantly demonstrated in animal experiments. The lymph nodes of bursectomized bird lack lymphoid follicles in the cortex; however, the diffuse paracortex is nor-

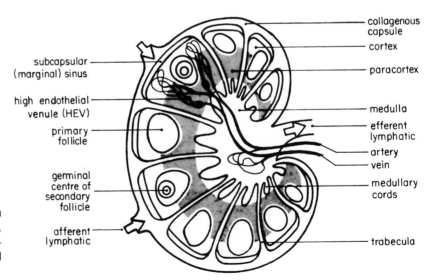

FIGURE 3-9. The structure of a lymph node. (From Roitt IM, Brostoff J, Male DK. Immunology. London, Gower Medical Publishing, 1985.)

subcapsular (marginal) sinus

high endothelial venule (HEV)

primary follicle

germinal centre of secondary follicle

afferent lymphatic

collagenous capsule

cortex

paracortex

medulla

efferent lymphatic

artery

vein

medullary cords

trabecula

mally populated with T cells. Conversely, thymectomy results in lymphocyte depletion in the diffuse paracortex area, but the follicles are normally populated by B cells. The preceding experimental observations indicate that the follicles are B-cell domain and that paracortex is T-cell domain. Thus, the functional duality of the immune system is reflected in the structural organization in the secondary lymphoid organs and tissues.

There are two types of follicles or nodules in a lymph node: primary and secondary follicles. A primary follicle is an aggregate of small B lymphocytes in a meshwork of dendritic cells. A secondary follicle develops from a primary follicle following antigenic stimulation. The secondary follicle has a germinal center surrounded by a mantle zone. The germinal center contains heterogeneous cell populations, including small and large lymphocytes, blast cells, macrophages, and dendritic cells. The mantle zone consists of small lymphocytes similar to primary follicles.

The diffuse paracortex contains small T lymphocytes, macrophages, interdigitating cells, and postcapillary venules. The inner medulla has an extensive medullary sinus and medullary cords that contain plasma cells and large lymphocytes.

Lymph nodes are strategically located at the junctions of lymphatic vessels throughout the body. The lymphatic vessels and the lymph nodes form a complete network that drains and filters the extravasated fluid (lymph) from the intercellular spaces of tissues. The lymph of tissue spaces is transported into the lymphatic vessels by osmotic pressure and muscular contractions. It is then directed into the subcapsular sinus of a lymph node through afferent lymphatic vessels. Once in the lymph node, the lymph travels through a series of sinusoids that percolate throughout the entire lymph node and exits the lymph node via efferent lymphatic vessels. Several efferent lymphatic vessels join to form a larger lymphatic duct that empties into the venous system by way of the thoracic duct. The antigens that enter the

tissue spaces are carried into the regional or draining lymph node by the lymphatic circulation described earlier. Normally, the majority of antigens are trapped in the regional lymph nodes, where they are phagocytized by the macrophages. Subsequently, some of the antigens are returned to the macrophage surface in a partially digested form and are presented to the lymphocytes during their passage through the lymph node.

Lymphocytes enter a lymph node from the bloodstream by way of the arterial blood supply to the lymph node. Both T and B cells adhere specifically to large specialized endothelial cells of postcapillary venules (also known as postcapillary high endothelial venule) and traverse these walls to enter the lymph node. These postcapillary high endothelial venules are located in the diffuse paracortical area. Thus, both T and B cells enter the diffuse paracortex, whereas T cells remain in the area of entrance, the B cells further migrate into the follicles. After traversing their special cortical areas, the lymphocytes enter the sinusoids of the medulla that lead to efferent lymphatic (see Fig. 3-9).

Spleen[11]

The spleen is the largest lymphoid organ that is specialized for filtering the blood. It is located in the left upper quadrant beneath the diaphragm and behind the stomach. The splenic tissue is organized into lymphoid white pulp and erythroid red pulp. The main function of the red pulp is to destroy degenerating red cells. The white pulp is the lymphoid tissue that surrounds the central arterioles and is also known as periarteriolar lymphoid sheath. The cellular organization of the white pulp is similar to a lymph node. The diffuse lymphoid tissue immediately surrounding the central arteriole is a T-cell area. Adjacent to the T-cell areas are lymphoid follicles, which are B-cell areas. Both primary and secondary follicles are found in a spleen. Each periarteriolar lymphoid sheath is surrounded by a marginal zone that con-

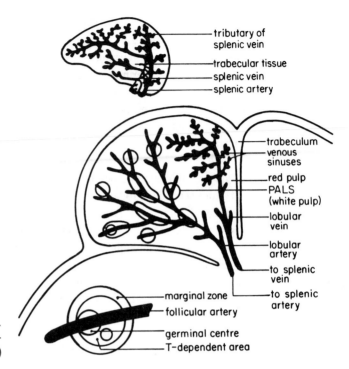

FIGURE 3-10. The structure of a spleen nodule. (From Roitt IM, Brostoff J, Male DK: Immunology. London, Gower Medical Publishing, 1985.)

tains blood vessels, macrophages, and lymphocytes (Fig. 3-10).

The lymphocytes enter and leave the white pulp through capillary branches of central arteriole in the marginal zone. While the entering T cells remain in the diffuse area, the B cells home to the follicles. Upon stimulation by antigen-charged APCs, the specific lymphocytes are retained in their respective domains and mount an immune response. Otherwise, the lymphocytes can freely leave the white pulp from the marginal zone. Some lymphocytes, especially the plasma cells, may travel across the marginal zone and enter the red pulp and the venous circulation.

Mucosal Associated Lymphoid Tissues

Mucosal-associated lymphoid tissues (MALT) are found in the submucosal areas along the gastrointestinal, respiratory, and urogenital tracts. These are noncapsulated lymphoid cell aggregates and are frequently organized into follicles containing germinal centers. The lamina propria of the intestinal wall usually contains diffuse lymphoid cells; the Peyer's patches of the ileum are often seen as prominent structures frequently containing follicles and germinal centers. The lymphoid tissues along the gastrointestinal tract are also known as gut-associated lymphoid tissue (GALT). Normally, MALT provides the first line of defense against microorganisms at the port of entry. Therefore, MALT is exceedingly important in the immune response at the mucosal surface.

Lymphocyte Circulation[1]

Once released from central lymphoid organs, the mature lymphocytes engage in a complex traffic pattern moving from one lymphoid organ to another by circulatory and lymphatic channels. Figure 3-11

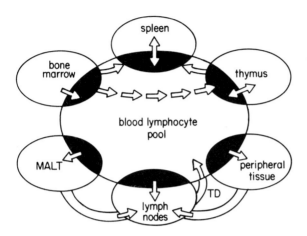

FIGURE 3-11. Lymphocyte recirculation. (From Roitt IM, Brostoff J, Male DK. Immunology. London, Gower Medical Publishing, 1985.)

represents a schematic diagram showing lymphocyte circulation pattern. After a short stay in the respective domains, both T and B cells leave the node through efferent lymphatics; the lymphatics empty into the peripheral blood through the thoracic duct, thus returning the lymphocytes to peripheral circulation. A slightly different lymphocyte traffic pattern takes place in the spleen: The lymphocytes leave the circulation by way of the capillaries in the marginal zone, and they leave the spleen by migrating into the sinusoid, which leads into the splenic vein.

Under normal conditions there is a continuous flow of lymphocytes between peripheral lymphoid organs and the circulation. However, during an antigenic stimulation the specific lymphocytes are preferentially retained in the lymphoid organ, which drain the areas of antigen entrance. The temporary sequestration of the antigen-specific lymphocytes in the antigen-draining lymphoid organ will provide opportunities for these lymphocytes to recognize and respond to the antigen. The constant lymphocyte

traffic between circulation and the peripheral lymphoid organs will ensure that every invading antigen will be encountered by the specific lymphocytes.

References

1. Roitt L, Brostoff J, Male D: Immunology, p 3.1. London, Gower Medical Publishing, 1985

2. Kimball JW: The structure of the immune system. In: Introduction to Immunology, p 127. New York, Macmillan, 1983

3. Osmond DG: Production and differentiation of B lymphocytes in the bone marrow. In Battisto J, Knight K, eds. Immunoglobulin Genes and B Cell Differentiation, p 135. New York, Elsevier North-Holland, 1980

4. Osmond DG, Batten SJ: Genesis of B lymphocytes in the bone marrow: Extravascular and intravascular localization of surface IgM-bearing cells in mouse bone marrow detected by electron-microscope radioautography after in vivo perfusion of anti-IgM antibody. Am J Anat 170:349, 1984

5. Osmond DG: The ontogeny and organization of the lymphoid system. J Invest Dermatol (Suppl) 85:2s, 1985

6. Reinherz EL, Schlossman S: The differentiation and function of human T lymphocytes. Cell 19:821, 1981

7. Platt WR: Maturation of leukocytes and the leukocyte count. In: Color Atlas and Textbook of Hematology, 2nd ed. p 83, Philadelphia, JB Lippincott, 1979

8. Nelson DA: Hematopoesis. In Henry JB (ed): Clinical Diagnosis and Management by Laboratory Method, 6th ed. p 918, Philadelphia, WB Saunders, 1979

9. Weiss L: The thymus. In: Histology: Cell and Tissue Biology, 5th ed. p 510, New York, Elsevier Biomedical, 1983

10. Weiss L: Lymphatic vessels and lymph nodes. In: Histology: Cell and Tissue Biology, 5th ed. p 527, New York, Elsevier Biomedical, 1983

11. Weiss L: The spleen. In: Histology: Cell and Tissue Biology, 5th ed. p 544, New York, Elsevier Biomedical, 1983

CHAPTER 4

Mechanisms of the Specific Immune Response

Suio-Ling Chen

Specific immune responses are traditionally classified as a humoral or cell-mediated immune response. The humoral immune response involves antibody production by the B lymphocytes, whereas the cell-mediated immune response involves mainly T lymphocytes and their mediators. The division of humoral and cell-mediated immune response is not absolute, and the occurrence of one type of response in the complete absence of the other is extremely rare. However, certain antigens may tend to elicit a predominantly antibody response with a minimal cell-mediated response, or vice versa.

An elaborate cascade of cellular interaction is required for a specific immune response to occur. Initially, the antigen needs to be processed by the antigen-presenting cells and presented to the specific lymphocytes. There are two functionally distinct types of specific lymphocytes: (1) the helper T lym-

phocytes (T_H) and suppressor T lymphocytes (T_S) with regulatory function and (2) the antigen-specific effector lymphocytes, which include the B lymphocytes for antibody production, cytotoxic T lymphocytes (T_C), and lymphokine-producing T cells. The interaction between the regulatory T_H or T_S cell and effector lymphocytes may require direct cell contact or soluble mediators.

Antigen Presentation

Antigen presentation, the initial step of an immune response, is carried out by a group of cells known as accessory cells or antigen-presenting cells (APCs). Among the well-characterized APCs are macrophages, dendritic cells, interdigitating cells, and Langerhans cells. The common characteristic of these APCs is that they are rich in surface MHC class II molecules, which play an important role in cellular interaction during an immune response.[1,2]

Upon entry to a host the antigens are first bound to the APCs. Although some of these antigens remain on the cell surface and are presented to the specific lymphocytes, most are internalized by the process of phagocytosis and digested by the hydrolytic enzymes. However, some partially digested antigens are returned to the cell surface, and it is in this form that the antigen is most efficiently recognized by the specific lymphocytes. In addition to antigen presentation, APCs release a soluble mediator, interleukin-1, which stimulates the antigen activated lymphocytes.

A subpopulation of the circulating T lymphocytes is endowed with a unique regulatory function that is to help other antigen specific T or B cells to proliferate and differentiate into functional effector cells, such as antibody-producing plasma cells or cytotoxic T cells. In humans these regulatory T lymphocytes are identified by their surface glycoprotein CD4 and are known as helper T cells (T_H cells).

Upon stimulation with antigen-charged APCs, the T_H cells undergo an activation process known as blast transformation. A series of cellular events occurs during this process. The noticeable changes in the cell morphology are increased cell size and the appearance of prominent nucleoli. At the molecular level the cell increases its mRNA and DNA synthesis, which leads to cell division and cell differentiation. Thus, the number of functional T_H cells increases. Direct contact between T_H cell and antigen-charged APC is necessary for T-cell activation.[3] Not only must the T_H cell recognize the antigen, but it must also recognize the MHC class II molecules presented on the APC surface. Such a dual recognition of antigen and MHC class II molecule is possible only when the two interacting cells are from the same host or genetically similar individuals. This phenomenon is known as MHC restriction. Thus, the T_H cell–APC interaction is MHC class II restricted.[2]

Two possible mechanisms are postulated for the interaction between a T_H cell and APC.[3] The independent recognition hypothesis states that the antigen and MHC class II molecule are expressed on the APC surface as independent entities; therefore, a T_H cell has two separate receptors, one for antigen and the other for a MHC class II molecule. The associate recognition hypothesis postulates that the antigen is presented in conjunction with the MHC class II molecule, and this antigen–MHC class II molecule complex is recognized by a single T_H cell receptor. There is evidence indicating that the CD4 glycoprotein on the T_H cell surface is the receptor for MHC class II molecule and that it is part of the T_H cell antigen receptor complex. Possible mechanisms of T_H cell–APC interaction are schematically represented in Fig. 4-1.[2,3]

The nature of the communication between the interacting T_H cell and APC is not completely elucidated. The T_H cell may transmit a signal or signals to the APC, resulting in the release of a soluble mediator, interleukin-1 (IL-1), by the APC. IL-1, in turn, activates a variety of antigen-sensitized lymphocytes, including T_H cells. T_H cells appear to play a central role in an immune response, because they release soluble mediators that promote proliferation and differentiation of the effector cells (Fig. 4-2).

Antibody Response

The mechanism of cellular interaction for the antibody response is demonstrated by the experiments using a constructed antigen, such as dinitrophenylated serum albumin. Dinitrophenol (DNP) alone does not elicit an antibody response. However, when conjugated to a protein molecule such as xenogenic serum albumin, an anti-DNP antibody response is generated. The term *hapten* is used to describe a substance, such as DNP, that is able to stimulate an antibody response only when it is conjugated to a larger molecule. A hapten is antigenic but not immunogenic. The molecule that renders a hapten im-

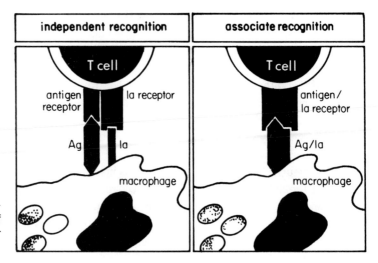

FIGURE 4-1. Mechanisms of T-cell-antigen recognition. (From Roitt IM, Brostoff J, Male DK. Immunology. London, Gower Medical Publishing, 1985.)

munogenic is known as a carrier. One may envision that a hapten is an antigenic determinant of a larger molecule and that naturally occurring antigens are composed of a carrier backbone to which numerous haptens are attached.

The Carrier Effect

The carrier effect in an antibody response is best demonstrated by the experiments in which the sec-

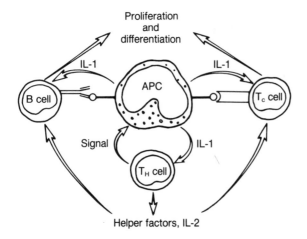

FIGURE 4-2. Cascade of cellular interaction in immune responses.

ondary antibody responses are measured.[2] For example, a mouse that is immunized with DNP conjugated with bovine serum albumin (DNP–BSA) for both primary and secondary challenges responds vigorously with anti-DNP antibodies. However, the animal responds poorly if DNP conjugated with ovalbumin (DNP-OA) is given in substitution for DNP-BSA during the secondary challenge. Thus, it is necessary to have the same carrier molecule for both primary and secondary challenge to elicit a strong anti-DNP antibody response (Table 4-1). This observation prompted further experimentation that involves cell transfer among genetically similar animals (syngeneic animals). In cell transfer experiments the recipient animals are irradiated to render their lymphocytes unresponsive to antigen while APCs remain functional. Thus, the functional role of lymphocyte populations can be evaluated within an irradiated recipient. A series of cell transfer experiments was conducted to define the role of T and B lymphocytes for antibody production. The following observations were made using the constructed antigens DNP-BSA and DNP-OA (Table 4-2):

1. A strong anti-DNP antibody response is made by the recipient when challenged with DNP-BSA and reconstituted with both T and B cells from the donor that had been primed with DNP-BSA.

Table 4-1: Carrier Effect

Antigen		Anti-DNP Response
Primary Challenge	Secondary Challenge	
DNP-BSA	DNP-BSA	++++
DNP-BSA	DNP-OA	+/−
DNP-OA	DNP-OA	++++
DNP-OA	DNP-BSA	+

2. A weak anti-DNP response or no anti-DNP response was made by the recipient when challenged with DNP-BSA and reconstituted with B lymphocytes from the donor that had been primed with DNP-BSA. In this experiment the donor lymphocytes were treated with antibody to T cells and complement to deplete the T-cell population.

3. A borderline anti-DNP antibody response was made by the recipient when challenged with DNP-OA and reconstituted with T and B cells from the donor that had been primed with DNP-BSA.

4. A strong anti-DNP antibody response was made by the recipient when challenged with DNP-OA and reconstituted with the B cells from a donor that had been primed with DNP-BSA and the T cells from another donor that had been primed with OA.

Table 4-2: T and B Cells Recognize Carrier and Hapten of an Antigen, Respectively

Source of Lymphocytes for Reconstitution					
DNP-BSA Primed Donor		OA Primed Donor		Challenging Antigen	Anti-DNP
B Cells	T Cells	B Cells	T Cells		
+	+	−	−	DNP-BSA	++++
+	−	−	−	DNP-BSA	+/−
+	+	−	−	DNP-OA	+/−
+	−	−	+	DNP-OA	++++
+	−	−/+	+	DNP-OA	+/−

In above cell transfer experiments, the recipients are irradiated such that their lymphocytes are not responsive to antigens but their APCs remain functional. When only B cells are needed for transfer, the donor lymphocytes are treated with anti–T-cell antibodies and complement for T-cell depletion.

Observations 1 and 2 indicate that both T and B cells are required in an antibody response, whereas observations 3 and 4 indicate that the T cells recognize the carrier portion of an antigen while the B cells recognize the hapten portion.

Mechanisms of T- and B-cell collaboration are currently debated. The need for direct cell contact has been suggested by some experimental data. In theory the antigen serves as a bridge between T and B cell. Thus, the T cell binds to the antigen through the carrier portion, whereas the B cell binds to the same antigen through the hapten portion. In addition, the MHC class II molecule is involved. The T-cell receptor for MHC class II molecule binds to the B-cell surface MHC class II antigen (Fig. 4-3). The preceding cellular contact appears to enhance the communication between two interacting cells.[2,4]

Communication between interacting T and B cells may be mediated by soluble factors released by the T cells and is suggested by cell culture experiments. *In vitro* antibody production is not inhibited when T and B cells are separated by a membrane; the membrane prevents cell contact yet allows antigen and soluble factors to diffuse freely (Fig. 4-4).[2] Two B-cell growth factors have been reported. B-cell growth factor 1 (also known as IL-4) stimulates proliferation of antigen-activated B cells, and B-cell growth factor 2 (also known as IL-6) induces differentiation of proliferating B cells.[5–9]

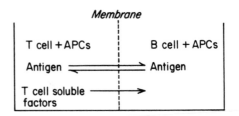

FIGURE 4-4. T–B-cell interaction mediated by soluble factors.

T-Cell Dependent and Independent Antigen

As discussed previously the antibody response to the majority of antigens requires helper T cells. These antigens are known as T-dependent antigens. There are, however, a small number of substances that are capable of activating B cells without the T-cell help; these are known as T-independent antigens. In general, T-independent antigens are large molecules with repeating antigenic determinants that elicit mainly IgM responses; the primary and secondary responses are indistinguishable, and immunologic memory and antibody affinity maturation do not occur.[3]

Antibody Responses in a Whole Animal

Primary and Secondary Antibody Response

The quality, magnitude, and tempo of an antibody response depend greatly on the host's experience with the antigen. A primary response is elicited when the antigen is introduced to an animal for the first time. During a primary response a latent phase occurs in which there is no detectable circulating antibody. The length of the latent phase is usually between 5 and 7 days; however, it may vary, depending on the individual and the antigen. The latent

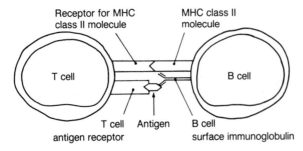

FIGURE 4-3. Mechanism of T–B-cell interaction by direct cell contact.

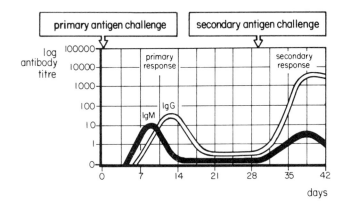

FIGURE 4-5. Primary and secondary antibody response. (From Roitt IM, Brostoff J, Male DK. Immunology. London, Gower Medical Publishing, 1985.)

phase is followed by a gradual rise, plateau, and final decline of the antibody titer. The final decline in the antibody titer is due to several factors, including the cessation of antibody production, clearance of antibody in the form of immune complexes, and catabolism of the antibody. The first immunoglobulin class to appear in a primary antibody response is IgM, which is followed by the production of IgG. Introduction of the same antigen for the second time evokes a secondary antibody response that differs from the primary response in many aspects (Fig. 4-5):

1. The latent phase is shorter.

2. The circulating antibody reaches higher titer.

3. IgG is the predominant immunoglobulin produced.

4. The antibody response tends to persist for a longer time period.

Thus, the secondary response is "faster" and "bigger" than the primary response. It is also called an anamnestic response because the immune system seems to remember the previous antigenic exposure. Presumably, both memory T and B cells are generated during the primary response.

Affinity Maturation

Antibodies produced during the secondary response have a higher affinity for the antigen than those produced during the primary response. This phenomenon is known as affinity maturation. Most likely, affinity maturation involves the selective activation of B cells that have high affinity receptors (*i.e.*, surface immunoglobulin with high affinity for the antigen). This is supported by both the biology of B cells and experimental observations.

Both the surface immunoglobulin of a B cell and the immunoglobulin secreted by the same B cell are coded by the same set of genes, which remain unchanged throughout the cell's life-span. Consequently, not only do the surface immunoglobulin and immunoglobulin secreted by a B cell have identical antigen specificity and affinity, but these biologic activities remain constant throughout the life-span of a B cell. Therefore, a B cell is able to make immunoglobulin molecules with one antigenic specificity whose antigen affinity remains a constant (*i.e.*, no affinity maturation within a single B cell). Affinity maturation must then rely upon heterogeneous clones of B cells that have similar antigenic specificity but different affinity for the antigen (high or low affinity). When the B cells with low-affinity surface immunoglobulin are activated, they produce low-affinity antibodies, and when only the B cells with high-affinity surface receptor (surface immunoglobulin) are activated, they produce high-affinity antibodies. This is supported by experimental observations: High antigen dose generally elicits antibodies that have low affinity for the antigen. In antigen excess, both B cells with high and low affinity have opportunity to interact with the antigen to become activated. On the contrary, at low antigen dose the B cells compete for the antigens, and only those B cells with high affinity will succeed in binding to the antigen, becoming activated, and producing high-affinity antibodies.[3,10]

Regulation of Antibody Production

The Regulatory Effect of Antibody

Antibody can have a negative feedback effect on its own production. Two possible mechanisms are suggested by which the antibody suppresses its further synthesis. Circulating antibodies and the B cell may compete for antigen binding. Thus, as the serum antibody titer increases, fewer B cells with the same antigen specificity will have the opportunity to become activated. Circulating antibodies may also bind to the B-cell surface by way of Fc receptors. Cross-linking between B-cell surface Fc receptor and surface immunoglobulin may occur when a multivalent antigen binds to the surface immunoglobulin and antibody that has been passively adsorbed by the Fc receptor. Such a cross-linkage of B-cell surface receptors will lead to B-cell inactivation, thus decreasing antibody synthesis (Fig. 4-6).[3]

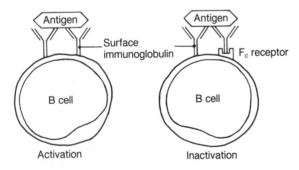

FIGURE 4-6. B-cell activation and inhibition.

The Regulatory Effect of Immune Complexes

Circulating immune complexes can either enhance or suppress antibody production. Antibody production is enhanced when immune complexes are fixed on the APC's surface by the Fc receptors. The surface-bound antigens are effectively presented to T cells. On the contrary, the B cells are inhibited when the immune complexes bind to the B cell by the Fc receptor; this leads to cross-linkage between B-cell surface immunoglobulin and Fc receptor, which inactivates B cells (see Fig. 4-6).[3]

The Regulatory Effect of Anti-idiotype Antibody

The variable region of an antibody molecule has unique antigenic characteristics that frequently elicit antibody responses in the same host. The antigenic determinants within the variable region or antigen binding site of an immunoglobulin molecule are known as idiotopes. Therefore, each immunoglobulin molecule can be categorized according to its idiotopes. The term *idiotype* is used to describe a group of antibody molecules that have similar idiotopes. In general, a B cell or B cells of the same clone produce antibodies with similar idiotype, because idiotopes of an antibody molecule are inherent properties of a B cell. The antibody produced against an idiotope is called anti-idiotypic antibody. During the course of an immune response anti-idiotypic antibodies are made by the host to regulate the response. The evidence for a suppressive effect of the anti-idiotypic antibody comes from murine experiments. A particular strain of mouse responds to the antigen phosphoryl choline (PC). Approximately 90% of the anti-PC antibodies produced belonged to the same idiotype. The antibody response to the antigen PC was suppressed in the animal that was given the antibodies that were raised against this idiotype (anti-idiotypic antibody). Furthermore, the suppression of anti-PC antibody was more pronounced in the production of this idiotype than other idiotypes. The plausible mechanism is that the anti-idiotype antibodies bind to the target idiotope on the B-cell surface immunoglobulin leading to the B-cell inactivation.[3]

The Regulatory Effect of Suppressor T Cells

Whereas T_H cells promote B-cell activation, suppressor T cells (T_S) down-regulate B-cell activity. T_S activity is demonstrated in cell transfer experiments. The antibody response to an antigen is suppressed in a recipient animal who received the T cells from an animal that has been rendered tolerant to the same antigen.[3]

Antibody Diversity

The immune system is capable of synthesizing different antibody molecules that collectively recognize an unlimited number of antigens. Such diversity has fascinated immunologists throughout history.

In 1930 the instructionist theory was proposed that stated that an antigen could serve as a template to which complementary antibody molecules were synthesized. This theory was ruled out when it was realized that the three-dimensional structure of an antibody molecule is determined by its amino acid sequence. The germline theory was formulated in 1960. It hypothesizes that antibody genes arise during vertebrate evolution by gene duplication, mutation, and selection. Thus, each individual is endowed with a complete antibody gene repertoire at conception, and antibody production merely requires antigen stimulus. On the contrary, the somatic mutation theory states that diversified antibody genes arise from a relatively small number of germline genes by mutation or recombination of the genes during development.

An understanding of structure and gene rearrangements of the antibody gene families offers good insight to the mechanism for generating antibody diversity. Antibody genes are located on three separate chromosomes: Heavy chain genes are located on chromosome 14, λ light chain genes are located on chromosome 22, and κ light chain genes are located on chromosome 2. The variable region of a heavy chain (V_H) is encoded by three genes, which are transcribed into three polypeptide segments: V_H, D, and J_H. The variable region of a light chain (V_L) is encoded by two separate genes that are transcribed into two polypeptide segments: V_L and J_L. These are known as variable-segment genes (V genes) of heavy and light chains. There are many different genes for each variable-segment gene. For example, there are about 100 different genes that encode for V_H segment, four for D segment, and six for J_H. Thus, a B cell is provided with an enormous gene library from which it selects the appropriate combination of V genes for V_H and V_L synthesis (Fig. 4-7). This process of V-gene recombination occurs early in B-cell development, allowing the emergence of diversified B-cell populations that collectively will recognize an unlimited number of antigens. Additional diversification comes from imprecision in joining the recombining genes. This phenomenon is known as *junctional diversity*. Furthermore, the high mutational rate of V genes also contributes to antibody diversity. In conclusion, the immune system is capable of responding to an unlimited number of antigens with exquisite specificity. Such a diversified response is made possible through gene recombination, junctional diversity, and V-gene mutation.[11–13]

Cell-Mediated Immune Response

The cell-mediated immune response involves primarily T lymphocytes, whereas antibody plays a subordinate role. The cytotoxic T cells (T_C) and lymphokines

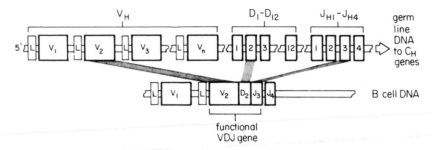

FIGURE 4-7. Heavy chain variable region g (V-gene) recombination: A sequence of gene rearrangement occurs in the stem cell that is destined to become a B cell. A given D gene translocates to a given J gene, forming DJ segment. This is followed by the translocation of a given V gene to the DJ segment. The light chain V-gene recombination occurs shortly after heavy chain gene rearrangement. (From Roitt IM, Brostoff J, Male DK: Immunology. London, Gower Medical Publishing, 1985.)

are important effectors of cell-mediated immune responses. Whereas the former destroy targets by direct cell contact, the latter recruit and activate other cells, such as macrophages, amplifying the response. In addition, lymphokines may be directly toxic to the target cells. Macrophages play dual roles in a cell-mediated immune response; they present antigen to the T cells during induction phase and become activated in response to lymphokines during effector phase. There is yet another group of lymphocytes known as natural killer (NK) cells that are able to destroy targets without previous sensitization. Finally, an effector mechanism that involves antibodies and cells for target destruction is known as antibody-dependent cell-mediated cytolysis (ADCC).

MHC Restriction of T-Cell Antigen Recognition

In general, T cells recognize antigen in association with MHC molecules. Free or soluble antigens do not usually stimulate T cells. Each T-cell population responds to antigens that are associated with either MHC class I or MHC class II molecules; T_H cells are MHC class II restricted and T_C cells are MHC class I

restricted. Biologically, this division of MHC restriction appears to make sense. Since the major function of T_C is to eliminate the virally infected cells, it needs to recognize the antigen in conjunction with MHC class I molecule, which is widely distributed on all nucleated cells in a host. On the other hand, the T_H cells are regulatory cells within the immune system, for such internal decision the T cells need to recognize antigens in association with the MHC class II molecule, which is limited to cells of the immune system.[14]

The T-Cell Antigen Receptor

The precise molecular structure of a T-cell receptor is still debated. The current understanding is that the T-cell receptor is a complex consisting of three components: antigen receptor, MHC molecule receptor, and a CD3 glycoprotein. The antigen receptor (Tr) is a heterodimer consisting of two polypeptide chains, α and β chains, which are linked by disulfide bonds. The Tr polypeptide chain and an immunoglobulin molecule are structurally similar. For example, both have variable and constant regions. Furthermore, the Tr may also have an idiotype. However, the genes

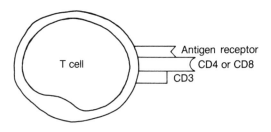

FIGURE 4-8. T-cell receptor.

that code for the Tr peptides are completely separated from immunoglobulin genes.

The second component of the T-cell receptor is the receptor for a MHC molecule. Either CD4 or CD8 is expressed, depending on the T-cell subpopulation. The third component, the CD3 molecule, is expressed by all T cells and is known to transmit the activation signal to the T cell. Therefore, the T-cell receptor is a complex structure consisting of three components:[14,15]

1. the antigen receptor, which consists of α and β chains;

2. the receptor for MHC molecule, CD4 or CD8; and

3. CD3, which transmits activation signals.

A schematic representation of a T-cell antigen receptor complex is depicted in Figure 4-8.

T-Cell Activation

T-cell activation requires both soluble mediators and direct cell contact. The well-characterized soluble mediators are interleukin-1 (IL-1) and interleukin-2 (IL-2). IL-1 is a cytokine synthesized by various cell sources, including macrophages. IL-2 is a lymphokine because it is made by antigen-sensitized T lymphocytes, whereas no other cell source has been identified. T-cell activation involves at least three cell populations (Fig. 4-9):

1. A macrophage or APC presents the antigen and provides IL-1.

2. A T_H cell recognizes the antigen in conjunction with an MHC class II molecule on the APC surface. During the cell contact, the APC may receive a signal or signals from the T_H cell and releases IL-1. IL-1 promotes the IL-2 receptor expression or IL-2 synthesis by T cells. Only T cells that are already sensitized by the antigen can respond to IL-1.

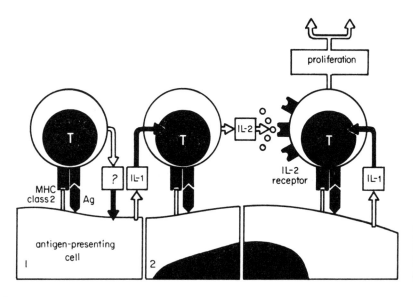

FIGURE 4-9. T-cell activation. (From Roitt IM, Brostoff J, Male DK. Immunology. London, Gower Medical Publishing, 1985.)

3. An effector T cell that is sensitized by the antigen and stimulated by IL-1 expresses IL-2 receptors. In the presence of IL-2 it undergoes blast transformation, cell division, and differentiation. The effector T cells may be cytotoxic or lymphokine-producing T cells.

Therefore, activation of an effector T cell requires three signals: antigenic stimulation, IL-1, and IL-2. Figure 4-9 outlines the sequence of T-cell activation.[14,16]

Effectors of Cell-Mediated Immune Response

The effectors of cell-mediated immune response include effector cells, which kill the target by direct cell contact, and soluble mediators, collectively known as cytokines (Table 4-3), which have direct cytolytic activity or enhance the cytolytic activity of the effector cells.

Table 4-3: Cytokines

Cytokines	Immunobiologic Activities
REGULATES OTHER LYMPHOCYTES	
IL-1	Stimulates antigen-activated T cells to express IL-2 receptors or produce IL-2
IL-2	Stimulates antigen-activated T-cell proliferation
IL-4 (B-cell growth factor 1)	Stimulates antigen-activated B-cell proliferation
IL-6 (B-cell growth factor 2)	Induces proliferating B-cell differentiation into a plasma cell
REGULATES HEMATOPOIESIS	
IL-3	Supports hematopoietic stem cell growth
Granulocyte–monocyte colony stimulating factor	Stimulates the growth of hematopoietic cells that are committed to granulocyte or monocyte lineage
REGULATES OTHER EFFECTOR CELLS	
MIF	Inhibits macrophage migration
MAF	Activates macrophages
γ interferon	Enhances NK cells' cytotoxicity, activates macrophages
DIRECT TOXICITY TO TARGETS	
TNF	Causes tumor cell death

Cytotoxic T Cells

Cytotoxic T cells (T_C) are capable of destroying target cells without involving antibody. Direct cell contact is required for target cell killing. This cell contact is achieved by the T-cell receptor, which binds to the target antigen and the MHC molecule on the target cell surface. This leads to the target cell swelling and destruction. A T_C can go through many cycles of target cell destruction; after killing one target cell, the T_C can attach to another target cell and repeat the killing activity.

The main function of T_C is to eliminate virally infected host cells. These T_C are CD8-positive cells with MHC class I restriction. A second type of T_C, found in patients undergoing graft rejection or in the tumor-infiltrating lymphocytes, is CD4 positive and MHC class II restricted.[14]

Macrophages

Macrophages are important inflammatory cells whose functions are often modulated by lymphokines. For example, macrophage migration inhibition factor (MIF) inhibits the migration of macrophages so that they are retained at the site of antigen response. Furthermore, their microbicidal and tumoricidal activities are greatly enhanced by yet another activated T-cell product, macrophage activation factor (MAF). However, the biologic activities of macrophages are not antigen specific. Lymphokines produced by the T cells sensitized to one antigen may activate macrophages that will destroy the sensitizing antigens as well as other unrelated targets. Therefore, the process of lymphokine production is antigen specific, whereas the biologic activity of lymphokine-activated macrophages is antigen nonspecific.[14]

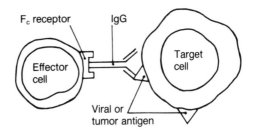

FIGURE 4-10. Antibody-dependent cell-mediated cytolysis.

Natural Killer Cells

A group of large lymphocytes with cytoplasmic granules is capable of killing virally infected cells or neoplastic cells without previous sensitization. These are known as natural killer (NK) cells. The cell lineage of NK cells is currently being debated. They do not express T- or B-cell markers; however, they consistently express Fc receptors on the cell surface. Their cellular activities are modulated by lymphokines. For example, IL-2 stimulates their proliferative activities, and interferon enhances their cytolytic activities.[14,17,18]

Antibody-Dependent Cell-Mediated Cytolysis

Effector cells with cytolytic activity and Fc receptors are able to lyse antibody-coated target cells (Fig. 4-10). This phenomenon is known as antibody-dependent cell-mediated cytolysis (ADCC). Direct effector–target cell contact is required for target cell lysis, and it probably involves the cytolytic mediator released by the effector cell. The antibody involved is usually IgG, which is directed against viral or tumor antigens on the target cell surface. Therefore, the antigen specificity in this cytolytic activity resides in antibody molecule. The effector cells are poorly defined. NK cells probably play an important role;

however, any Fc receptor–positive cells—including macrophages, monocytes, and neutrophils—have potential to be effector cells.[14]

Cytokines

Cytokines are protein molecules that essentially transmit messages between cells. Recent experimental data suggest that the primary biologic activities of cytokines are regulation of cell growth and cellular differentiation. The cytokines that are produced by lymphocytes are known as lymphokines, whereas those produced by monocytes are known as monokines.

Lymphokines are primarily produced by activated T cells. IL-2 is a T-cell growth factor that induces proliferation of antigen-activated T cells and enhance NK cells' cytolytic activities. There are two well-characterized lymphokines that affect hematopoiesis: interleukin-3 (IL-3) and granulocyte–macrophage colony stimulating factor. IL-3 supports the growth of pluripotential stem cells of the hematopoietic system, whereas granulocyte–macrophage colony stimulating factor induces the growth of hematopoietic cells that are differentiated and committed to become granulocytes or macrophages. Activated T cells also produce B-cell growth factors; interleukin-4 (IL-4, also known as B-cell growth factor 1) stimulates proliferation of antigen-activated B cells, and B-cell growth factor 2 induces differentiation of proliferating B cells into antibody-secreting plasma cells. MIF and MAF are activated T-cell products that regulate macrophage functions described in the previous section. Gamma interferon is also a lymphokine that is known to have biologic functions, including enhancement of NK cells' cytolytic activities and activation of macrophages.[9]

The two well-characterized monokines are IL-1 and tumor necrosis factor (TNF). IL-1 stimulates IL-2 receptor expression and IL-2 synthesis by antigen-activated T cells. TNF has direct cytolytic activity against tumor cells.[19]

Idiotypic Network in Regulation of Immune Response

Jerne proposed the theory of idiotypic network based on the observations made by two independent groups: Kunkle et al, and Oudin and Michel.[20] The theory postulates that the immune system consists of a network of idiotypes. Antibodies generated in response to an antigen constitute the first wave of antibody response. The second wave of antibody response is initiated by the idiotypes of the first-wave antibodies. The second-wave antibodies are known as anti-idiotypic antibodies and express idiotopes that generate a third wave of antibody response (anti–anti-idiotypic antibody). In theory, the preceding idiotype–anti-idiotype response can continue indefinitely; however, the circuit is ended when one of the antibody's idiotopes resembles that of an earlier antibody's idiotopes. The idiotypic network can be enormous, because each antibody molecule has more than one idiotope.[21,22]

The implications of the idiotypic network in immune regulation are many. Antibody production may be enhanced or suppressed by anti-idiotypic antibody. Anti-idiotypic antibody may mimic the challenging antigen, resulting in B-cell activation. Conversely, anti-idiotypic antibody may suppress the B-cell clone with a specific idiotype (see "The Regulatory Effect of Anti-idiotype Antibody" earlier in this chapter).

In principle, T and B cells should share similar regulatory mechanisms. The search for T-cell idiotypes has proved to be rewarding: The existence of an idiotope profile of the variable regions of T-cell antigen receptor is well documented. Thus, the potential for the T cells to be regulated by way of the idiotypic network exists.[23,24] The idiotypic network of T-cell antigen receptor is likely to be more complex than the antibody idiotypic network because two types of regulatory T cells, inducer and suppressor T cells, exist.

In conclusion, the idiotypic network is probably widely utilized by the immune system for regulation of its response. Experimental data imply that regulation of both T- and B-cell responses involve idiotypic network.

References

1. Thiele DI, Lipsky PE: The accessory function of phagocytic cells in human T-cell and B-cell responses. J Immunol 129:1033, 1982

2. Schwartz RH: T-lymphocyte recognition of antigen in association with gene products of the major histocompatibility complex. Annu Rev Immunol 3:237, 1985

3. Roitt I, Brostoff J, Male D: Immunology, p 8.1. London, Gower Medical Publishing, 1985

4. Mehta SR, Sandler RS, Ford RJ, et al: Cellular interaction between B and T lymphocytes: enhanced release of B cell growth factor. Lymphokine Res 5:49, 1986

5. Howaed M, Paul WE: Interleukins for B lymphocytes. Lymphokine Res 1:1, 1982

6. Maizel AI, Sahasrabuddhe C, Mehta S, et al: Characterization of B-cell growth factor. Lymphokine Res 1:9, 1982

7. Sharma S, Mehta S, Morgan J, Maizel A: Molecular cloning and expression of a B-cell growth factor gene in *Escherichia coli*. Science 235:1489, 1987

8. Yokoda T, Otsuka T, Mosmann T, et al: Isolation and characterization of a human interleukin cDNA clone, homologous to mouse B-cell stimulatory factor 1, that expresses B-cell and T-cell stimulating activities. Proc Natl Acad Sci USA 83:5894, 1986

9. Dinarello CA, Mier JW: Lymphokines. N Engl J Med 317:940, 1987

10. Hood LE, Weissman IL, Wood WB, et al: The immune response: Affinity maturation and immunologic memory. In: Immunology, 2nd ed. p 287, Menlo Park, CA, Benjamin/Cummings, 1984

11. Roitt I, Brostoff J, Male D: Immunology, p 8.1. London, Gower Medical Publishing, 1985

12. Yancopoulus GD, Alt FW: Regulation of the assembly and expression of variable-region genes. Annu Rev Immunol 4:339, 1986

13. Griffiths GM, Berek C, Kaartinen M, et al: Somatic mutations of immune response to 2-phenyl oxazolone. Nature 312:271, 1984

14. Roitt I, Brostoff J, Male D: Immunology, p 11.1. London, Gower Medical Publishing, 1985

15. Kronenberg M, Siu G, Hood LE, Shastri N: The molecular genetics of the T-cell antigen receptor and T-cell antigen-recognition. Annu Rev Immunol 4:529, 1986

16. Schwab R, Crow MK, Russo C, Weksler HE: Requirements for T-cell activations by OK3 monoclonal antibody: Role of T3 molecules and interleukin-1. J Immunol 135:1714, 1985

17. Lazarus AH, Baines MG: Studies on the mechanism of specificity of human natural killer cells for tumor cells: correlation between target cell transferin receptor expression and competitive activity. Cell Immunol 96:255, 1985

18. MacDougall SL, Shustik C, Sullivan AK: Target cell specificity of human natural killer cells. Cell Immunol 103:352, 1986

19. Le J, Vilcek J: Tumor necrosis factor and interleukin-1: Cytokines with multiple overlapping biological activities. Lab Invest 36:234, 1987

20. Jerne NK: Idiotypic network and other preconceived ideas. Immunol Rev 79:5, 1984

21. Burdette S, Schwartz RS: Idiotypes and idiotypic networks. N Engl J Med 317:219, 1987

22. Rajewsky K, Takemori T: Genetics, expression, and function of idiotypes. Annu Rev Immunol 1:569, 1983

23. Geha RS: Idiotypic determination on human T cells and modulation of human T cell receptors by anti-idiotypic antibodies. J Immunol 133:1846, 1984

24. Sim GK, Mackneil A, Augustin AA: T helper receptors; idiotypes and repertoire. Immunol Rev 90:49, 1986

CHAPTER 5

Mechanisms of the Nonspecific Immune Response

Karen James

Cellular Mechanisms of the Nonspecific Immune Response

Barrier Epithelial Cells

The body's first line of defense is an intact barrier of epithelial cells. This includes the skin and the mucous membrane linings of the respiratory, urinary, and gastrointestinal tracts. The skin is the largest single organ of the body; one of its primary functions is protection from the external environment.[1] The layers of the skin are essentially continuous with the mucous membranes of the digestive, respiratory, and genitourinary tracts. When epithelial structures are damaged (e.g., cuts or punctures) or destroyed (severe burns), the protective effect of the epithelial barrier has been broken and the danger of an infectious process has been significantly increased. Most infections enter the body through the mucous membranes, which are protected not only by barrier epithelial cells, but also by biochemical defense mechanisms in the secretions (e.g., lysozyme, stomach acid, secretory immunoglobulins).

Polymorphonuclear Neutrophils

Polymorphonuclear neutrophils (PMNs) comprise the largest percentage of leukocytes in the peripheral blood of humans. The mature PMN is a phagocytic cell with distinct granules.[2] The granules contain acid hydrolases, myeloperoxidase, lysozyme, lactoferrin, and cationic proteins. Each of these biochemical components performs either a bactericidal function or serves to degrade the organic materials that remain after bacteria are killed.[3]

PMNs are involved in the nonspecific immune response through a series of steps: (1) adherence or attachment to the damaged epithelium, (2) locomotion or ameboid movement, (3) diapedesis or emigration through the wall of the blood vessel, (4) chemotaxis or directed movement toward the particles to be engulfed, (5) phagocytosis or ingestion of the particles, (6) increased metabolism through glycolysis, (7) degranulation, and (8) digestion of the foreign material.[4,5]

Adherence of PMNs to the vascular endothelial cells is a poorly understood phenomenon. These cells become "sticky" after exposure to chemotactic factors *in vitro* (outside the body, as in a test tube or petri dish) or *in vivo* (inside the body, as in experimental animals).

Locomotion of PMNs is similar to the movements of amebae.[5] These cells can crawl about on the surfaces of blood vessel walls, changing direction every 20 μm or so by sending out pseudopods from a different part of the cell surface. In the absence of specific stimuli, this locomotion is not in a straight line and is not directed toward anything particular.

For diapedesis to occur, locomotion is necessary, as is adherence to the walls of the capillaries.

Diapedesis, or emigration through the wall of the blood vessel, occurs following adherence to the endothelium (Fig. 5-1). The PMN inserts pseudopods between the endothelial cell junctions, disrupting the basement membrane at that location so that the PMN can "squeeze" itself out of the blood vessel into the surrounding tissue spaces.[5]

Chemotaxis is the directed movement of phagocytic cells either toward or away from particles in the environment.[5] Directed migration of PMNs is mediated primarily by fluid phase components of the complement system, particularly C5a, which will be discussed later in this chapter. Other factors that are known to be chemotactic include certain products of the coagulation or fibrinolytic pathways and certain bacterial products.[2]

Phagocytosis has been studied for over 75 years. The external cell wall of the PMN adheres to and completely surrounds the offending bacterium or other particle, encapsulating the foreign substance with a layer of inside-out membrane called a phagosome (Fig. 5-2). Opsonins such as C3b and IgG clearly increase the rate and quantity of particle up-

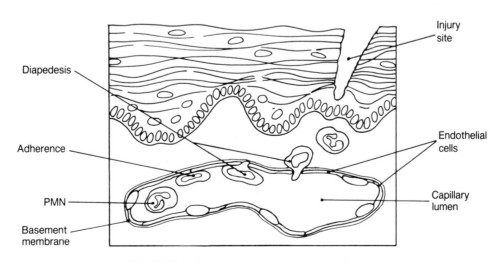

FIGURE 5-1. Adherence and diapedesis of PMNs.

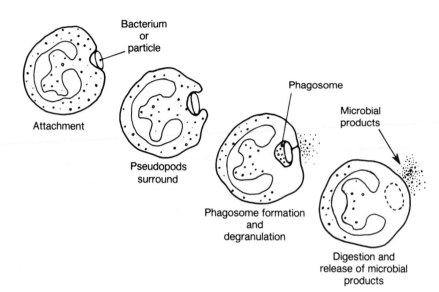

FIGURE 5-2. Phagocytosis.

take. Opsonins have been described as the "butter on the bread" that makes the particle more "appetizing" to the phagocytic cell. C3b and IgG function as opsonins because PMNs and other phagocytic cells have receptors on their surface that specifically recognize the exposed portions of those molecules when they coat bacteria or other particles.

During phagocytosis, the metabolism of leukocytes changes rather dramatically. O_2 and glucose are consumed, primarily through the hexose monophosphate shunt. H_2O_2 is produced in the respiratory burst that occurs as the phagocytosed particle is digested.

Degranulation of granulocytes involves the fusion of intracellular granules with the plasma membrane. The contents of the granules are then released either into the phagosome or into the accumulated fluid outside of the cell.[3,5] As will be discussed in the section on inflammation, much of the tissue damage associated with injury can be attributed to the contents of the granules that are released during degranulation of PMNs.

Digestion occurs following the degranulation step. When the granules are fused with the vacuole containing the phagocytosed particle, the particle is exposed to the lytic action of the enzymes. The mechanism by which many types of bacteria are killed following ingestion by phagocytes requires H_2O_2 and the enzyme myeloperoxidase.

Dysfunctions of PMNs

Diseases associated with dysfunctions of PMNs include chronic granulomatous disease (CGD), glucose-6-phosphate dehydrogenase (G6PD) deficiency, myeloperoxidase (MPO) deficiency, and Chediak-Higashi syndrome.[6]

CGD is an X-linked, inherited disease with clinical manifestations appearing during the first 2 years of life. These patients are susceptible to severe infections with organisms that are catalase positive but are normally not pathogenic (*e.g.*, *Staphylococcus epidermidis*, *Escherichia coli*, *Serratia marcescens*). Patients with CGD have an enzymatic deficiency that results in an absence of hexose monophosphate (HMP) shunt activity, causing a decreased production of H_2O_2 necessary for the killing of these bacteria after they have been phagocytosed. Catalase-negative organisms can still be killed by their own H_2O_2 production inside the digestive vacuole. However, catalase-positive organisms can detoxify the bacterial peroxide and the organism survives.

The laboratory test most useful in the diagnosis of CGD is the nitroblue tetrazolium (NBT) test. NBT is a yellow, water-soluble compound that turns blue upon reduction. The dye is ingested in the presence of latex particles. When H_2O_2 is produced along with other events associated with the respiratory burst, the dye is reduced by the normal PMN, and blue granules can be seen morphologically, or the NBT can be extracted and the reaction read at OD_{580} to measure NBT reduction as a ratio to ingestion.[7,8] The normal ratio is ≥ 2.5. In the absence of bacteria, the CGD PMN cannot produce H_2O_2, so the dye remains yellow, with a resulting NBT reduction–ingestion ratio ≤ 1.5. Females with a ratio between 1.5 and 2.5 have a subpopulation of PMNs of cells that do not reduce NBT and may be carriers of the X-linked disease.[9]

G6PD deficiency is an X-linked recessive disorder resulting in a defective enzyme rather than an absence of the enzyme. Several hundred variants of the enzyme have been described, only a few of which lead to severe hemolysis in the absence of defined oxidative stress. The form of G6PD deficiency seen in blacks from the United States does not result in hemolysis unless stimulated by a drug (*e.g.*, quinine) or (rarely) by a febrile illness or diabetic ketoacidosis.[9] The G6PD enzyme is the first in the hexose monophosphate shunt pathway. Only in recent years has it been realized that these patients also have a defect in leukocyte function.[6] Although G6PD deficiency is inherited in an X-linked manner, leukocyte function in both males and females can be affected. The susceptibility to organisms is similar to that of CGD patients, but the onset of the disease is usually later in life and associated with anemia. Laboratory diagnosis is by the NBT test and by detection of the G6PD enzyme deficiency.

MPO deficiency and Chediak-Higashi (CH) syndrome are relatively rare disorders.[6] Functional and immunochemical absence of the enzyme MPO from granules of neutrophils and monocytes but not from eosinophils is inherited as an autosomal recessive trait.[9] MPO potentiates the microbicidal effectiveness of H_2O_2 in the phagosome, which is necessary for killing certain organisms, particularly *Candida* species and staphylococcal species. MPO deficiency can be diagnosed in the laboratory by peroxidase staining of peripheral blood leukocytes.

CH syndrome is a rare, genetically determined disease manifested clinically by abnormal leukocyte granulation, defective pigmentation, and increased susceptibility to infections.[10] Morphologically, CH syndrome is characterized by giant cytoplasmic granular inclusions in PMNs and platelets that are discernible by light microscopy. The metabolic and biochemical pathways associated with other enzyme deficiencies appear to be normal, but the PMNs of these patients have abnormal intracellular killing of certain organisms, including streptococcal and pneumococcal species as well as those listed earlier for MPO deficiency. Recently, Chediak-Higashi syndrome patients have been shown also to have defective natural killer (NK) cells,[10] a defect that can be partially reversed *in vitro* by substances known to increase cyclic GMP or decrease cyclic AMP. Such substances have normalized both bacterial killing and NK response.[10,11] The laboratory diagnosis of CH syndrome can be made by light microscopic examination of PMNs and platelets.

Eosinophils

The eosinophilic granulocytes constitute less than 3% of the circulating leukocytes in the blood of normal humans. Eosinophils arise from a common progenitor cell with PMNs but are much less efficient at phagocytosis. The granules of eosinophils do not contain lysozyme, but are rich in acid phosphatase and peroxidase activity.[12] Although the role of eosinophils is not known, two roles have been postulated: ingestion of immune complexes and limiting inflammatory reactions by antagonizing the effects of mediators (discussed later). Eosinophil granules also have a unique protein called eosinophilic basic protein, which has been found to be toxic to certain parasites, the clearance of which is also attributed to eosinophils.[12] Eosinophilia (>10% of leukocytes in peripheral blood) is found in association with allergic reactions as well as parasitic infections.

Mediator Cells

Cells that participate in immunologic reactions by release of biochemical substances (mediators) include mast cells, basophils, and platelets.[12] The biologic activities of these mediators include increased vascular permeability, smooth muscle contraction, and augmentation of the inflammatory response (Fig. 5-3). Blood platelets contain serotonin and lysosomal enzymes that are released from the granules during platelet aggregation. Serotonin apparently does not have a pharmacologic role in humans, but lysosomal enzymes participate in digestion of foreign materials.

Human skin and the gastrointestinal tract are particularly rich in mast cells. Granules containing the potent mediators are released from mast cells upon injury to these tissues.[13] The biochemical components of these granules include heparin, histamine, serotonin, hyaluronic acid, and eosinophil chemotactic factor of anaphylaxis (ECF-A). Immunologic reactions involving IgG or IgE, which bind to receptors on the surface of mast cells and basophils, can trigger degranulation and release of the mediators into the circulation (Fig. 5-4). Mast cells can be stimulated to degranulate by nonimmunologic mechanisms (*e.g.*, infections of the skin or mucous membranes, surgical incisions, and certain other agents, including opiates).[13]

Basophilic granulocytes make up 0.5% to 2% of circulating leukocytes. At one time it was thought that basophils were circulating mast cells (or that mast cells were stationary basophils), but further study has shown these two cell types do differ in the structure and content of their granules. Basophilic granules contain primarily histamine and a group of sulfidopeptide leukotrienes LTC_4, LTD_4, and LTE_4 (formerly called slow-reacting substance of anaphylaxis [SRS-A]), which are potent spasmogenic agents causing constriction of smooth muscle.[14] *

---

* LTC_4 = 5S-hydroxy-6R-S-glutathionyl-7,9-*trans*-11,14-*cis*-eicosatetraenoic acid (leukotriene C_4).

LTD_4 = LTC_4 cleaved by γ glutamyl transpeptidase to 5S-hydroxy-6R-S-cysteinylglycyl-7,9-*trans*-11,14-*cis*-eicosatetraenoic acid (leukotriene D_4).

LTE_4 = LTD_4 cleaved by a dipeptidase to 5S-hydroxy-6R-S-cysteinyl-7,9-*trans*-11,14-*cis*-eicosatetraenoic acid (leukotriene E_4).

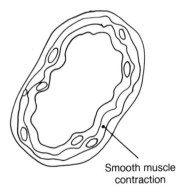
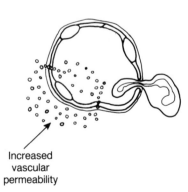

Smooth muscle contraction   Increased vascular permeability

FIGURE 5-3. Biologic activities of mediator substances.

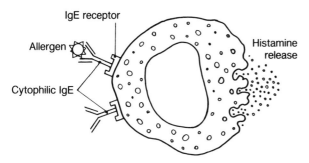

FIGURE 5-4. Basophil/mast cell histamine release.

Like mast cells, basophils respond to IgE-containing immune complexes that bind to the IgE receptors on the basophils to stimulate degranulation. The primary function of the basophil appears to be to amplify the reaction that starts with the mast cells at the site of entry of the antigen. For example, contact sensitivity with the antigenic substances from poison ivy first cause a rash on the surface of the skin or mucous membranes, but a severe case of exposure to poison ivy can result in disseminated effects from the histamine released from basophils within the circulation. Rare cases of basophil leukemia have been reported, but no specific diseases have been associated with a general basophilia.

Mononuclear Phagocyte System

The term *reticuloendothelial system* (RES) was introduced by Aschoff in 1924 to designate all actively phagocytic cells.[5] The current definition of the RES limited to mononuclear phagocytic cells has been renamed the *mononuclear phagocyte system* (MPS). Mononuclear phagocytes include tissue macrophages located primarily in the reticular connective tissue framework of the spleen, liver, and lymphoid tissues[7] and their immature circulating form as blood monocytes.[15] Debris removed by the MPS include old or injured red cells, white cells and platelets, bacteria, antigen–antibody complexes, and degenerated or damaged cell membranes.[16] The Kupffer cells of the liver are the most actively phagocytic cells in the MPS. Other histiocytes (tissue macrophages) actively involved in phagocytosis include alveolar (pulmonary) macrophages, splenic macrophages, and macrophages of the lymph nodes, peritoneum, and other areas (Fig. 5-5). At times when the MPS is actively involved in eliminating debris from circulation, organs that are rich in tissue macrophages become involved, resulting in lymphadenopathy (enlarged lymph nodes), splenomegaly (enlarged

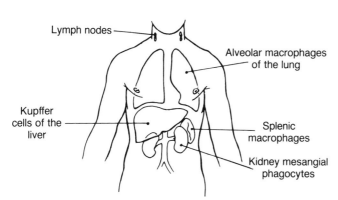

FIGURE 5-5. Organs and cells of the MPS.

spleen), or hepatomegaly (enlarged liver). It is the intent of the body's defense mechanisms that these secondary barriers stop the spread of infection, but in some cases, even the MPS becomes overwhelmed.

Mechanisms of phagocytosis that were described earlier for PMNs also occur with monocytes and macrophages. Circulating PMNs, however, are end stage cells (i.e., after phagocytosis and degranulation, these cells die). Macrophages, conversely, appear to be stimulated by the processes involved with phagocytosis, become secretory cells, synthesize acute phase proteins, and may even proliferate locally within the tissues.[15]

Mononuclear phagocytes respond to the same chemotactic factors that attract PMNs (e.g., the C5a peptide of complement). The primary chemotactic materials to which macrophages respond, however, are soluble factors released from T lymphocytes, such as migration inhibitory factor (MIF), which will be discussed in more detail in a later chapter. Peripheral blood monocytes are much less efficient at phagocytosis and killing bacteria than are PMNs. Macrophages utilize predominantly the oxygen-dependent metabolic pathways to provide energy for the cell.

Mononuclear phagocytes are less efficient than PMNs at killing bacteria, and the mechanisms of killing are not as well understood. When macrophages are stimulated by phagocytic events, they become secretory cells that produce and secrete a wide variety of biologically active factors that influence the activities of lymphocytes.[17] One factor, interleukin-1 (IL-1), has specificity for activating T cells, but most of the factors secreted by macrophages nonspecifically suppress the activities of lymphocytes. These include interferon, prostaglandins, complement components, and certain other acute phase proteins.

Antigen presentation is another very important function of a subset of macrophages that have HLA-DR (or Ia) antigens on their surface.[17] The HLA-DR (or Ia) molecule appears to interact with the antigen

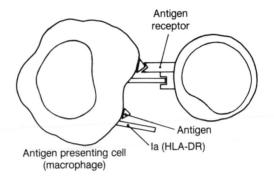

FIGURE 5-6. HLA-DR (Ia)$^+$ monocyte-bound antigen.

molecules that are tightly bound to the surface of the macrophages, with this "complex" of HLA-DR (or Ia) and antigen being recognized by lymphocytes as immunogenic (Fig. 5-6). It has been shown that macrophage-bound antigen is significantly more antigenic than is an equivalent amount of free antigen.

Humoral Mechanisms of the Nonspecific Immune Response

Complement

The complement system consists of 14 components that are involved in two separate pathways of activation. The five proteins that are unique to the classical pathway include the trimolecular complex of C1 (C1q, C1r, C1s), C4, and C2. Three proteins are unique to the alternative pathway, including Factor B, Factor D, and P (properdin). Six components that participate in both the classical and alternative pathway include C3, C5, C6, C7, C8, and C9. These components were named in the order in which they were described; consequently, the sequence of activation is not in numerical order. Although complement activation is complex, the components interact in a specific cascading sequence. Both pathways can be divided into three units (recognition, activation, and membrane attack), which simplifies the study of complement.[18]

Classical Pathway

Recognition Unit. The C1q molecule consists of a collagenous region with six globular head groups. This component appears to be like a flower pot with six flowers. When a specific antibody interacts with its corresponding antigen, binding sites for the globular head groups of C1q are exposed on the Fc region of the antibody molecule (Fig. 5-7). At least two molecules of IgG or C-reactive protein (CRP) or one molecule of IgM are required for binding C1q.[19] When circulating in plasma, the collagen portion of C1q is surrounded by two molecules of C1r and two molecules of C1s. When C1q binds to the Fc region of IgG or IgM or the equivalent region of CRP, a conformational change occurs in C1q. This change in C1q causes the proenzyme C1r to become the enzymatically active $\overline{C1r}$. The substrate for the enzyme $\overline{C1r}$ is C1s, which is then cleaved to become the serine esterase, $\overline{C1s}$.

Activation Unit. The active enzyme of $\overline{C1s}$ cleaves two proteins, C4 (into C4a and C4b) and C2 (into C2a and C2b), in a magnesium-dependent reaction. C4b and C2a combine to form an active enzyme,

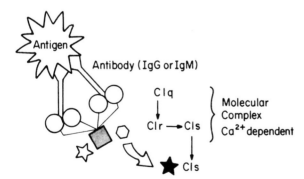

FIGURE 5-7. The classical pathway recognition unit. (From James K. Complement: activation, consequences, and control. Am J Med Technol 1982; 48: 735.)

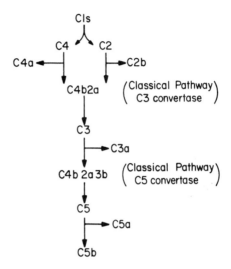

FIGURE 5-8. The classical pathway activation unit. (From James K. Complement: Activation, consequences, and control. Am J Med Technol 1982; 48: 735.)

C4b2a, which is the classical pathway C3 convertase (Fig. 5-8). C4a and C2b are by-products of the process of activation of the classical pathway. The enzymatically active C4b2a complex can cleave many molecules of C3 into C3a and C3b. The C3b then either can form a covalent bond with the antigen or with bystander surfaces (*e.g.,* erythrocytes) in immune adherence (to be discussed later) or can bind to C4b2a to form C4b2a3b, an enzyme with specificity for C5. The final enzymatic step of the classical complement pathway is the cleavage of C5 into C5a and C5b by the C5 convertase, C4b2a3b. At this point, the classical pathway and the alternative pathway converge, with both pathways using the same membrane attack unit.

Membrane Attack Unit. C5b binds to one molecule of C6 to form a stable bimolecular complex, C5b6. If C7 is present, a trimolecular complex is formed, C5b67. C5b67 binds hydrophobically to a membrane (Fig. 5-9). Once C5b67 is bound, C8 can attach to form a functional transmembrane channel. Up to six molecules of C9 can surround the puncture

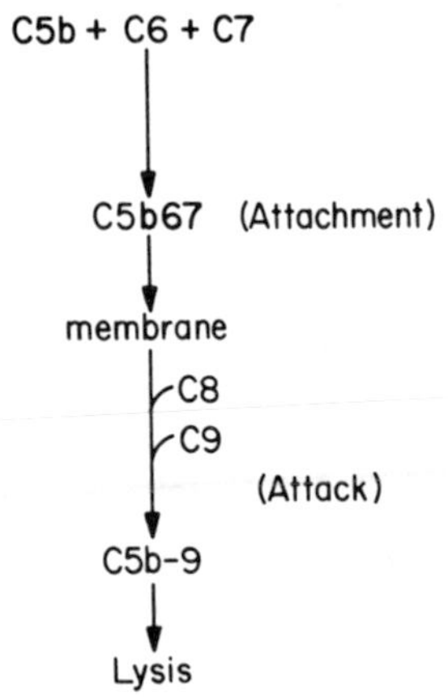

FIGURE 5-9. The membrane attack unit, common to both pathways. (From James K. Complement: activation, consequences, and control. Am J Med Technol 1982; 48: 735.)

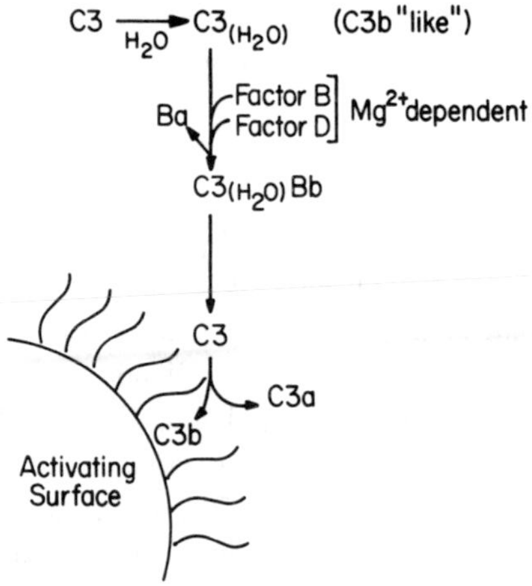

FIGURE 5-10. The alternative pathway recognition unit. (From James K. Complement: activation, consequences, and control. Am J Med Technol 1982; 48: 735.)

site, which effectively prevents the channel from being resealed. C9 is not essential for the lytic event, but it does accelerate lysis.

Alternative Pathway

Recognition Unit. Efficient activation of the alternative pathway is dependent upon the availability of an activating surface. Substances known to provide an activation surface are bacterial cell walls, bacterial lipopolysaccharide, fungal cell walls, some virus-infected cells, and rabbit erythrocytes.[20] It has recently been shown that the "activating surface" is actually a protective surface, protecting spontaneously hydrolyzed C3 (nonenzymatically cleaved into C3a and C3b) from being inactivated by the control proteins.[21] Hydrolyzed C3 becomes C3b-like (Fig. 5-10). In the presence of Factor D and magnesium, this C3b-like molecule can cleave Factor B into Ba and Bb. Ba becomes a by-product and Bb binds to the C3b to form an alternative pathway C3 convertase, C3bBb. By itself C3bBb is a very unstable molecule and would be quickly inactivated by control proteins (discussed later) unless it is bound to an activating surface such as those listed previously.

Activation Unit. When protected by an activating surface and stabilized by P (properdin), the C3bBbP enzymatic complex can cleave additional molecules of C3. If a second C3b molecule is inserted into the C3 convertase to become C3bBb3bP, this becomes a C5 convertase that can cleave C5 into C5a and C5b (Fig. 5-11).

Membrane Attack Unit. The membrane attack unit for the alternative pathway begins with C5b and progresses through C6, C7, C8, and C9 in exactly the same sequence as it does for the classical pathway.

Biologic Consequences of Complement Activation

Amplification. C3b can be generated either by the classical pathway C3 convertase (C4b2a) or by the alternative pathway C3 convertase (C3bBbP). This provides a feedback loop that uses the alternative pathway components (B,D,P) in both pathways to amplify the activation of the C3 through C9 components of activation and membrane attack (Fig. 5-12).

Anaphylatoxin. The cleavage of C4, C3, and C5 results in the release of the biologically active pep-

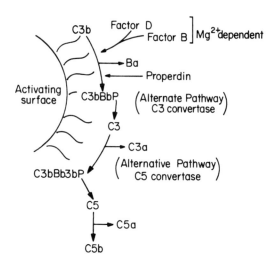

FIGURE 5-11. The alternative pathway activation unit. (From James K. Complement: activation, consequences, and control. Am J Med Technol 1982; 48: 735.)

tides C4a, C3a, and C5a (Fig. 5-13). These anaphylatoxins mediate inflammation by inducing the release of histamine from basophils and mast cells, by causing smooth muscle to contract, and by increasing vascular permeability.[22]

Immune Adherence. Immune adherence is the covalent bonding between the cleaved form of C3 (C3b) and nearby soluble immune complexes or particulate surfaces (Fig. 5-14). The portion of the C3b that does not adhere is exposed and available for binding to the receptor for C3b on human erythrocytes, B lymphocytes, monocytes, glomerular epithelial cells, or mast cells. B lymphocytes and macrophages also have receptors for C3d, which is formed by cleaving C3b into C3c and C3d. Many of the cells with receptors for C3b also have receptors for C4b. One biologic purpose for immune adherence is to facilitate removal of soluble immune complexes. Immune adherence provides a mechanism for the soluble complexes to bind to erythrocytes, facilitating removal of the complexes by the MPS.

Opsonization. Immune adherence is the covalent binding of C3b to a surface; however, once C3b and

IgG are present on that surface it becomes opsonized for more effective phagocytosis by PMNs or monocytes. The C3b receptors on these cells bind to the exposed C3b on the surface of the particle. The membrane of the phagocytic cell surrounds the opsonized particle, much like the two sides of a zipper fusing together. When the particle is completely surrounded, the cell membrane fuses together, thereby engulfing or phagocytosing the particle (see Fig. 5-2).

Chemotaxis. The by-product resulting from the cleavage of C5 by either the classical or alternative pathway C5 convertase is C5a (Fig. 5-15). C5a is a potent chemotactic factor as well as an anaphylotoxin. It induces the directed migration of neutrophils and monocytes into the area of inflammation.[22]

Kinin Activation. The fragment of C2 (C2b) released during cleavage by C1s interacts with plasmin to produce kinin-like activity (Fig. 5-16). The biologic activity of C2b results in smooth muscle contraction, mucous gland secretion, increased vascular permeability, and pain.[23]

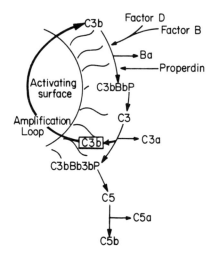

FIGURE 5-12. The amplification loop of the alternative pathway. (From James K. Complement: activation, consequences, and control. Am J Med Technol 1982; 48: 735.)

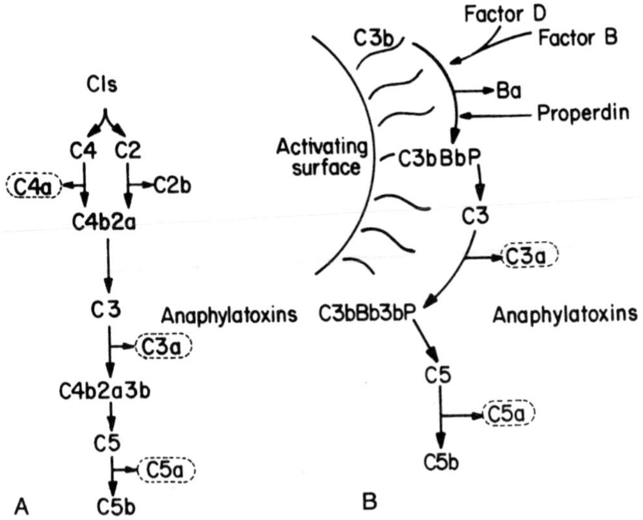

FIGURE 5-13. The anaphylatoxins are biologically active cleavage products resulting from the cleavage of C4, C3, and C5. (From James K. Complement: activation, consequences, and control. Am J Med Technol 1982; 48: 735.)

Lysis. In the laboratory the activity of complement is studied by measuring the degree of lysis of sheep red blood cells that occurs. Lysis, however, plays a relatively minor biologic role. One example of lysis as the biologic consequence of complement activation is an antibody-mediated transfusion reaction. The lytic function of complement also appears to be necessary for host defense against *Neisseria,* which will be discussed later in this chapter.

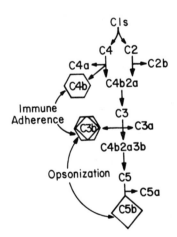

FIGURE 5-14. Immune adherence, mediated by C3b and C4b. Opsonization, mediated by C3b and C5b. (From James K. Complement: activation, consequences, and control. Am J Med Technol 1982; 48: 735.)

Deficiencies of Complement Components

Hereditary deficiencies reported for most of the complement components are summarized in Table 5-1.[24] The complement components are inherited as autosomal codominants, with each of two genes contributing 50% of normal protein levels. Consequently, a normal human with two functioning production genes will have 100% of the normal levels of each complement component. A heterozygote-deficient patient (with one defective gene and one normal gene) will have 50% of the normal level of the protein. A homozygote-deficient patient (with two deficient or defective genes) will have 0% to 10% of the normal level of the protein both quantitatively and functionally. The heterozygous state is usually not associated with any disease process unless the patient is compromised by some other medical problem. An exception to this is the increased incidence of juvenile rheumatoid arthritis (JRA) associated with the heterozygous C2-deficient state.[24] Since C2 deficiency is also associated with the HLA haplotype A25, B18, Dw2, the JRA association could be a genetic predisposition to disease.

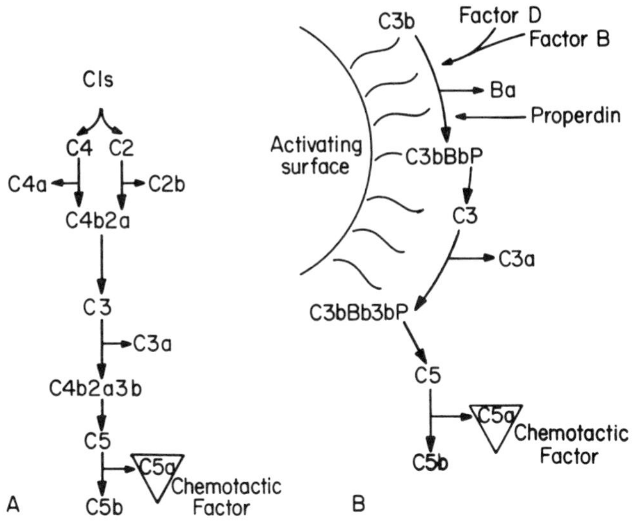

FIGURE 5-15. Chemotactic attraction of phago-cytic cells, mediated by C5a. (From James K. Complement: activation, consequences, and control. Am J Med Technol 1982; 48: 735.)

Patients with homozygotic deficiencies of complement proteins have an increased incidence of collagen vascular diseases.[24] Deficiencies of the early complement proteins of the classical pathway (C1, C4, C2) have a significantly higher incidence of lupus-like disease.

C2 deficiency is the most common hereditary complement component deficiency, occurring in one in 10^5 individuals.[24] The gene for Factor B appears to be closely associated with the gene for C2, since C2-deficient patients have been reported to have decreased levels of Factor B. The gene for C4 is also

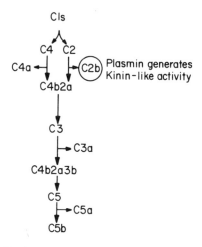

FIGURE 5-16. Kinin-like activity, mediated by a fragment of activated C2. (From James K. Complement: activation, consequences, and control. Am J Med Technol 1982; 48: 735.)

Table 5-1: Deficiencies of Complement Components

Deficient Component	Disease Association
C1 (q, r, or s)	Lupus-like disease
C4	Lupus-like disease
C2	Lupus-like disease
C3	Overwhelming infection
C5, C6, C7	Neisserial infections
C9	No known disease association
C1INH	Angioedema
H or I	Recurrent bacterial infections

linked to the histocompatibility complex, but to antigens A2, Bw44 (12) Dw2 (maternal) and A2, Bw62 (15) (paternal).[6]

Other complement component deficiencies are rare. Deficiencies of control proteins for C3 have been reported as well as the pathologic protein C3 nephritic factor (both described later), both of which result in markedly decreased levels of C3 due to activation or consumption of C3. No true deficiency of C3 has been found, suggesting that absence of C3 would be incompatible with life.

Deficiencies of the complement components involved in the membrane attack complex (C5, C6, C7) have a high incidence of infections, particularly with *Neisseria* organisms. These patients have recurrent gonococcal or meningococcal infections, organisms that require complement-dependent lysis to be destroyed. C9 deficiencies do not appear to be associated with any particular disease state.

Control Mechanisms

If any or all of the biologic consequences of complement activation were to go uncontrolled, the effects of even minor inflammatory processes involving activation of either complement pathway would be potentially devastating. The body, however, does not leave a reaction uncontrolled.

The first means of control is the extreme lability of activated complement components. If an activated enzyme does not combine with its substrate within milliseconds, the activity is lost or markedly decayed.[20] "Innocent bystander" cells in the vicinity of activated complement would be rapidly destroyed if the activated components were not so highly labile. Additionally, several proteins serve as inhibitors or inactivators of specific reactions or products involved in the complement cascade.

C1 Inhibitor (C1INH). C1INH forms an irreversible complex with both $\overline{C1r}$ and $\overline{C1s}$ (Fig. 5-17) that blocks their enzymatic activities and dissociates them from C1q.[25] The hereditary or acquired deficiency of this protein results in uncontrolled activation of the classical pathway. Control proteins that exercise their activity at the level of C3 or later are still functioning, retarding the amplification loop and other biologic consequences of C3–C9 activation. $\overline{C1s}$, in the absence of C1INH, continues to cleave C4 and C2 unchecked, resulting in release of C2b kinin-like activity and C4a anaphylatoxin activity.

The disease process associated with C1INH deficiency is angioedema (*angio-*, denoting relationship to blood vessels; *-edema*, indicating the presence of extraordinary amounts of fluid in the tissue spaces). C2b and C4a can both stimulate smooth muscle to contract and cause increased vascular permeability, which allows the fluid parts of the blood to leak out into the extravascular spaces, causing edema. The hereditary form of the disease, hereditary angioedema (HAE), is transmitted as an autosomal dominant trait and occurs in approximately one in 10^6

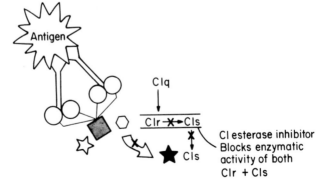

FIGURE 5-17. C1INH controls C1 activation by blocking the enzymatic activity of $\overline{C1r}$ and $\overline{C1s}$. (From James K. Complement: activation, consequences, and control. Am J Med Technol 1982; 48: 735.)

individuals.[26] The C2b also causes excess mucous membrane secretions, reflected in HAE when the episodes involve the respiratory tract (which can be life-threatening), and by intense gastrointestinal pain. Acquired forms of angioedema are much rarer and are usually associated with lymphoproliferative diseases.[27] Both forms of the disease are treated with an anabolic steroid, danazol, which appears to stimulate the liver to produce C1INH as well as other proteins. The most effective screening test for C1INH is a serum C4 level, since C4 is decreased because of activation of C4 and C2. The protein C1INH can be quantitatively analyzed by radial immunodiffusion or nephelometry or qualitatively evaluated by a modification of the total hemolytic complement assay. A small but significant percentage (15%) of individuals with HAE have normal levels of nonfunctional protein. In such cases the level of C1INH is normal to elevated but the qualitative or functional assay shows deficiency in activity.

β1H (H) and C3b Inactivator (I). The most important biologic consequence of complement activation is the feedback loop amplification mediated by C3b. Proteins H and I serve to control tightly the enzymes that cleave C3 and C5 (Fig. 5-18). I inactivates C3b and C4b, whereas H accelerates the decay of the alternative pathway C3 convertase by disso-

ciating Bb from the enzyme.[28] H and I are both involved in cleaving C3b into its hemolytically inactive form, C3bi, which is further cleaved into C3c and C3d. Fluid phase C3b is rapidly inactivated by H and I. Consequently, activation of the alternative pathway is dependent upon the presence of a protective (activating) surface that shelters C3b from these two control proteins.

In patients with deficiencies of I or H, a very low serum C3 is found because of the uncontrolled formation of the alternative pathway C3 convertase that results in a rapid catabolism of C3 and Factor B.[28,29] These patients are subject to recurrent bacterial infections because of poor opsonization or chemotaxis. A serum C3 level effectively screens for the deficiencies of H and I control proteins.

C4 Binding Protein (C4BP). C3b inactivator (I) can also cleave and inactivate C4 but requires an accessory protein, C4BP (Fig. 5-18).

Anaphylatoxin Inactivator. Carboxypeptidase controls the effects of C4a, C3a, and C5a by removing a single amino acid, a carboxyterminal arginine.[22] Cleavage of this amino acid destroys the anaphylatoxin activity of these peptides (Fig. 5-19).

MAC Inhibitor. Several serum proteins can bind to fluid phase C5b67, preventing attachment of this trimolecular complex to membranes (Fig. 5-20). Li-

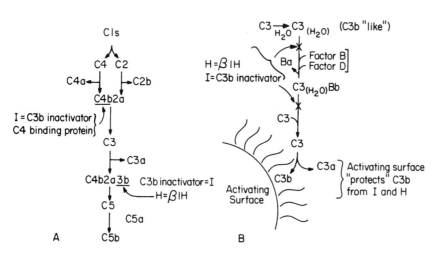

FIGURE 5-18. H and I control the amplification loop by dissociating Bb from the C3 convertase and inactivating C3b. (From James K. Complement: activation, consequences, and control. Am J Med Technol 1982; 48: 735.)

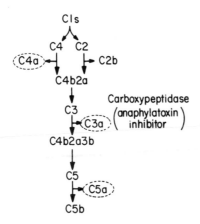

FIGURE 5-19. Carboxypeptidase inactivates anaphylatoxins. (From James K. Complement: activation, consequences, and control. Am J Med Technol 1982; 48: 735.)

poproteins or C8 bound to the MAC prior to its attachment to a cell surface can prevent that attachment.[30,31]

Properdin. The preceding control mechanisms are all inhibitors. Properdin (P) is an enhancer. Although not required for the activation sequence of

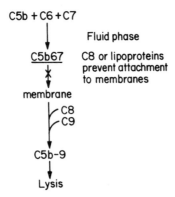

FIGURE 5-20. The membrane attack complex is prevented from attaching to membranes when C8 or lipoproteins bind to fluid phase C5b67. (From James K. Complement: activation, consequences, and control. Am J Med Technol 1982; 48: 735.)

the alternative pathway, P stabilizes the C3 and C5 convertases to prolong their activity.

C3 Nephritic Factor. Nephritic factor (NF) is a pathologic enhancing protein. NF is an IgG antibody with specificity for the alternative pathway C3 convertase.[32] NF binds to the C3 convertase so that it prevents inactivation by the control proteins H and I. When NF is present, C3 activation proceeds uncontrolled, thereby markedly depleting C3.

Patients with C3NF present with recurrent bacterial infections and frequently also have partial lipodystrophy, which is a disturbance in fat metabolism that leaves people appearing emaciated.[29] Serum C3 levels are markedly depleted, whereas C4 levels are normal. To distinguish C3NF from alternative pathway activation or deficiency of H or I, Factor B levels are helpful. Factor B levels are normal in C3NF, but decreased in alternative pathway activation, H deficiency, or I deficiency.

Synthesis of Complement Components

Most complement components are synthesized in the liver, with the exception of C1, which is synthesized in the epithelial cells of the intestine.[33] Limited quantities of most complement components, including C1q, can be synthesized by activated macrophages–monocytes. Synthesis by these mononuclear phagocytes takes place at the site of inflammation, providing for a microenvironment that perpetuates the inflammatory process.

The level of C1q parallels the relative levels of the immunoglobulins (*i.e.*, in hypogammaglobulinemia, C1q is also low, and in hypergammaglobulinemia, C1q is present in high levels). Several of the other complement components (especially C3 and Factor B) are acute phase reactants (*i.e.*, elevate in response to inflammation). For that reason the levels of these proteins should be interpreted in light of other measurements of inflammation such as erythrocyte sedimentation rate or C-reactive protein.[34] Levels that are in the "normal range" may reflect activation or depletion if the patient is in the acute phase.

Summary

The activation of complement provides the humoral (fluid-phase) effector mechanism most responsible for immune-mediated injury. The classical pathway is activated by an antigen–antibody reaction. The binding of C1q initiates the sequential activation of the 11 proteins. The classical pathway has a calcium-dependent step (C1q, C1r, C1s) and a magnesium-dependent reaction, the enzymatic action of $\overline{C1s}$ on C4 and C2.

The alternative pathway appears to be spontaneously activated, but the perpetuation of that activation is dependent upon the availability of an activating (or protective) surface that interferes with the inactivation of C3b by control proteins. The alternative pathway has a magnesium-dependent step, the binding of B to C3b to form the C3 convertase. Once initiated, the alternative pathway activation results in the sequential activation of nine proteins, six of which are common to both pathways.

The activation of complement results in a variety of biologic consequences that can cause injury to the host. The potential destructiveness of the effects of complement activation is modulated by a series of control proteins.

Deficiencies of complement component or control proteins are not as uncommon as once thought. Patients with homozygotic deficiencies appear to have an increased incidence of collagen vascular diseases. Deficiencies in C3 or control proteins that regulate C3 result in life-threatening diseases such as fulminant or recurrent bacterial infections. Patients with deficiencies in complement components involved in the MAC have a high incidence of infections with Neisserial organisms that appear to require complement-induced lysis of the organisms.[35]

The Acute Phase Response

When the body is injured, among the many ways it responds is by increasing the hepatic synthesis of a number of plasma proteins. This increased synthesis results in an increase in the concentration of these proteins in the plasma and at the site of injury. Experimental evidence indicates that these acute phase proteins play a major role in wound healing.[36]

From a teleological (adapting to the environment) perspective, the systemic acute phase response helps to ensure survival during the period immediately following injury. The systemic response must help to achieve the same goals as the localized inflammatory response (*i.e.*, to contain or destroy infectious agents, to remove damaged tissue, and to repair the affected organ).[37] Studies of the acute phase response have involved infections, surgical wounds or other traumas with definite onsets, burns, and myocardial infarctions. Certain of the acute phase proteins are elevated in pregnancy and in neoplasia (malignancies).

One of the first acute phase responses recognized was fever, which may occur following many types of inflammatory stimuli, including noninfectious states. Fever reflects the effects of endogenous pyrogens that elevate the set point of the hypothalamic center for body temperature.[37] The monokine (soluble factor released from monocytes during activation) interleukin-1 (IL-1) is believed to be identical to endogenous pyrogen.[37] Another long recognized, but variable, acute phase response is an increase in the granulocyte count in the blood. This initially reflects release from the storage pool and later reflects increased production by the bone marrow.

The best-studied acute phase proteins in humans differ markedly in the magnitude of their rise after onset of injury. They may be classified into three groups based on the degree of elevation during the acute phase response (Table 5-2).

C-Reactive Protein (CRP)

The discovery of C-reactive protein in 1930 focused attention on the acute phase response and the role of the proteins produced as a result of an injury to the body. CRP was recognized because of its ability to

Table 5-2: Acute Phase Proteins Listed by Relative Change

Concentration usually increases about 50%

α_2-Macroglobulin

Ceruloplasmin

C3 (and other complement components)

Concentration usually increases twofold to fourfold

α_1-Antitrypsin

Fibrinogen

Haptoglobin

Concentration usually increases several hundred times

C-reactive protein (CRP)

Concentration usually decreases

Albumin

---

precipitate with the C-polysaccharide extract of pneumococcus.[38] CRP did not appear to be a typical antibody to pneumococcus for several reasons: (1) the concentration of CRP rapidly decreased in the sera from patients who had recovered from pneumonia, in contrast to the typical antibody response (to the type-specific capsular polysaccharides) that gradually elevated; (2) CRP was also present in the sera from patients with other bacterial illness of nonpneumococcal origin; and (3) CRP was not detectable in the sera from normal individuals.[39] Subsequently it has been shown that CRP is normally present in nanogram (ng/mL) quantities[40] but may increase dramatically to hundreds of micrograms/mL within 3 days following tissue injury.[41] This represents a 100- to 1000-fold increase within hours of tissue damage.

Although CRP was recognized as being distinct from antibody, many parallels between the two molecules are evident. Like antibody, CRP will react with its substrate to cause lattice formation and precipitation. Both CRP and antibody participate in passive agglutination of red blood cells to which their substrate has been attached. CRP can induce capsular swelling of pneumococcus. Two of the most striking examples of the similarity between CRP and immunoglobulins include the initiation of the complement cascade through C1 activation by complexed CRP in a manner analogous to antibody–antigen complexes, and the ability of CRP to opsonize red cells coated with C-polysaccharide for ingestion by phagocytic cells.[39]

The functional similarities between CRP and antibody are striking, but CRP is produced by liver hepatocytes, unlike antibody which is synthesized by lymphoid tissue and plasma cells. Additionally, there is little physical or biochemical resemblance between CRP and antibody (Fig. 5-21). The binding of CRP to C-polysaccharide or other phosphocholine-containing compounds is calcium-dependent. Approximately one phosphate is bound per CRP subunit (of which there are five), requiring two calcium ions per CRP subunit.

CRP may be considered a primitive form of an antibody molecule with specificity for components found in cell membranes of microorganisms such as bacteria and fungi as well as for damaged membranes of cells from normal humans. When complexed to a binding specificity, CRP can activate complement to enhance opsonization and clearance of the microorganisms *prior* to the production of specific IgM or IgG. Complexed CRP can bind to natural killer (NK) cells and to monocytes and may make these cells tumoricidal.[42,43] CRP is produced early in the inflammatory response and may also play a role in tumor surveillance prior to the production of antibody or the activation of specific cytotoxic T cells.

Haptoglobin

The principal biologic function of haptoglobin is to bind to and remove free hemoglobin released by intravascular hemolysis. Haptoglobin irreversibly

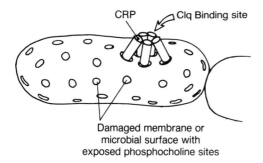

CRP

Clq Binding site

Damaged membrane or
microbial surface with
exposed phosphocholine sites

FIGURE 5-21. Schematic drawing of C-reactive protein bound to exposed phosphocholine (PC).

binds to free hemoglobin, forming a complex that is rapidly cleared by hepatocytes.[44] Following injury, haptoglobin increases twofold to fourfold and is frequently found in inflammatory exudates. The rise in plasma haptoglobin in response to inflammation is due to the *de novo* synthesis of the protein by the liver and does not involve the release of previously formed haptoglobin from other sites.[44]

Low haptoglobin levels are always clinically significant after the first year of life. In some cases, the cause may be decreased synthesis due to liver disease, but in the majority of patients the cause is intravascular hemolysis and rapid clearance of the haptoglobin–hemoglobin complex. No quantitative correlation is possible between the plasma haptoglobin content and the severity of hemolysis, because relatively minor hemolytic events have the potential of markedly depleting the haptoglobin in the absence of an inflammatory response.[44] Conversely, infections or inflammation may lead to a twofold to tenfold increase in haptoglobin. In such situations a "normal" haptoglobin level does not rule out the diagnosis of intravascular hemolysis. The haptoglobin level should be interpreted in light of the levels of another acute phase protein (*e.g.*, CRP).[34]

Fibrinogen

Fibrinogen accumulates at the site of injury for the first or second week after a surgical incision. In the presence of enzymes released from PMNs and plate-

lets, fibrin is formed.[36] Fibrin increases the tensile strength of the wound and stimulates fibroblast proliferation and growth. Fibrinogen synthesis, but not haptoglobin synthesis, by hepatocytes can be stimulated by fibrinogen or fibrin degradation products (FDP), suggesting a feedback amplification loop.[45] The macrophage is necessary in this loop, since FDP does not directly stimulate hepatocytic synthesis of fibrinogen but does promote the production of IL-1 by peripheral blood monocytes or Kupffer cells.

α_1-Antitrypsin

α_1-Antitrypsin is one of a family of serine protease inhibitors in human plasma. Although named antitrypsin, the physiologic targets are the proteases (*e.g.*, elastase) released from leukocytes rather than trypsin.[46] Elastase is an endogenous enzyme capable of degrading elastin and collagen. In chronic pulmonary inflammation, lung tissue is damaged because of the activities of these leukocyte proteases released during phagocytosis and digestion of microorganisms and other debris. Once bound to α_1-antitrypsin, the activity of the proteases is completely inhibited, being later removed and catabolized. α_1-Antitrypsin is synthesized by the liver, which can increase synthesis fourfold when stimulated by an inflammatory process. In contrast to complexes of proteases with α_2-macroglobulin, α_1-antitrypsin–protease complexes are not taken up by macrophages.[36] There is experimental evidence that proteases can be transferred between α_1-antitrypsin and α_2-macroglobulin.

A loss of lung elasticity is a normal feature of aging, but this loss can be accelerated and cause premature emphysema in either the smoker or the patient with homozygous α_1-antitrypsin deficiency. When the two were combined (smoking *and* α_1-antitrypsin deficiency), emphysema onset occurred as early as 30 years of age, with death by the age of 50. Air pollution or respiratory infections are also detrimental to the α_1-antitrypsin–deficient patient.

α_1-Antitrypsin deficiency is also associated with liver disease.[46] Homozygous-deficient infants may develop neonatal cholestasis, which can progress to cirrhosis as children. Adults who are homozygous-deficient invariably show histologic evidence of liver damage, with about one fifth of these individuals developing cirrhosis.

Heterozygous individuals are at more risk than normal individuals of developing liver disease, connective tissue disease (e.g., rheumatoid arthritis), inflammatory eye disease, and glomerulonephritis.[47] α_1-Antitrypsin has a role in several mediator pathways involved in the inflammatory response; consequently, in the absence of this protein these proteases attack the tissue surrounding the inflammatory process and cause damage that may lead to chronic inflammation.

Ceruloplasmin

Ceruloplasmin is a glycoprotein that is the principal copper-transporting protein in human plasma.[36] Eighty percent to 95% of the total circulating copper is bound to ceruloplasmin, the rest being bound more loosely to albumin and amino acids. Ceruloplasmin appears to be the primary copper transport protein for transferring copper to cytochrome C oxidase, vital to aerobic energy production, which, along with glycolysis, increases during wound healing.[48] Ceruloplasmin and the copper it carries are essential to collagen formation and the extracellular cross-linking and maturation of collagen and elastin.[36] Ceruloplasmin and the copper it contains may also serve to protect the matrix of healing tissue against superoxide ions, generated by phagocytes in the course of clearing tissue debris or microorganisms.

An absence or marked depletion of ceruloplasmin is associated with a degenerative process named Wilson's disease, which is an autosomal recessive trait and is relatively rare.[49] There is a gastrointestinal absorption defect that allows copper to be taken up in excessive amounts. In the absence of ceruloplasmin, copper is massively increased in the tissues. The disease is also characterized by massive renal tubular reabsorption defects, which results in excessive urinary excretion of proteins, glucose, and other elements.

α_2-Macroglobulin

α_2-Macroglobulin is one of two principal protease inhibitors in human plasma, the other being α_1-antitrypsin. Proteolytic enzymes released from damaged tissues as well as from phagocytic cells have their activity inhibited partially by being bound by α_2-macroglobulin. These complexes of proteases and α_2 macroglobulin are rapidly phagocytosed by macrophages and fibroblasts.[50] α_2-Macroglobulin appears to be a scavenger protease inhibitor that binds excess molecules that cannot be handled by the intended inhibitor. In that role, it functions in hemostasis, coagulation, fibrinolysis, and complement pathways.[51] No diseases have been associated with a deficiency in α_2-macroglobulin, so deficiency in this protein may be incompatible with life.

Inflammation

The preceding chapters have provided a foundation of knowledge about each of the specific systems (cellular and humoral) involved in the inflammatory process. Celsus of Rome first described the famous "four cardinal signs" of inflammation: redness, swelling, heat, and pain.[52,53] Loss of function was later recognized as another sign of inflammation. Inflammation appears to represent an orderly sequence of coordinated events designed to protect the host from a foreign invader, minimizing damage to the host tissue. In addition to killing off the adversary, the inflammatory process is intended also to eliminate the debris and to repair the damaged tissues.[52,53] The localized inflammatory reaction can be divided into four stages: increased vascular permeability, emigration of neutrophils, emigration of mononuclear cells, and cellular proliferation.

Vascular Permeability

The vascular phase of the inflammatory response primarily involves the microcirculation (i.e., the capillaries, the arterioles, and the venules). Following injury, the first phase is hyperemia (a rush of blood

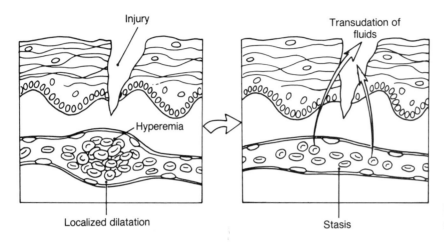

FIGURE 5-22. Vascular phase of inflammation.

into the affected area) initially confined to the vicinity of the site of the injury (Fig. 5-22). This is facilitated by the localized dilatation (dilated or stretched beyond normal dimensions) of capillaries and venules resulting from the chemical mediators released as a direct result of the injury (*e.g.*, histamine released from mast cells in skin that has been punctured).

After the hyperemia phase, transudation begins. Transudation is the passage of serum or other body fluids through a membrane. A transudate, in contrast to an exudate, is characterized by a low protein content and few cells. Transudation is brought about by chemical mediators, such as histamine and kinins, which increase vascular permeability by causing the endothelial cells' smooth muscle to contract. As the endothelial cells contract, adjacent cells separate from one another, creating gaps where fluids and even diapedetic PMNs can escape through the basement membrane and move into the tissues. If fibrinogen is extravasated into the tissues, the clotting mechanism is activated and fibrin forms from fibrinogen, the body's effort to "plug the leak."

As transudation proceeds, the blood flow in the dilated capillaries and venules slows. In severe injury the blood flow may cease completely (stasis), caused by hemoconcentration when the fluids are lost by transudation. During stasis the red blood cells, which normally repel each other, clump into tight stacks. Stasis (in contrast to thrombosis) is completely re-

versible; that is, when blood flow is restored, the red cell aggregates break up and normalcy resumes. Depending upon the type and severity of the inflammation, microthrombus formation and platelet aggregation may also occur and may not be reversible.

Emigration of Neutrophils

Shortly after the initial injury, the endothelial cells become "sticky" and circulating PMNs begin to adhere to the endothelium. Initially, the numbers of cells involved are small and the adherence seems transitory, but soon the endothelial surface becomes completely "pavemented" by leukocytes. PMNs are the most conspicuous, but eosinophils and basophils, platelets, and even erythrocytes do participate.

Following pavementing, the leukocytes exhibit ameboid movement and actively migrate through the wall of the blood vessel by the process called diapedesis (see Fig. 5-1). Erythrocytes that appear in the tissues apparently have been passively forced through the gaps in damaged epithelium. It is the hemoglobin breakdown products that result in the purple, then green, and finally yellow color of a bruise. Bruise spots can occur following the most minor of injuries and are probably explainable by extravasating red blood cells rather than actual blood vessel damage and spilling of blood into the tissues.

The emigration of significant numbers of neutrophils into the area of inflammation is dependent upon chemotactic factors. If immune complexes are involved in initiating the inflammation, the chemotactic factors released during complement activation (C5a) will attract PMNs. Neutrophil granules themselves, when released from the PMNs arriving first on the scene, are chemotactic for other PMNs. Certain bacterial products are also chemotactic for neutrophils. The intensity and duration of the neutrophil emigration may last 24 to 48 hours and are proportional to the amount of chemotactic factor present in the inflamed area.

Neutrophils participate in the inflammatory process in many ways. They are actively phagocytic for microorganisms and other foreign material. Their lysosomes contain a number of biologically active macromolecules. The active aerobic glycolysis of PMNs is responsible for formation of large amounts of lactic acid (which causes pain) found in inflamed tissues. When the amount of foreign material attracts a large number of neutrophils, it also stimulates the accumulation of fibroblasts, the prolifera-

tion and synthesis of collagen, and it may result in the formation of a walled-off abscess that may require drainage before healing can occur.[53]

Emigration of Mononuclear Cells

The third stage of the inflammatory response is the emigration of mononuclear cells into the affected area. This begins about 4 hours after the initial stimulus and may reach a peak (during a defined and single injury) of 16 to 24 hours. A few mononuclear cells may be found along with the PMNs early in the cellular phase of the response. These few monocytes either are directly stimulated by phagocytosis of the debris or are indirectly stimulated by products of PMN phagocytosis and degranulation to produce monokines (e.g., IL-1).[54] IL-1 is also released from neutrophils, epithelial cells, fibroblasts, and many other cell types. IL-1 (endogenous pyrogen) is associated with many of the manifestations of inflammatory reactions, such as fever, elevation of acute phase proteins, and infiltration of inflammatory sites by

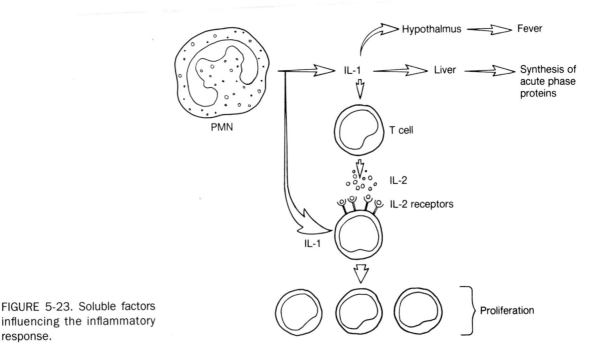

FIGURE 5-23. Soluble factors influencing the inflammatory response.

leukocytes. Thus, another feedback amplification loop has begun. IL-1 attracts and activates other monocytes–macrophages as well as lymphocytes into the area of inflammation (IL-1 was first described as lymphocyte-activating factor [LAF]). IL-1 can stimulate (or activate) T lymphocytes to produce interleukin-2 (IL-2), which in turn enhances the proliferation of T lymphocytes (Fig. 5-23).

Cellular Proliferation and Repair

Resolution and repair are the final stages of the inflammatory process.[53] Fibroblast proliferation begins within 18 hours and peaks by 48 to 72 hours. During proliferation, fibroblasts produce acidic mucopolysaccharides, which may neutralize the effects of some of the chemical mediators that are still being released by damaged mast cells and basophils. The end stage of inflammation may involve complete repair and restoration of function of the affected area. Alternatively, an injury may lead to formation of an abscess with at least some loss of function. Another end stage of inflammation may be formation of a granuloma, which is a tightly-packed pocket of inflammatory cells that die and degenerate (necrosis) from the center out. Granuloma formation is a typical end stage result of delayed hypersensitivity of cell-mediated immunity and will be described in a later chapter.

References

1. Mescon H, Grots IA: The skin. In Robbins SL (ed): Pathologic Basis of Disease, p 1374. Philadelphia, WB Saunders, 1974

2. Werb Z, Goldstein IM: Phagocytic cells: Chemotaxis and effector functions of macrophages and granulocytes. In Stites DP, Stobo JD, Wells JV (eds): Basic and Clinical Immunology, 6th ed, p 96. Norwalk, Appleton and Lange, 1987

3. Hammond WS: Immunologic protection. In Abramoff P, LaVia MF (eds): Biology of the Immune Response, p 374. New York, McGraw-Hill, 1970

4. Cooper EL: Granulocytes and mast cells. In: General Immunology, p 92. New York, Pergamon Press, 1982

5. Park BH, Good RA: Phagocytosis and host resistance. In: Principles of Modern Immunobiology, p 159. Philadelphia, Lea & Febiger, 1974

6. Ammann AJ: Immunodeficiency disease. In Stites DP, Stobo JD, Wells JV (eds): Basic and Clinical Immunology, 6th ed, p 317. Norwalk, Appleton and Lange, 1987

7. Stites DP: Clinical laboratory methods for detection of cellular immune function. In Stites DP, Stobo JD, Wells JV (eds): Basic and Clinical Immunology, 6th ed, p 285. Norwalk, Appleton and Lange, 1987

8. Southwick FS, Stossel TP: Phagocytosis. In Rose NR, Friedman H, Fahey JL (eds): Manual of Clinical Laboratory Immunology, p 326. Washington DC, American Society for Microbiology, 1986

9. Boxer LA, Stossel TP: Neutrophil disorders—qualitative abnormalities of neutrophils. In Williams WJ, Beutler E, Erslev AJ, et al (eds): Hematology, p 809. New York: McGraw-Hill, 1983

10. Roder JC, Haliotis T, Klein M, et al: A new immunodeficiency disorder in humans involving NK cells. Nature 284:553, 1980

11. Hayward A: Immunodeficiency. In Lachmann PJ, Peters DK (eds): Clinical Aspects of Immunology, p 1691. Oxford, Blackwell Scientific, 1982

12. Bellanti JA, Kadlec JV: General immunobiology. In Bellanti JA (ed): Immunology III, p 16. Philadelphia, WB Saunders, 1985

13. Frick OL: Immediate hypersensitivity. In Stites DP, Stobo JD, Wells JV (eds): Basic and Clinical Immunology, 6th ed, p 197. Norwalk, Appleton and Lange, 1987

14. Lee TH, Austen F: Arachidonic acid metabolism by the 5-lipogenase pathway, and the effects of alternative dietary fatty acids. Adv Immunol 39:145, 1986

15. Drutz DJ, Mills J: Immunity and infection. In Stites DP, Stobo JD, Wells JV (eds): Basic and Clinical Immunology, 6th ed, p 167. Norwalk, Appleton and Lange, 1987

16. Robbins SL: Inflammation and repair. In Robbins SL (ed): Pathologic Basis of Disease, p 55. Philadelphia, WB Saunders, 1974

17. Herscowitz HB: Immunophysiology: Cell functions and cellular interactions in antibody formation. In Bellanti,

JA (ed): Immunology III, p 16. Philadelphia, WB Saunders, 1985

18. James K: Complement: Activation, consequences, and control. Am J Med Technol 48:735, 1982

19. Gewurz H, Lint TF: Alternative modes and pathways of complement activation. In Day NK, Good RA (eds): Comprehensive Immunology, Vol 2, Biological Amplification Systems in Immunology, p 17. New York, Plenum Press, 1977

20. Lint TF, Gewurz H: Testing for complement defects. Clinics in Immunology and Allergy 1:561, 1981

21. Pangburn MK, Schreiber RD, Muller-Eberhard HJ: Formation of the initial C3 convertase of the alternative complement pathway: acquisition of the C3b-like activities of spontaneous hydrolysis of the putative thioester in native C3. J Exp Med 154:856, 1981

22. Hugli TE, Muller-Eberhard HJ: Anaphylotoxins: C3a and C5a. Adv Immunol 26:1, 1978

23. Donaldson VH, Rosen FS, Bing DH: Role of the second component of complement (C2) and plasmin in kinin release in hereditary angioneurotic edema (H.A.N.E.) plasma. Trans Assoc Am Phys 90:174, 1977

24. Agnello V: Complement deficiency states. Medicine (Baltimore) 57:1, 1978

25. Ziccardi RJ, Cooper NR: Active disassembly of the first component of complement, C1, by C1 inactivator. J Immunol 123:788, 1979

26. Frank MM, Gelfand JA, Atkinson JP: Hereditary angioedema: the clinical syndrome and its management. Ann Intern Med 84:580, 1976

27. Luskin AT, Tobin MC: Alterations of complement components in disease. Am J Med Technol 48:749, 1982

28. Pangburn MK, Muller-Eberhard HJ: Relation of a putative thioester bond in C3 to activation of the alternative pathway and the binding of C3 to biological targets of complement. J Exp Med 152:1102, 1980

29. Lint TF, Gewurz H: Testing for complement defects. Clinics in Immunology and Allergy 1:561, 1981

30. Lint TF, Behrends CL, Gewurz H: Serum lipoproteins and C567-INH activity. J Immunol 127:1261, 1981

31. Nemerow GR, Yamamoto KI, Lint TF: Restriction of complement-mediated membrane damage by the eighth component of complement: A dual role for C8 in the complement attack sequence. J Immunol 123:1245, 1979

32. Davis AE, Ziegler JB, et al: Heterogeneity of nephritic factor and its identification as an immunoglobulin. Proc Natl Acad Sci (USA) 74:3980, 1977

33. Colten HR: Biosynthesis of complement. Adv Immunol 22:67, 1976

34. Witte DA: Laboratory tests to confirm or exclude iron deficiency. Lab Med 16:671, 1985

35. Nicholson A, Lepow IH: Host defense against *Neisseria meningitidis* requires a complement-dependent bactericidal activity. Science 205:298, 1979

36. Powanda MC, Moyer ED: Plasma proteins and wound healing. Surg Gynecol Obstet 153:749, 1981

37. Kushner I: The phenomenon of the acute phase response. In Kushner I, Volanakis JE, Gewurz H (eds): C-reactive protein and the plasma protein response to tissue injury. Ann NY Acad Sci 389:39, 1982

38. Tillett W, Francis T: Serological reactions in pneumonia with nonprotein somatic fraction of pneumococcus. J Exp Med 52:561, 1930

39. James KK: Studies of the interaction of C-reactive protein with mononuclear leukocytes, p 1. Thesis, 1980

40. Claus D, Osmand A, Gewurz H: Radioimmunoassay of human C-reactive protein and levels in normal sera. J Lab Clin Med 87:120, 1976

41. Fischer C, Gill C, Forrester M, et al: Quantitation of "acute phase proteins" post-operatively. Am J Clin Pathol 66:840, 1976

42. James K, Baum L, Adamowski C, et al: C-reactive protein antigenicity on the surface of human lymphocytes. J Immunol 131:2930, 1983

43. Deodhar SD, James K, Chiang T, et al: Inhibition of lung metastases in mice bearing a malignant fibrosarcoma by treatment with liposomes containing human C-reactive protein. Cancer Res 42:5084, 1982

44. Javid J: Human haptoglobin. Curr Top Hematol 1:151, 1978

45. Fuller GM, Ritchie DG: A regulatory pathway for fibrinogen biosynthesis involving an indirect feedback loop. In Kushner I, Volanakis JE, Gewurz H (eds): C-reactive Protein and the Plasma Protein Response to Tissue Injury. Ann NY Acad Sci 389:308, 1982

46. Carrell RW: Alpha-1 antitrypsin: Molecular pathology, leukocytes, and tissue damage. J Clin Invest 78:1427, 1986

47. Breit SN, Wakefield D, Robinson JP, et al: The role

of alpha-1 antitrypsin deficiency in the pathogenesis of immune disorders. Clin Immunol Immunopathol 35:363, 1985

48.   Goldstein IM, Kaplan HB, Edelson HS, et al: Ceruloplasmin: An acute phase reactant that scavenges oxygen-derived free radicals. In Kushner I, Volanakis JE, Gewurz H (eds): C-reactive protein and the plasma protein response to tissue injury. Ann NY Acad Sci 389:368, 1982

49.   Foley JM: The nervous system: Degenerative diseases. In Robbins SL (ed): Pathologic Basis of Disease, p 1539. Philadelphia, WB Saunders, 1974

50.   Van Leuven F, Cassiman JJ, Van-den Berghe H: Uptake and degradation of alpha-2 macroglobulin protease complexes in human cells in culture. Exp Cell Res 117:273, 1978

51.   Roberts RC: Protease inhibitors of human plasma: Alpha-2 macroglobulin. J Med 16:149, 1985

52.   Park BH, Good RA: Inflammation and mechanisms of immunologic injury. In: Principles of Modern Immunobiology, p 165. Philadelphia, Lea & Febiger, 1974

53.   Bach FH, Good RA: Inflammation. In Bach FH (ed): Clinical Immunobiology, p 139. New York, Academic Press, 1980

54.   Oppenheim JJ, Ruscetti FW, Faltynek CV: Interleukin and interferons. In Stites DP, Stobo JD, Wells JV (eds): Basic and Clinical Immunology, 6th ed, p 82. Norwalk, Appleton and Lange, 1987

CHAPTER 6

Hypersensitivity

Suio-Ling Chen

Traditionally, immune responses were thought to develop only for the benefit of the host. It is now clear that the protective immune response can also have deleterious effects. Thus, immune responses may eradicate the infecting microorganism; at the same time, they can cause significant tissue damages. To distinguish between the beneficial and deleterious effects of the immune responses, the term *hypersensitivity* is used to describe an exaggerated response that causes tissue damage in a host. Such a response usually occurs in a sensitized host when it encounters the same antigen for the second time. Gell and Coombs classified the mechanisms of tissue injury resulting from hypersensitivity into four categories[1]:

Type I: anaphylactic
Type II: cytotoxic
Type III: immune complex disorders
Type IV: delayed hypersensitivity

The first three are antibody mediated, whereas type IV hypersensitivity involves T cells and macro-phages. The major characteristics of four mechanisms of tissue injury are listed in Table 6-1. This classification, however, is not absolute; frequently there is an overlap in the type of hypersensitivity response. Some substances can cause more than one type of reaction in a sensitive individual. For example, penicillin can cause a fatal type I anaphylactic reaction, type II hemolytic anemia, type III immune complex disorder, and type IV delayed hypersensitivity reaction. These reactions may occur simultaneously or at different stages during a disease process.

Type I Hypersensitivity

Type I hypersensitivity is also known as immediate hypersensitivity because the reaction occurs within minutes of contact with the antigen or allergen. An allergic individual has circulating basophils or tissue mast cells that are sensitized by the cytotrophic an-

Table 6-1: Characteristics of Hypersensitivities

Hypersensitivity	Effector Cells	Immunoglobulin	Complement Activation	Example
Type I, anaphylactic hypersensitivity	Basophils Mast cells	IgE	No	Ragweed hay fever Insect allergy
Type II, cytotoxic antibody	—	IgG or IgM	Yes	Goodpasture's syndrome Graves' disease Myasthenia gravis
Type III, immune complex disorders	—	IgG or IgM	Yes	SLE, rheumatoid arthritis
Type IV, delayed-type hypersensitivity	T cells Macrophages	—	No	Contact sensitivity to poison ivy, PPD skin test

tibody, IgE (Fig. 6-1). Upon subsequent exposure to the allergen, these sensitized cells are triggered to release vasoactive amines that produce allergic symptoms (Fig. 6-2). The extent of an allergic response is partly influenced by the port of entry of the allergen. For example, a bee sting will introduce the allergen into circulation, causing a systemic anaphylaxis, and the inhaled antigen can cause respiratory symptoms, such as rhinitis and asthma. Various clinical conditions, including asthma, eczema, and hay fever, are collectively known as atopy, because they share many common features.

Approximately 5% to 10% of the population exposed to airborne allergens becomes sensitized. Family studies have indicated a strong hereditary linkage associated with allergy.[2]

Mechanism of Vasoactive Amine Release

The effector cells involved in an allergic response are basophils and mast cells. In general, basophils are found in circulation, whereas mast cells are distrib-

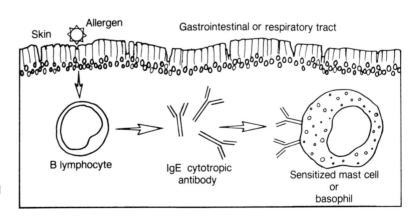

FIGURE 6-1. Mast cell or basophil sensitization.

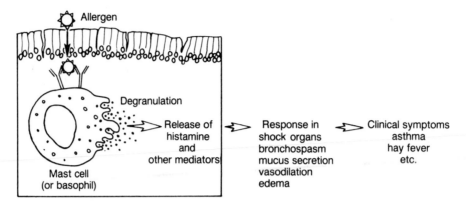

FIGURE 6-2. Allergic reaction.

uted in the tissue of shock organs. The two cell types are indistinguishable in many of their biologic characteristics:

1. They express cell surface Fc receptors for IgE.

2. They have cytoplasmic granules containing vasoactive amines.

3. They are triggered to release vasoactive amines by similar mechanisms.

IgE antibodies produced by the plasma cells are bound to the cell surface of a basophil or mast cell by way of Fc receptors. Subsequent exposure to the same allergen will cause immune complex formation on the cell surface, leading to the release of vasoactive amines.[3,4] The crucial event appears to be cross-linking of the effector cell surface Fc receptors.[5,6] It is possible to trigger the vasoactive amine release experimentally. For example, effector cells are triggered by cross-linking the Fc receptors using an antibody to the Fc receptor, or an antibody to IgE heavy chain (Fig. 6-3). Thus, the physiologic conditions required for effector cell triggering are as follows: At least two IgE molecules are occupying the adjacent Fc receptors on a effector cell, and the al-

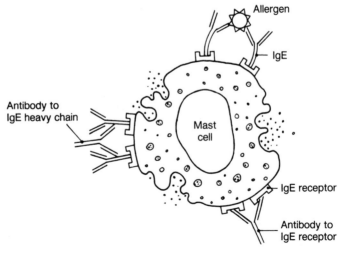

FIGURE 6-3. Granule release triggered by cross-linking of the cell surface Fc receptors.

lergen is multivalent, such that it is able to cross-link the two IgE molecules on the effector cell (see Fig. 6-3). Whereas the released vasoactive amines cause general symptoms of an allergic response, the IgE molecules convey the specificity of an allergic response. One of the biologic events resulting from receptor cross-linking is the fusion of granular membranes and cell membranes, which leads to the release of stored, preformed granular contents. Therefore, the effector cells become degranulated. Receptor cross-linking also results in the synthesis of mediators from arachidonic acid.

Allergens

Allergens are the antigens that are able to elicit IgE antibody responses in certain individuals. Most naturally occurring allergens have a molecular weight of 10,000 to 70,000 d. Small antigens may not have sufficient numbers of epitopes to facilitate the Fc receptor cross-linking to trigger a basophil or mast cell, while a larger molecule may not be able to diffuse across the mucosal surface to reach the sensitized effector cells. Various modes of exposure to allergens are identified:

1. The respiratory airway is constantly exposed to airborne particles that may cause allergic responses. The most common inhalant allergens are plant pollens, fungal spores, and animal danders.

2. Absorption of allergen from the digestive tract can also cause allergic responses.

3. Direct skin contact with pollen or other allergen can cause localized urticaria or even systemic symptoms in a highly sensitive individual.

Immunoglobulin E

Immunoglobulin E (IgE) is also known as reaginic antibody. The control mechanism for IgE synthesis by plasma cells is currently being investigated. IgE antibody differs from other immunoglobulin classes:

It has five heavy chain domains, and it is cytotrophic for basophils and mast cells. The binding of IgE molecules to the Fc receptors is mediated by heavy chain constant domains 3 and 4. This cytotrophic activity is heat sensitive; heating at 56°C for 30 minutes will abolish this activity. The serum half-life of IgE is approximately 2.5 days. However, once bound to the effector cell surface by the Fc receptor, the half-life increases to 6 to 12 weeks.[7]

Pharmacologic Roles of the Mediators[6,8]

The primary role of the mediators appears to be defense against injury. For example, during nematode infection in rats, the sensitized tissue mast cells are triggered by the parasite antigen to release vasoactive amines. The increased vascular permeability causes the leakage of plasma proteins. Among these proteins are antibodies against the parasite. The antibodies neutralize the parasites, which are cleared from the host as a form of immune complex. Thus, in this case vasodilation is beneficial to the host. However, in an allergic response, the similar normal defense mechanism is exaggerated, causing extensive tissue damages.

The mediators of allergic response may be divided into two categories: preformed and newly synthesized mediators. Preformed mediators are stored in the granules, and the newly formed mediators are synthesized after the effector cells are triggered.

Preformed Mediators

Histamine

Histamine (molecular weight 111 d) causes contraction of the bronchioles and smooth muscle of blood vessels, increases capillary permeability, and increases mucous gland secretion in the airway. This preformed mediator is stored in the granules and can be released 1 to 2 minutes after allergen–antibody reaction. The duration of histamine activity is approximately 10 minutes.

Eosinophil Chemotactic Factor of Anaphylaxis

Eosinophil chemotactic factor of anaphylaxis (ECF-A) has a molecular weight of 500 d. This is a pre-formed mediator released during degranulation. It stimulates eosinophils to migrate to the site of an antigen–antibody reaction. Eosinophils are known to have several functions, which include (1) phagocytosis and disposal of antigen–antibody complexes and (2) release of the enzymes histaminase and arylsulfatase. These enzymes dampen the allergic reaction caused by allergic mediators.

Newly Synthesized Mediators

Following activation the newly synthesized mediators are derived from membrane lipid of basophils and mast cells. Arachidonic acid is liberated from the membrane lipid by the action of the enzymes phospholipase A or phospholipase C and diacylglycerol lipase. The freed arachidonic acid is then processed by one of two metabolic pathways: the cyclooxygenase (prostaglandin synthetase) pathway, or the 5-lipoxygenase pathway. Whereas the former pathway leads to prostaglandin production, the latter leads to leukotriene production (Fig. 6-4).

Prostaglandin D_2

Prostaglandin D_2 causes vasodilation and increases vascular permeability. The clinical symptoms caused by this compound are similar to those seen with histamine—erythematous wheal and flare reaction. However, the prostaglandin D_2 effect can persist for as long as 2 hours; the histamine effect lasts approximately 10 minutes.

Leukotrienes

Leukotrienes C_4, D_4, or E_4 cause erythema and wheal formation. When inhaled, they cause bronchospasm. Furthermore, their bronchoconstrictic potency is 30 to 1000 times that of histamine. Leukotrienes C_4 and D_4 have also been shown to stimulate mucous secretion by human airway tissue.

Type II Hypersensitivity

Type II hypersensitivity involves IgG or IgM antibody against cell surface molecules or tissue compo-

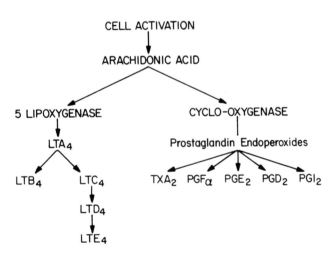

FIGURE 6-4. Pathway of oxidative metabolism of arachidonic acid.

nents. The tissue damage may be mediated by one of the following mechanisms: (1) accelerated clearance of the antibody-sensitized target cells by the mono-nuclear phagocytic system (reticuloendothelial system), (2) blockade of normal cellular function because of antibody binding to the target cells, (3) complement-mediated lysis of the target cells, or (4) the damage of innocent by-stander cells or tissue by the lysosomal enzymes released by the neutrophils present at the site of antigen–antibody reactions.

Antibody-Mediated Tissue Damage

Hemolytic anemia from a warm antibody is frequently associated with antibody production against red cell antigen of the Rh system, such as C, D, and E antigen. The sensitized red blood cells are cleared by the macrophages at an accelerated rate, causing anemia in the afflicted individual. The etiology of this disease is unknown, but it is frequently associated with other autoimmune disorders.[9]

Patients with Graves' disease have circulating antibodies specific for thyroid stimulating hormone (TSH) receptor. When bound to the TSH receptors, these antibodies will stimulate the thyroid epithelial cells to produce thyroglobulin, independent of the normal feedback control mechanism. Persistent stimulation of the thyroid gland causes hyperthyroidism. These antibodies are known as long-acting thyroid stimulator (LATS).[10]

Antibodies against cell surface structure can also block the normal cellular activities. For example, the antibody against acetylcholine receptors prevents the neurotransmitter, acetylcholine, from binding to the receptor at the neuromuscular junction. This type of antibody is associated with myasthenia gravis, a disease with muscular paralysis as the clinical manifestation.[11]

Complement-Mediated Cell Lysis

When the antibody–antigen complex is able to activate the complement cascade, direct cell lysis occurs. Transfusion reactions are the most important clinical manifestation of this type of hypersensitivity. Transfusion of ABO-incompatible blood will result in lysis of the donor's red blood cells because the recipient has antibodies to nonself ABO antigens. For example, a recipient with type A blood will have antibody to the B antigen, a type B recipient will have antibody to A antigen, and a type O individual will have antibodies to both A and B antigens. These pre-existing antibodies against nonself ABO red cell antigens are also known as naturally occurring red cell antibodies. The production of such antibodies is thought to occur during bacterial infections because the infecting microorganisms coincidentally express antigens that are similar to the ABO blood group antigens.

Hemolytic disease of the newborn (HDNB) is due to maternal–fetal red cell incompatibility. The Rhesus D (RhD) antigen is the most frequently involved red cell antigen. An RhD-negative mother becomes immunized to the D antigen on fetal red blood cells because of maternal–fetal blood mixing during delivery. The mother synthesizes IgG antibodies against the D antigen. In a subsequent pregnancy with an RhD-positive fetus, the IgG antibodies cross the placenta and circulate in fetal circulation, causing complement-mediated lysis of the fetal red blood cells. Prophylactic RhD immune globulin treatment given to the mother immediately after delivery can prevent the HDNB in the subsequent pregnancy. The RhD antibodies in the Rh immune globulin will prevent maternal RhD antibody production by neutralizing the fetal RhD-positive red blood cells that leak into maternal circulation during delivery.[12]

Formed blood elements other than red blood cells can also be the target of cytotoxic antibody lysis. For example, antibody against platelets causes idiopathic thrombocytopenic purpura, antibody to neutrophils causes granulocytopenia, and antibody to T cells is associated with systemic lupus erythematosus.

Cytotoxic Antibodies to Tissue Components

Cytotoxic antibodies to tissue components frequently cause inflammatory responses. The sequence of events includes antibody–antigen reaction, complement activation, generation of such chemotactic factors as C3a and C5a, infiltration of the tissue by neutrophils, and release of lysosomal enzymes by the neutrophils, which eventually leads to tissue damage. The classic example is Goodpasture's syndrome. The patient develops antibodies against glomerular and pulmonary basement membranes. Binding of these antibodies to the basement membrane initiates the sequence of events described earlier. Direct immunofluorescent study of a kidney biopsy shows linear deposition of antibodies and complement along the glomerular basement membrane. The inflammatory reactions produced by anti–basement membrane antibody deposition account for the clinical symptoms observed in these patients. The symptoms include hematuria, renal failure, and hemoptysis.[13]

Type III Hypersensitivity

Type III reactions are triggered by the deposition of circulating immune complexes in tissues, causing inflammation. The antibody involved is predominantly IgG or IgM, and the antigens can be infecting microorganisms, drugs, or self-antigens. Complement is usually activated, which greatly amplifies the inflammatory response.

Fate of Circulating Immune Complexes

Under normal conditions circulating immune complexes are rapidly cleared by the mononuclear phagocytic system, preventing tissue deposition and associated damage. The physicochemical property, especially the molecular size of immune complexes, appears to affect their clearance directly; large immune complexes are cleared rapidly by the host, whereas small soluble complexes tend to have a prolonged plasma half-life and are associated with tissue deposition, which causes inflammatory responses. Various factors that affect the size of immune complexes are identified here; the principles of antibody–antigen binding are discussed in Chapter 10.

Ratio of Antigen (Ag) to Antibody (Ab)

The ratio of Ag to Ab has a direct effect on the size of immune complexes. Small immune complexes are usually formed in antigen excess (an excess of 5 to 60 times). These small complexes usually have Ag–Ab ratio in the range of 1.2 to 1.25, and molecular formulas of Ag_1Ab_1, Ag_2Ab_2, or possibly Ag_2Ab_1. Studies of the rate of immune complex clearance in animals indicate that immune complexes with a density of less than 19S and an Ag–Ab ratio greater than 2:5 tend to have a prolonged plasma half-life. Conversely, immune complexes with a density greater than 19S and Ag–Ab ratio of 2:5 or less are cleared rapidly by the animal (Fig. 6-5).[14-16]

Antigen Valency

The number of antigenic determinants of an antigen may have an effect on the size of immune complexes. This is demonstrated experimentally using constructed hapten–protein conjugates; conjugates with less than four hapten molecules form small soluble immune complexes with a density of less than 19S,

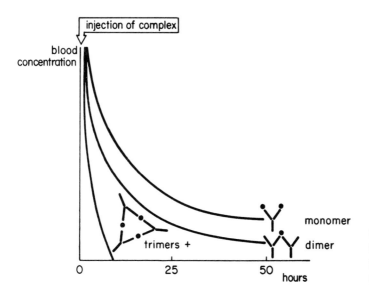

FIGURE 6-5. Immune complex clearance by the reticuloendothelial system. (From Roitt IM, Brostoff J, Male DK. Immunology. London: Gower Medical Publishing, 1985.)

an Ag–Ab ratio greater than 2:5, and a tendency to prolonged plasma half-life.[15]

Antibody Affinity

Antibody with low affinity tends to form immune complexes that are easily dissociated and become small soluble immune complexes.

The Fc receptors of phagocytic cells also play an important role in immune complex clearance, because the receptors enable the phagocytic cells to attach to the immune complexes (opsonization), enhancing phagocytosis. Normally, the immune complex needs to have at least two IgG molecules to be cleared efficiently by the reticuloendothelial system. When the host is overloaded with a high concentration of immune complexes, the Fc receptors of the mononuclear phagocytic system can become saturated, which results in persistent circulating immune complexes.[14,15]

Complement activation by immune complexes also has an impact on their clearance. Complement receptors (C3b) on the mononuclear phagocytic cells appear to mediate immune adherence, promoting

phagocytosis of the immune complexes that fix complement.[15]

Site of Immune Complex Deposition

The site of immune complex deposition is mainly determined by the hemodynamics and the concentration of the circulating immune complexes. The area of great blood flow and turbulence appears to have marked predilection for complex deposition; the arterial bifurcation of the heart valve and the renal glomeruli are frequently involved. The renal glomeruli seem to be the prime targets, and several factors may contribute to this predilection: (1) Filtration occurs in this site, (2) they are subjected to unusual hydrodynamic stress, and (3) glomerular endothelial cells have a high affinity for certain antigens, such as DNA.[14,16]

Localized immune complex formation can also result in type III hypersensitivity. Inflammation of the joint seen in rheumatoid arthritis exemplifies the condition in which tissue damage occurs at the site of immune complex formation.

Pathogenesis

In experimental animals, systemically injected immune complexes do not always lead to tissue deposition. However, if histamine is injected with immune complexes, tissue deposition occurs. Furthermore, administration of antihistamine can abrogate the histamine effect, suggesting that increased vascular permeability plays an important role in immune complex deposition. There are several sources of vasoactive amines. These include basophils, mast cells, platelets, and complement fragments.

Inflammatory responses are triggered as a result of complement activation by immune complexes. Complement activation products, such as C3a and C5a, have anaphylatoxic activities (anaphylatoxins). These anaphylatoxins will trigger vasoactive amine release from basophils and mast cells, leading to in-

creased vascular permeability that will enhance the immune complex deposition and neutrophil infiltration. Furthermore, neutrophils are attracted to the site of inflammation by C3a and C5a. Lysosomal enzymes are released by the neutrophils as they attempt to phagocytize the immune complexes, leading to the damage to adjacent cells and tissues. The immune complexes can also interact with Fc receptors on platelets and trigger vasoactive amine release by the platelets, thus perpetuating the cycle described earlier (Fig. 6-6).

Examples of Type III Hypersensitivity

Arthus Reaction

The Arthus reaction is induced experimentally by intradermal injection of the antigen into a sensitized animal. The local antigen–antibody interaction (immune complex formation) results in destructive in-

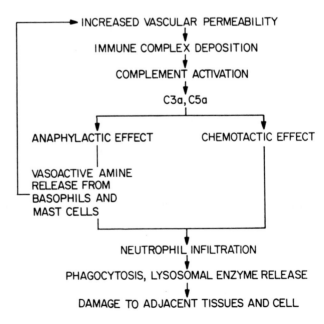

FIGURE 6-6. Pathogenesis of immune complex disorders.

flammation of small blood vessels, called vasculitis. Local swelling and erythema appear within 1 to 2 hours and subside within 10 to 12 hours. Microscopic examination of the tissue reveals neutrophil infiltration initially, followed by mononuclear cells and eosinophil infiltration. The mononuclear cells and eosinophils degrade the immune complexes.

Hypersensitive pneumonitis or extrinsic allergic alveolitis is probably the clinical counterpart of the Arthus reaction. The inhaled antigens may be fungal spores, avian proteins (the cause of bird handler's pneumonitis), or insect antigens. The clinical symptoms include chills, cough, dyspnea, and fever. Usually resolution of symptoms occurs in 12 to 18 hours once the source of antigen is eliminated.

Immune Complex Disorders

The term *immune complex disorder* is used to describe the diseases associated with clinical features secondary to immune complex deposition. The classic example is serum sickness, which frequently develops in patients who receive heterologous serum as a form of passive immunotherapy or immunosuppressive therapy. For example, horse antisera to diphtheria, tetanus, or other microorganisms were used in the past as a form of prophylactic immunotherapy, and heterologous antilymphocyte antibodies were given to renal transplant recipients to suppress tissue rejection. The patients make antibodies against the heterologous serum proteins and develop immune complex disorders.

Glomerulonephritis

Deposition of immune complexes in the renal glomeruli causes inflammatory responses that present with clinical symptoms of glomerulonephritis. For example, systemic lupus erythematosus (SLE) is an autoimmune disorder in which autoantibody to double-stranded DNA plays an important role in pathogenesis. The pathogenic role of antibody–DNA immune complexes is indicated by experimental observations: Antibody–DNA immune complexes have been eluted from the diseased kidney, and immunofluorescent study of kidney biopsy demonstrates immunoglobulin and C3 deposition in the glomeruli. The immunofluorescent staining pattern of SLE kidney biopsy differs from that of glomerulonephritis associated with Goodpasture's syndrome. Whereas the latter demonstrates smooth, linear staining of the glomerular basement membrane, the SLE lesion shows granular or "lumpy" staining, which may be confined to the mesangium, extended to the subendothelium or the basement membrane.[14,17,18]

Glomerulonephritis due to immune complex deposition is also associated with such infections as streptococcal infection and hepatitis B viral infection.[19,20] Malignancies also appear to cause nephritis occasionally.

Vasculitis

Vasculitis is a group of syndromes that have common clinicopathologic features associated with the inflammatory reaction in vessel walls. The classification of vasculitis is based on the type and size of affected vessels, organs involved (lung, kidney, skin, etc.), the characteristic of inflammatory reaction, and the clinical features.

Polyarteritis nodosa is characterized by the inflammation of small and medium-sized arteries. Approximately 50% of the patients with polyarteritis nodosa are found to have hepatitis B infections. Hepatitis B surface antigens (HBsAg), either alone or with immunoglobulin and complement, have been demonstrated in the vessel walls in the patient with polyarteritis nodosa.

Vasculitis is also seen in patients with rheumatoid arthritis. Immunofluorescent study of the lesion shows the deposition of immunoglobulin and C3 in the arterial walls in a granular pattern.[17,18]

Destruction of Innocent Bystanders

Circulating immune complexes can nonspecifically adhere to the elements of blood, initiating their destruction and that of innocent bystanders. Drug administration often elicits an antibody response that results in circulating antibody–drug immune complexes. These antibody–drug immune complexes become adsorbed onto the surface of red blood cells, causing intravascular hemolysis. The absorption of immune complexes is thought to be mediated by the red blood cell surface C3b receptors. Quinidine, quinine, and phenacetin are known to cause red blood cell lysis by this mechanism.[14]

Type IV Hypersensitivity

Type IV hypersensitivity, cell-mediated immune reaction or delayed hypersensitivity, is mediated by soluble factors or lymphokines released by the sensitized T lymphocytes. The characteristic histology of the lesion is a mononuclear cell infiltration. Such lesions appear 24 to 48 hours following antigen challenge and peak within 72 hours. Antibody and complement are usually not directly involved in type IV hypersensitivity.

Mechanism of Pathogenesis

The response is initiated by interactions between the antigen and a small number of sensitized T lymphocytes. Lymphokines are produced by these T lymphocytes following activation. The lymphokines have biologic activities affecting various cell types, such as macrophages, neutrophils, and other lymphocytes. These secondary cells are recruited to the site of reaction. For example, macrophages that respond to the lymphokine, migration inhibition factor (MIF), are prevented from leaving the lesion and become activated.[21] The overall function of lymphokines is to amplify the response that is initiated by a small number of T lymphocytes. This is achieved by recruiting and directing the secondary cells, macrophages, neutrophils, and other lymphocytes, both T and B cells. Normal control mechanisms lead to resolution of the reaction; however, multiple antigenic challenges in a hypersensitive individual may lead to the ulceration and necrosis of the lesion. Usually the symptoms develop over a period of 24 to 48 hours after antigen exposure, and the histologic examination shows characteristic mononuclear infiltration.

Examples of Type IV Hypersensitivity

Tuberculin-Type Hypersensitivity

Tuberculin-type hypersensitivity is induced by subcutaneous injection of the antigen in a sensitized individual. The area of induration and swelling at the site of injection appears within 24 to 72 hours. Microscopic examination reveals intense mononuclear cell infiltration around the blood vessels and disruption of the organization of the collagen bundles in the dermis. The classic example is the tuberculin skin test in which purified protein derivative (PPD) prepared from the culture filtrate of *Mycobacterium tuberculosis* is administered intradermally. A positive response consists of 10 mm or greater erythema and induration between 48 and 72 hours. A positive test indicates that the individual has been exposed to *Mycobacterium tuberculosis* or related organisms. A negative test signifies either no infection or a false negative due to immunosuppression associated with severe infection. A false negative test result may also be caused by immune suppressive conditions, including corticosteroid therapy, lymphoid malignancies, viral infections, and sarcoidosis.[22]

Contact Sensitivity

Certain compounds can cause systemic sensitization through direct skin contact. A second encounter with the same antigen by skin contact results in edema of the epidermis with formation of microvesicles. The microscopic observation of the lesion indicates a mononuclear cell infiltrate that first appears at 6 to 8 hours and peaks at 12 to 15 hours after exposure to the antigen. The most common antigens that induce contact sensitivity are poison ivy and poison oak.[23]

Granulomatous Hypersensitivity

Granulomatous hypersensitivity results from the persistent presence of microorganisms within the macrophages that the cell is unable to destroy. Inert substances, such as talc, may also cause granulomatous hypersensitivity. In both cases the macrophages are unable to digest the phagocytized substance. The characteristic cells found in a granulomatous lesion are lymphocytes, macrophages, epithelioid cells, and multinucleated giant cells. Epithelioid cells are poorly understood. The giant cells are multinucleated with little endoplasmic reticulum, degenerated mitochondria, and lysosomes. Thus, it is likely a terminally differentiated macrophage. Granulomatous hypersensitivity is seen in tuberculosis, leprosy, and sarcoidosis.[24]

References

1. Wells JV: Antibody-mediated tissue injury. In Stite DP, Stobo JD, Fudenberg HH, et al (eds): Basic and Clinical Immunology, 5th ed, p 132. Los Altos, Lange Medical Publications, 1984

2. Marsh DG, Meyers DA, Bias WB: The epidemiology and genetics of atopic allergy. N Engl J Med 305:1551, 1981

3. Ishizaka T, Soto CS, Ishizaka K: Mechanisms of passive sensitization. III. Number of IgE molecules and their receptor sites on human basophil granulocytes. J Immunol 111:500, 1973

4. Schleimer RP, MacGlashan DW Jr, Shuiman FS, et al: Human mast cell and basophil-structure, function, pharmacology, and biochemistry. Clin Rev Allergy 1:327, 1983

5. Ishizaka T: Biochemical analysis of triggering signals induced by bridging of IgE receptors. Fed Proc 41:17, 1982

6. Schleimer RP, MacGlashan DW Jr, Peter SP, et al: Inflammatory mediators and mechanisms of release from purified human basophils and mast cells. J Clin Immunol 74:473, 1984

7. Bennich H: Structure of IgE. Prog Immunol 2:49, 1974

8. Serafin WE, Austin KF: Mediators of immediate hypersensitivity reactions. N Engl J Med 317:30, 1987

9. Petz LD, Garratty G: Specificity of autoantibodies: Specificity of autoantibodies associated with warm-antibody type autoimmune hemolytic anemia. In: Acquired Immune Hemolytic Anemia, p 232. New York, Churchill Livingstone, 1980

10. Volpe R: Autoimmunity in the endocrine system, Vol 20, Monographs in Endocrinology. New York, Springer-Verlag, 1981

11. Lindstrom J: Autoimmune response to acetylcholine receptors in myasthenia gravis and its animal model. Adv Immunol 27:1, 1979

12. Leikola J: Blood banking and immunopathology. In Stites DP, Stobo JD, Wells JV (eds): Basic and Clinical Immunology, p 304. Norwalk, Appleton & Lange, 1987

13. Briggs WA, Johnson JP, Teichnab S, et al: Antiglomerular basement membrane antibody-mediated glomerulonephritis and Goodpasture's syndrome. Medicine 58:348, 1975

14. Thaler MS, Klausner RD, Cohen HJ: Immune complex disease. In: Medical Immunology, p 139. Philadelphia, JB Lippincott, 1977

15. Wells JV: Immune mechanisms in tissue damage. In Fudenberg HH, Stite DP, Caldwell JL, et al (eds): Basic and Clinical Immunology, 2nd ed, p 274. Los Altos, Lange Medical, 1978

16. Roitt I, Brostoff J, Male D: Hypersensitivity-type III. In: Immunology, p 21.1. London, Gower Medical Publishing, 1985

17. Inman RD, Day NK: Immunologic and clinical

aspects of immune complex diseases. Am J Med 70:1097, 1981

18. Inman RD: Immune complexes in SLE. Clin Rheum Dis 8:49, 1982

19. Gutman RA, Striker GE, Gillard BC, et al: The immune complex glomerulonephritis of bacterial endocarditis. Medicine 51:1, 1972

20. Shusterman N, London WT: Hepatitis B and immune-complex disease. N Engl J Med 310:43, 1984

21. Sergent JS: Vasculitis with hepatitis B antigene-mia: long-term observation in nine patients. Medicine 55:1, 1976

22. Snider DE: The tuberculin skin test. Annu Rev Respir Dis (Suppl) 125:102, 1982

23. Diaz LA, Provast TT: Dermatologic diseases. In Stite DP, Stobo JD, Wells JV (eds): Basic and Clinical Immunology, 6th ed, p 516. Norwalk, Appleton & Lange, 1987

24. Roitt I, Brostoff J, Male D: Hypersensitivity—Type IV. In: Immunology, p 22.1. London, Gower Medical Publishing, 1985

7

Tumor Immunology

Karen James

Neoplasia means new growth; a "neoplasm is an abnormal mass of tissue, the growth of which exceeds and is uncoordinated with that of normal tissues and persists in the same excessive manner after cessation of the stimuli which evoked the change."[1]

The terms *tumor* and *cancer* are used by the general public when referring to neoplastic diseases. The word *tumor* actually refers to swelling or to a defined mass of tissue distinct from normal physiologic growth; thus, a scar would by definition be a tumor.[2] The Latin word for *tumor* is *oncos;* thus, the origin of the word *oncology*, the study and treatment of tumors or neoplasms. The commonly used term for all malignant tumors or neoplasms is *cancer.*

A neoplasm is essentially a parasite that establishes a relationship with the host, referred to as tumor–host interactions.[2] Benign tumors may cause clinical disease by interfering with the functions of normal tissues or by producing hormones with functional activity. Malignant tumors cause similar symptoms of disease; however, they also invade nor-

mal tissue, grow rapidly, and use nutrients that normal tissues need to survive. In contrast, the host also develops a response to the tumor, referred to as tumor immunity.

Scientists have long hypothesized that the immune system has a role in tumor immunity. Key evidence is that solid tumors removed from humans during surgery invariably have a mononuclear cell infiltrate, implying an immune response to the cancer. Only since the 1960s, however, have the mechanisms of lymphocyte-mediated immunity been understood.

Cellular Immunity to Tumors

T-cell-mediated immunity to tumor antigens is analogous to the body's response to other T-dependent antigens, such as transplantation antigens. In *in vitro* experiments, tumor antigens provoke the pro-

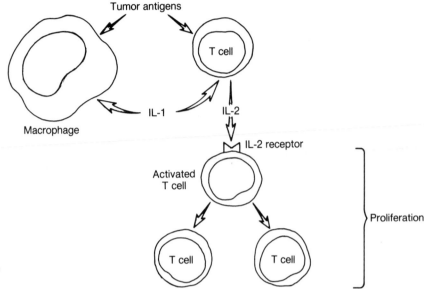

FIGURE 7-1. Amplification of effector functions of T cells.

liferation of T cells of all subpopulations (helper, suppressor, and cytotoxic). The amplification of effector functions (Fig. 7-1) of these cells requires the production of antigen nonspecific, low-molecular-weight, mediator molecules released from nucleated cells, which are called cytokines or cytotoxins. Specific cytokines are secreted by activated T cells (lymphokines) and macrophages (monokines).

The most significant cytokine is interleukin-1 (IL-1). IL-1 promotes the proliferation and activation of T cells, B cells, and natural killer (NK) cells. IL-1 is the endogenous pyrogen that elicits the fever response to inflammation, stimulates the production of acute phase proteins, and is responsible for many other activities.[3] The monokine, tumor necrosis factor (TNF), which is identical to cachectin, mediates inflammation to promote resistance to tumor cells and induces IL-1 secretion.[4] Several lymphokines important to the cell-mediated immune response to tumors[6] are found in Display 1.

T-Cell-Mediated Cytotoxicity

Cytotoxic T lymphocytes (CTL) have the capacity to directly lyse tumor cells that bear antigens to which these immune T cells have been previously exposed (also referred to as "primed"). The first step in the CTL response is recognition of the tumor antigens by cell surface interactions (Table 7-1). The primary pathway of interactions between CTL and tumor cells involves the recognition of the class II antigens

---

Display 1: Lymphokines Involved in Tumor Immunity

1. Interleukin-2 (IL-2) stimulates the proliferation of activated T cells and NK cells and enhances the cytotoxic activity of both cell types.

2. Migration inhibition factor (MIF) appears to immobilize macrophages at the tumor site.

3. Macrophage-activating factor (MAF) serves to stimulate macrophages to be cytotoxic for tumor cells.

4. Tumor necrosis factor (TNF) induces an inflammatory response that destroys tumor cells.

5. Interferon gamma (type II IFN) activates macrophages and augments cytocidal activities of natural killer cells.

Table 7-1: Surface Markers of Cells Involved in Tumor Immunology

Surface Marker	T Cells	NK Cells	Macrophages	Mechanism of Interaction With Tumor Cells
HLA-DR (Ia)	Activated (not resting)	–	Activated (not resting)	Recognition of self for proliferation (T cells) for tumor antigen presentation (macrophages)
IgG Fc receptors	CD8+	+	+	Recognition of antibody complexed to tumor antigens that stimulates proliferation (T cells and NK cells) and facilitates tumor antigen presentation (macrophages)
Complement receptors	–	–	+	Anchoring mechanism or second signal in addition to antibody for activating macrophages
CD3	+	–	–	T-cell antigen receptor; interaction with antigen stimulates proliferation, generation of HLA-DR, and synthesis of lymphokines
CD2	+	+	–	Sheep erythrocyte receptor that may regulate the signals received from other surface markers during tumor antigen recognition
C-Reactive protein (CRP) receptor	–	+	+	Recognition of tumor antigens at the early stages of the inflammatory process prior to the production of specific antibody

(HLA-DR) of the major histocompatibility complex (MHC), identifying those tumor antigens as self through an interaction with the CD3 T-cell receptor (Fig. 7-2). Tumor-specific antigens are primarily glycoprotein moieties on the surface of neoplastic cells, which, in combination with Ia (HLA-DR) molecules, comprise the distinguishing components that elicit a CTL response to the tumor cells.[5] (Tumor antigens will be further described later.)

The second step in the T-cell-mediated response to tumors is specific proliferation of the activated (primed) T cells. Concomitant with this clonal proliferation is the production of lymphokines. Simultaneously, the cytotoxic T cells seek out the tumor cells, which contain the tumor-specific antigen and the recognizable HLA-DR antigen, and cause lysis. The lytic step is not yet well understood, but this phenomenon can be reproduced *in vitro* as well as in adoptive transfer studies.

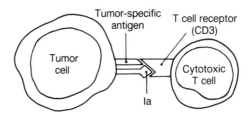

FIGURE 7-2. MHC involvement in recognition of tumor antigens as self.

Natural Immunity to Tumors

Natural immunity is present spontaneously in normal individuals, analogous to the innate immunity of the acute phase response to inflammation. Natural immunity does not depend upon previous exposure to tumor cells; its activity can be augmented very rapidly (within hours or a few days) and may be the first line of defense against tumors. Cells that are involved in natural immunity include macrophages, natural killer (NK) cells, killer (K) cells, and lymphokine-activated killer (LAK) cells.[6]

Macrophage-mediated cytotoxicity is the tumoricidal function of activated macrophages.[9] Macrophages from normal individuals (not activated) display only minimal levels of tumor cytotoxicity and have characteristic surface markers (see Table 7-1). Activated macrophages, however, can differentiate between tumor cells and normal cells and can selectively kill tumor cells, leaving normal cells unscathed. This provides evidence that there are unique antigens that are associated with tumor cells. These tumor-specific antigens are specifically recognized by cells that evoke natural immunity. Unlike cytotoxic T cells, macrophage tumoricidal activity is not dependent upon recognition of HLA-DR molecules or other self constituents. Macrophage-mediated tumor cytotoxicity occurs independently of genetic factors, including species barriers.

A variety of factors or events activate macrophages, including infections with intracellular organisms, such as *Mycobacteria, Listeria,* and *Toxoplasma.*[7] Endotoxins (lipopolysaccharides), soluble products of bacteria, also can activate macrophages.[8] The lymphokines MIF, MAF, and IFN significantly enhance tumor cytotoxicity by macrophages *in vitro* and presumably also play a role *in vivo.* Immune complexes (antigen–antibody) and complexes containing C-reactive protein have also been shown to stimulate macrophage-mediated cytotoxicity *in vitro.*[9]

Destruction of tumor cells by macrophages requires close physical contact between the macro-

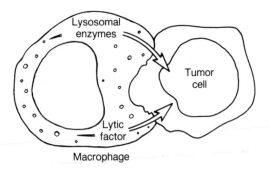

FIGURE 7-3. Macrophage-mediated tumor cytotoxicity.

phage and the tumor cell (Fig. 7-3). *In vitro* studies using labeled lysosomes indicate that the cytotoxic macrophage directly transfers its lysosomal contents to the tumor cell while the membranes of the two cells are fused.[7] Activated macrophages contain increased numbers of lysosomes, which may contribute to the effectiveness of the killing by these cells.

One of the leading causes of death from malignancies is metastases (*i.e.,* release of cells from the primary tumor site to initiate growth of a tumor). The metastasized cells have the same surface antigens and other characteristics as the primary tumor had in another, previously normal area of the body. The principal sites of metastasis are the lymph nodes, lung, and liver. Activated macrophages have been shown in animal studies to be very effective at decreasing the incidence of metastasis in several tumor models.[9]

Natural killer (NK) *cells* can recognize and lyse a number of tumor cells and other cell lines *in vitro.* There is a broad specificity for the NK effector function that may include target cells from the following sources[6]: syngeneic (*e.g.,* identical twins), allogeneic (same animal species, different genetic background), and xenogeneic (different species with different genetic background). The lineage of NK cells is still a topic of debate, but most of the evidence indicates a lymphoid origin. NK cells are also called LGL (large granular lymphocytes) because of the azurophilic granules in the cytoplasm and the high cytoplasm:nucleus ratio. NK cells lack surface immunoglobulin

(SIg) or C3 receptors but do have IgG Fc receptors and low levels of CD2 and CD8 antigens, which are characteristically found on T cells (see Table 7-1). However, mice that are congenitally athymic or that have been thymectomized as neonates and have no detectable T cells do have detectable and functional NK cells. NK cells share some surface antigens in common with monocytes but are not phagocytic.

Similar to activation of macrophages, NK cells can also be activated by the lymphokines IFN and IL-2.[5] In contrast to T cells and B cells, activation of NK cells does not induce immunologic memory.[6] There is no primary or secondary response detectable for NK cells, only a proliferative response that appears to be triggered by IL-1 during the acute inflammatory process. NK cells are also subject to suppression by certain factors known to be produced by tumor cells as well as by macrophages (*e.g.*, prostaglandin E_2). NK activity changes with age, from low levels in the neonates, peaking at puberty, and steadily declining with advancing age. NK effector function appears to play no role in immunity to established solid tumors. The experimental evidence supports the hypothesis that the antitumor effects of NK cells are likely to be the first line of defense against developing tumors[8] and metastasis.[9]

Display 2: Stages of Natural Killer Effector Function

1. Target cell binding when physical contact is made between effector cells and target cells.

2. Programming for lysis, during which the effector cell cytoskeletal components and Golgi apparatus move within the cytoplasm to the area of the effector cell that has physical contact with the target cell.

3. Secretion of factors such as NK cell cytotoxic factor (NKCF), granule cytolysin, and IL-1 by the LGL effector cell.

4. The cell-independent phase of the lytic event where the NK cells are no longer needed; soluble factors complete the killing process.

The lytic action of NK cells involves a complex sequence of events leading to the destruction of target cells. The lytic action of NK cells can be divided into at least four distinct stages,[10] listed in Display 2 and illustrated in Fig. 7-4.

Lymphokine-activated killer (LAK) cells, which specifically respond to IL-2, appear to have many of the same cell surface antigens as NK cells and may be unstimulated NK cells.[11] Like NK cells, LAK cells are LGLs that do not express the T-cell CD3 receptor. The LAK activity reflects the potent ability of IL-2 both to stimulate cytotoxic activity and to expand the population(s) of natural effector cells.

Humoral Immunity to Tumors

Neoplastic changes involve the loss of certain normal antigens from the cell surface and the appearance of new (neo-) antigens that were not detectable on the normal cells. NK cells and cytotoxic macrophages recognize these neoantigens (*in vitro*, at least) and apparently use them to differentiate tumor cells from normal cells. Spontaneously occurring tumors show minimal antigenic changes, whereas chemically-induced tumors express definite neoantigens that are capable of eliciting an antibody response. It is well documented that tumor cells can change their neoantigens (*i.e.*, can modulate the expression of these antigens in response to their environment).

Tumor-Specific Antigens

Antigens associated with solid tumors fall into four classes (Fig. 7-5):

1. Antigens that are absolutely restricted to one tumor are not found in association with any other tumors. Chemically-induced tumors have unique antigens even when the same chemical induces different tumors at different sites in the same individual.

2. Shared tumor antigens are found on the tumor cells of different individuals. Many virally induced tumors share common antigens.

3. Antigens that are widely distributed and found associated with different tumors as well as

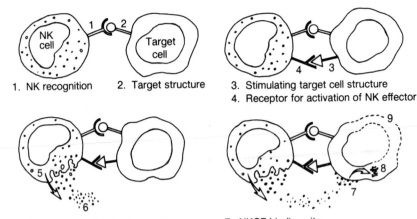

1. NK recognition   2. Target structure

3. Stimulating target cell structure
4. Receptor for activation of NK effector

5. Secretion of granule contents
6. Release of NK cytotoxic factor

7. NKCF binding site
8. NKCF induced polymerization pore-
   forming protein
9. Pore formation → lysis → killing

FIGURE 7-4. Stages of natural
killer effector functions.

with normal cells have been referred to as "illegiti-mate" antigens. One example is the presence of the blood group antigens MN in certain brain tumors.[5]

4. Retrogenetic antigens are normally expressed only by fetal tissue, not by adult tissues. These antigens are also referred to as oncodevelopmental or oncofetal antigens. With very sensitive assays these antigens can be found in small quantities on normal adult tissues.

The two most common oncofetal antigens are carcinoembryonic antigen (CEA) and alpha-fetoprotein (AFP). The appearance of these oncofetal antigens suggests their presence is a result of gene derepression and loss of synthesis control rather than

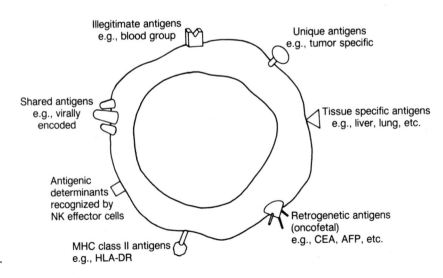

Illegitimate antigens
e.g., blood group

Unique antigens
e.g., tumor specific

Shared antigens
e.g., virally
encoded

Tissue specific antigens
e.g., liver, lung, etc.

Antigenic
determinants
recognized by
NK effector cells

Retrogenetic antigens
(oncofetal)
e.g., CEA, AFP, etc.

MHC class II antigens
e.g., HLA-DR

FIGURE 7-5. Tumor antigens.

the appearance of new gene products following a mutation.

CEA is found in serum in association with gastrointestinal tumors, particularly colon cancer. CEA is a glycoprotein that is normally synthesized and secreted by cells lining the gastrointestinal (GI) tract. In normal situations CEA is eliminated through the bowel. CEA can be found in circulation in disorders of the GI tract where there has been damage to the mucosal surface, which allows CEA into the bloodstream. Such GI disturbances include inflammatory bowel disease, ulcerative colitis, Crohn's disease, multiple polyps, and tumors of the GI tract. Certain types of tumors have been shown to secrete CEA, including adenocarcinoma of the colon, pancreas, liver, and lung, especially when there is metastasis to the liver. If the tumor is a CEA-secreting tumor, CEA can be used to monitor the effectiveness of surgical removal of the tumor as well as to monitor for recurrence of disease.[12] CEA is not recommended for use as a screening test for cancer, however, because of the incidence of CEA elevations in inflammatory but not neoplastic diseases.

AFP is a major plasma glycoprotein of the early human fetus. The fetal liver is the principal site of synthesis. AFP is found in high concentrations in fetal serum, maternal serum, and serum of adults with hepatomas (liver cancer) and testicular teratoblastomas.[5] Not all hepatomas or teratoblastomas produce AFP, but those that do synthesize this glycoprotein do so in very large amounts. Elevated levels of AFP are not always associated with malignancy; AFP can be elevated in inflammatory diseases of the liver, such as viral hepatitis, chronic hepatitis, and cirrhosis. High levels of AFP can also occur in inflammatory diseases of the bowel, such as Crohn's disease and ulcerative colitis, that also produce elevated levels of CEA. AFP, like CEA, is not useful as a screening test for cancer because elevated levels are associated with inflammatory processes.

AFP levels are useful in obstetrics, where high levels are found in amniotic fluid associated with neural tube defects.[13] Maternal serum can be screened for elevated levels of AFP in patients who are at higher risk for having a baby with certain forms of nephrosis or with neural tube defects such as spina bifida.

Antibody-Dependent Cell-Mediated Cytotoxicity

Immune complex activation of cellular immunity is also referred to as antibody-dependent cellular cytotoxicity (ADCC). Three cell types that contain IgG Fc receptors can evoke ADCC *in vitro:* granulocytes, macrophages, and killer (K) cells. ADCC requires an antibody-coated target (tumor) cell (Fig. 7-6). This antibody coating facilitates the effector–target cell interaction by way of the Fc receptor, which is necessary for cytolysis of the target cell. Indeed, macrophages that participate in ADCC are referred to as "armed macrophages." It appears that ADCC is most effective in killing the tumor cells that are resistant to macrophage-mediated cytotoxicity or NK activity. It is not known whether there are any differences between granulocytes and macrophages that participate in ADCC and those cells that can be directly cytotoxic to tumor cells. It is also debatable whether there are any differences between K cells, NK cells, and LAK cells, since these cells have similar surface markers and LGL appearance.

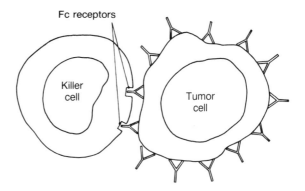

FIGURE 7-6. Antibody-dependent cell-mediated cytotoxicity.

Immune Surveillance

The term *immune surveillance* has its origins in the works of Paul Ehrlich, who, in 1909, proposed that the immune system was responsible not only for defending the body against bacterial infections, but also for eliminating "altered constituents" that have since been termed cancer cells.[14] Thomas,[15] and others later postulated the "immune surveillance theory," which stipulates that the immune response of normal individuals regularly eliminates malignant or potentially malignant cells, thereby preventing the establishment and growth of tumors. The immune surveillance theory has been the subject of much controversy. Patients who have immunodeficiency diseases or are immunosuppressed by drug treatments are significantly more vulnerable to both neoplasia and infections, a fact that tends to support the immune surveillance theory. The concept of immune surveillance states that malignant disorders occur when there is a *failure* of the immune system to recognize and destroy tumor cells before they become established.[16] When cancer is initially diagnosed, most cancer patients, however, have an intact immune response to their tumors, as measured by laboratory techniques *in vitro.* If "immune surveillance" is indeed responsible for immunity to tumors, why does anyone with a "normal" immune system ever get cancer?

Mechanisms of Immunologic Escape

Escape from immune surveillance mechanisms (see Table 7-2) occurs when the balance between tumor growth and tumor immunity is altered. Tumor immunity, which controls tumor growth or destroys the tumor, is overcome by factors that favor tumor growth.[16]

Most of the escape mechanisms can be demonstrated in experimental animals, but it is still only

Table 7-2: Factors That Contribute to Escape From Immune Surveillance

Tumor growth kinetics	Lymphocyte trapping
Antigenic modulation	Genetic factors
Antigen masking	Blocking factors
Antigen shedding	Tumor products
Tolerance	Growth factors

hypothetical that immunologic escape occurs in humans. Tumor kinetics is probably an important escape mechanism for many types of tumors. Tumor kinetics has also been referred to as "sneaking through." The tumor has to start somewhere. If it starts with just a few cells, the tumor may not be recognized as abnormal by the body until growth is established and the immune system has already been overwhelmed. In experimental animals if larger doses of the same tumor cells are injected, the tumor cells are destroyed. Low doses of the same tumor cells may be tolerated by the host and render the host nonresponsive.

The three mechanisms that involve antigen presentation are ways that tumors "protect" themselves from host immunity. As discussed earlier, many tumors have the capacity to modulate their surface antigens, expressing different antigens if the original antigens have been recognized and antibody has been developed to them. Tumors can also produce substances, such as sialomucin, that can bind to the surface of tumor cells and "mask" any antigens that may be present. Antigens that have apparently been shed from the tumor have been detected in human serum and urine as well as the body fluids of experimental animals. These soluble antigens may saturate the receptors on T cells or B cells and yet be too small to be cross-linked to stimulate the proliferative response or the effector function.

Lymphocytes that are sensitized to the tumor antigen(s) may get trapped in the lymph node or lymph organ that drains the affected site. This may result in a proliferative response within a single lymph node, trapping the effector cells in the node, preventing them from entering the peripheral circulation.

Genetically determined unresponsiveness has been shown with certain viruses in association with several histocompatibility antigens. This generally involves haplotypes of certain HLA antigens that seem to render that individual unable to respond to virally infected cells. Families have been described who are genetically unresponsive to Epstein-Barr virus–infected cells.[17]

Blocking factors have been hypothesized for many years but have not conclusively and consistently been shown to exist. The shed antigens described earlier may be considered to be blocking factors. Tumor-specific antigens may also elicit an immune response resulting in the formation of antibody. The antibody may complex with shed antigens, or may bind to still-bound antigen and be modulated off the tumor cell surface (Fig. 7-7). These complexes theoretically can block T-cell cytotoxicity either by directly binding to the cytotoxic T cells, preventing them from binding to the tumor cells, or by binding to the helper T cells, preventing them from recognizing the tumor cells and providing help for the cytotoxic T cells.

Tumor cells have been shown to secrete many products that enhance their own environment or depress the immune response. Certain types of tumors that tend to invade bone and cartilage have been shown to secrete collagenase, which causes lytic destruction of those components that would otherwise be impermeable to growth of a soft tissue.[18] Other tumors can secrete prostaglandins, which negatively regulate NK and K cells.[19] Clonal proliferation of primed or sensitized T cells or NK cells is crucial to the amplification of their function. Tumors that produce substances that interfere with the production of IL-1 by macrophages or IL-2 by T-cell subsets would limit the overall responsiveness to tumors.

Therapeutic Approaches to Tumors

There are basically four approaches to therapy of cancer in general: surgery, radiotherapy, chemotherapy, and immunotherapy. In many situations a combination of therapeutic approaches is necessary to eliminate or limit the tumor burden.

Surgery is the first and necessary therapeutic modality to decrease the solid tumor burden in early stages of breast cancer, colon cancer, lung cancer, and prostate cancer—the four major cancers in man

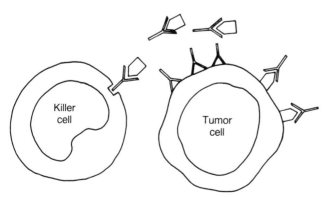

FIGURE 7-7. Blocking factors affect tumor immunity.

representing more than 50% of solid tumors.[20] In these and other types of cancers, the tumor may grow in an unnoticed "parasitic-type" of relationship with the host until it restricts a necessary function of the body and signals its presence. By then it may be necessary to remove the tumor surgically to prevent loss of function of a body part.

Radiotherapy can either be a primary therapy or an adjuvant (supplementary) therapy. Primary radiotherapy is most useful in cancers of the head and neck and in Hodgkin's disease (HD). In HD the radiotherapy is targeted to affected lymph nodes in various portions of the body. Radiotherapy is less disfiguring and more efficacious in tumors of the soft tissue in areas adjacent to the jaw and nasal passages. In many other solid tumors radiotherapy to draining lymph nodes after surgical excision of the primary tumor has been found to increase the 5-year survival rate.[21] The ultimate in radiotherapy is, however, whole body radiation, which is used prior to bone marrow transplantation as an effective treatment for certain types of acute leukemias that are refractory to chemotherapy.

Chemotherapy generally consists of treatment with drugs that are antimetabolites (*i.e.*, interfere with nucleic acid or protein synthesis). The approach to chemotherapy is to treat with as much of a single drug or combination of drugs as a person can tolerate. The rationale of chemotherapy is to kill the tumor cells, which are faster growing than normal cells.[22] The general approach is to give chemotherapy in "courses," allowing time for the normal body cells to recover before subsequent courses are administered. Leukemias are most effectively treated with chemotherapy. Acute leukemias of childhood are quite responsive to appropriate regimens of chemotherapy that are administered according to the cellular classification of the leukemia. Chemotherapy is also administered as adjuvant therapy to either surgery or radiotherapy.

Most therapeutic regimens have been arrived at by trial and error of various combinations of drugs or therapies. Large study groups (oncology groups) have been formed with regional institutions cooperating by inputing data.[23] The study groups can then generate a statistical approach to each combination. The cancer is "staged" prior to any therapy; that is, the extent of disease is ascertained by extensive evaluations that are consistently applied between institutions. Clinical trials are performed, randomly giving patients treatment A or treatment B. Within 2 years it is usually possible to determine which treatment is better. The statistically significantly "better" treatment is then later compared to treatment C, and the process is repeated.

Immunotherapy of cancer attempts to destroy tumor cells using manipulations of the immune system. Various modalities of immunotherapy have been explored, including immunoprophylaxis, active and passive immunotherapy, *in vitro* stimulation of the patient's lymphocytes, adoptive transfer, and mediator factor stimulation *in vivo*.[24]

Immunoprophylaxis with vaccines to certain viruses has been a successful therapeutic approach in animals.[25] Marek's disease, caused by a herpes virus, is a lymphoproliferative disease in chickens for which a vaccine has been highly successful. The incidence of feline leukemia has also been significantly decreased as a result of a vaccination program for cats. To date no vaccine is available to protect against any human tumors, primarily because no virus has been conclusively proved to cause specific forms of cancer.

Active immunotherapy can be specific, nonspecific, or a combination of both.[26] Specific immunotherapy involves injecting attenuated tumor cells or membrane components that bear the tumor-specific antigens to stimulate the immune system directly. Nonspecific immunotherapy uses adjuvants, substances that are known to enhance the body's own immune response. The two most widely used adjuvants are BCG* and a nonviable form of *Corynebacterium parvum*. Both produce a generalized enhancement of immune responsiveness against a

---

* BCG = bacille Calmette-Guérin (an attenuated strain of *Mycobacterium bovis*).

variety of antigens that can be demonstrated *in vitro*. BCG treatment has been most successful in treating melanoma skin lesions where statistically significant tumor regression can actually be measured. *C. parvum* also is most successful when it is injected directly into the tumor site. *C. parvum* has had limited but important clinical effects in treating lung cancer. Recombinant cytotoxins have recently been used in clinical trials of nonspecific immunotherapy. Several lymphokines or monokines have been purified, sequenced, and cloned, including IL-1, IL-2, IFN, and TNF. Although results are still preliminary, it appears that a single purified cytotoxin is not effective in arresting the progression of tumors; combinations of recombinant molecules hold promise as immunotherapeutic agents.[4]

Passive immunotherapy was first attempted by injecting tumor cells from a patient into an animal, raising antisera to the tumor, and injecting the antisera into the patient. This approach not only had no demonstrable effect, but also caused the patient to develop antibodies to the animal sera, resulting in serum sickness immune complex disease.

More recently, monoclonal antibodies (MAb) to certain tumor antigens have been used in a variety of approaches.[27] One use has been to enhance detection of metastatic lesions, facilitating their destruction by directed chemotherapy or by radiotherapy. Another method of potentiation targets MAb to micrometastases of cancer patients. When MAb to the CD3 receptor on T cells is used as immunosuppressive therapy in allograft recipients, these transplant patients become highly sensitized against the xenogeneic protein and produce antibodies to the MAb.[28]

The antibodies produced are of two types: those that recognize the isotypic (immunoglobulin subclass specificity) regions and the idiotypic determinants (areas of the variable Fab region that confer the unique specificity to each antigen). The anti-idiotypic antibodies are of major clinical importance, since they can block the ability of the MAb to bind to its target antigen. Consequently, although theoretically the use of MAb in passive immunotherapy looked promising, in practical application it may not be effective because of the specificity of the host's immune response.

In vitro stimulation of the patient's lymphocytes, NK cells, or macrophages has been developed as an alternative approach to adoptive immunotherapy. Rosenberg *et al*[29] have recently shown limited success with systemic administration of autologous LAK cells plus recombinant IL-2 in achieving tumor regression in certain cancer patients. The toxic effects of this type of immunotherapy, however, may preclude its use in all but the most resistant forms of cancer that cannot be cured by conventional therapies.

Molecular biologic approaches to cancer will supplant tumor immunology in the future. The approach to cancer therapy is changing, largely as a result of the discovery of oncogenes. These genes (oncogenes) cause cancer and are very similar to the normal genes that control cell differentiation, proliferation, and expression of their protein products.[30] The oncogenic proteins appear to act on normal cells at different stages of differentiation, "freezing" their development to one specific stage. Chromosomal translocations (rearrangements) that may be induced by carcinogens, viruses, irradiation, and so on, have been shown to be involved in certain B-cell malignancies.[31] The protein products (monoclonal immunoglobulins) of B-cell neoplasms are helpful in identifying the stage at which differentiation of the abnormal cells was arrested. The therapy can then be specifically directed toward known susceptibilities of cells at that single stage of differentiation. As other protein products of oncogenes are identified and characterized, more rational approaches to cancer therapy can be developed.

References

1. Willis RA: The Spread of Tumors in the Human Body. London, Butterworth and Co, 1952

2. Robbins SL: Pathologic basis of disease, p 106. Philadelphia, WB Saunders, 1974

3. Oppenheim JJ, Kovacs EJ, Matsushima K, et al: There is more than one interleukin 1. Immunol Today 7:45, 1986

4. Ruddle NH: Tumor necrosis factor and related cytotoxins. Immunol Today 8:129, 1987

5. Roitt IM, Brostoff J, Male DK: Immunity to tumors. In: Immunology, p 18.8. London, Gower Medical Publishing, 1985

6. Hersey P, Bolhius R: "Nonspecific" MHC-unrestricted killer cells and their receptors. Immunol Today 8:233, 1987

7. Adams DO, Nathan CF: Molecular mechanisms in tumor cell killing by activated macrophages. Immunol Today 4:166, 1983

8. Taramelli D, Holden HT, Varesio L: Endotoxin requirement for macrophage activation by lymphokines in a rapid microcytotoxicity assay. J Immunol Methods 37:225, 1980

9. Deodhar SD, Barna BP: Macrophage activation: potential for cancer therapy. Clev Clin Quart 53:223, 1986

10. Wright S, Bonavida B: Studies on the mechanisms of natural killer cell cytotoxicity. III. Activation of NK cells by interferon augments the lytic activity of released natural killer cytotoxic factors (NKCF). J Immunol 130:2960, 1984

11. Herberman RB, Balch C, Golub S, et al: Lymphokine-activated killer cell activity: Characteristics of effector cells and their progenitors in blood and spleen. Immunol Today 8:178, 1987

12. Martin EW, James KK, Minton JP: The use of CEA as an early indicator for gastrointestinal tumor recurrence and second-look procedures. Cancer 29:440, 1977

13. Greenberg PD: Tumor immunology. In Stites DP, Stobo JD, Wells JV (eds): Basic and Clinical Immunology, 6th ed, p 186. Norwalk, Appleton and Lange, 1987

14. Ehrlich P: In Himmelweit F (ed): The Collected Papers of Paul Ehrlich, Vol II, p 550. London, Pergamon Press, 1957

15. Thomas L: In Lawrence HS (ed): Cellular and Humoral Aspects of the Hypersensitive States, p 529. New York, Hoeber Publishers, 1959

16. Roitt IM, Brostoff J, Male DK: Immunity to tumors. In: Immunology. p 18.12. London, Gower Medical Publishing, 1985

17. Provisor AJ, Iacuone JJ, Chilcote RR, et al: Acquired agammaglobulinemia after a life-threatening illness with clinical and laboratory features of infectious mononucleosis in three related male children. N Engl J Med 293:62, 1975

18. Salo T, Liotta LA, et al: Secretion of basement membrane collagen-degrading enzyme and plasminogen activator by transformed cells. Role in metastasis. Int J Cancer 30:669, 1982

19. Fontana A, Kristensen F, Dubo R, et al: Production of prostaglandin E and interleukin-a like factor by cultured astrocytes and C6 glioma cells. J Immunol 129:2413, 1982

20. Silverberg E, Lubera J: Cancer statistics, 1987. Ca-A Cancer Journal for Clinicians 37:2, 1987

21. Harris JR, Hellman S, Kinne DW: Limited surgery and radiotherapy for breast cancer. Ca-A Cancer J Clin 36:120, 1986

22. Krakoff IH: Cancer chemotherapeutic agents. Ca-A Cancer Journal for Clinicians 37:92, 1987

23. Bennett JM: Basic concepts in investigational therapeutics. In Rubin P (ed): Clinical Oncology, p 96. Rochester, American Cancer Society, 1978

24. Hollingshead A, Stewart HM, Takita H, et al: Adjuvant specific active lung cancer immunotherapy trials. Cancer 60:1249, 1987

25. Jarrett W, Mackey L, Jarrett O, et al: Antibody response and virus survival in cats vaccinated against malignant lymphoma. Nature 253:71, 1975

26. Crispen RG (ed): Neoplasm Immunity: Solid Tumor Therapy. Chicago, Franklin Institute Press, 1977

27. Beverley PCL, Riethmuller G: Immunological intervention with monoclonal antibodies. Immunol Today 8:101, 1987

28. Chatenoud L: The immune response against therapeutic monoclonal antibodies. Immunol Today 7:367, 1986

29. Rosenberg SA, Lotze MT, Muul LM, et al: Special report: Observations on the systemic administration of autologous lymphokine-activated killer cells and recombinant interleukin-2 to patients with metastatic cancer. N Engl J Med 313:1485, 1985

30. Hunter T: The proteins of oncogenes. Scientific American 251:70, 1984

31. Marcu K, Melchers F, Morse HC, et al: Mechanisms in B cell neoplasia. Immunol Today 7:249, 1986

CHAPTER 8

Antibody Structure and Function

Dorothy J. Fike

General Structure of the Antibody Molecule

Antibody or immunoglobulin molecules are the major component of the specific humoral response to an antigenic challenge. Although antibodies have been divided into five classes—depending on their molecular weight, chemical composition, amino acid sequence, and function—all antibodies are protein molecules. All classes use the abbreviation Ig, which stands for *Immunoglobulin*.

When serum protein is separated during electrophoresis, most of the γ globulin region is immunoglobulin. Likewise, most, but not all, immunoglobulin migrates to the γ region (Fig. 8-1). The IgG class migrates to the γ region. IgA migrates to the γ and β globulin regions, with the majority to the γ region. IgM migrates to the γ, β, and α_2 regions, but the

majority of this class is in the β globulin region. IgD and IgE both migrate in the β globulin region.[1]

All immunoglobulins have the basic immunoglobulin structure composed of four polypeptide chains, two heavy and two light. Varying amounts of carbohydrate are attached; the amount of carbohydrate varies from 4% to 18% of the total composition of the immunoglobulin molecule (Fig. 8-2). The four chains are usually joined together by disulfide bonds; the number of disulfide bonds between heavy chains varies from one to 14.[2] Only one disulfide bond joins a heavy and light chain in most classes and subclasses.

The heavy and light chains have the amino terminus at the same end. The amino terminus is the variable region of the immunoglobulin molecule and is encoded by the V-D (light chains) or V-D-J (heavy chains) genes (see Chap. 4). It is called the variable region, since the amino acid sequence of each immu-

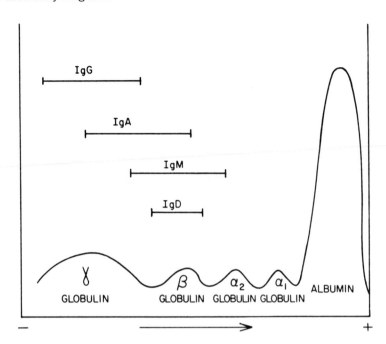

FIGURE 8-1. Serum proteins may be separated based on their electrical charge. Immunoglobulins may migrate in the α_2, β, or γ globulin regions.

noglobulin molecule varies and gives the antibody molecule its specificity to a particular epitope (antigenic determinant). Within the variable region there are some areas that exhibit even more variability and are the hypervariable regions.

The constant region is the same for all immunoglobulin polypeptide chains of a particular class or type. On the heavy chain, there are three or four subregions or domains. Each domain is coded for by a different exon of the immunoglobulin constant gene and has approximately 110 amino acids. Each domain has specific function for the immunoglobulin molecule.

The first and second constant domains of the heavy chain define the hinge region. This region allows an immunoglobulin molecule to change its configuration from a free-floating immunoglobulin molecule with a T configuration to a Y shape when the immunoglobulin molecule binds to the antigen (Fig. 8-3). The Y configuration exposes the complement recognition site on the heavy chain of IgM and

IgG that initiates the classical pathway of complement when CIq attaches to the site.

Certain enzymes degrade the immunoglobulin at specific points on the heavy chain. Two enzymes, papain and pepsin, have been useful in determining the function of specific areas. Papain splits the immunoglobulin molecule in the hinge region adjacent to disulfide bonds that hold the two heavy chains together (Fig. 8-4). This degradation yields three fragments. Two identical fragments consist of an entire light chain plus the variable domain and part of the constant domain of the heavy chain. This fragment of the immunoglobulin molecule can bind to the antigen and is called Fab (fragment antigen binding). The third fragment produced by papain cleavage consists of the remainder of the constant region of the two heavy chains linked by disulfide bonds. This fragment crystallizes and is called Fc (fragment crystallizable). Fc receptors found on other cells will bind to this region of the immunoglobulin molecule.[3]

A Variable and Constant Regions

B Heavy Chain Domains

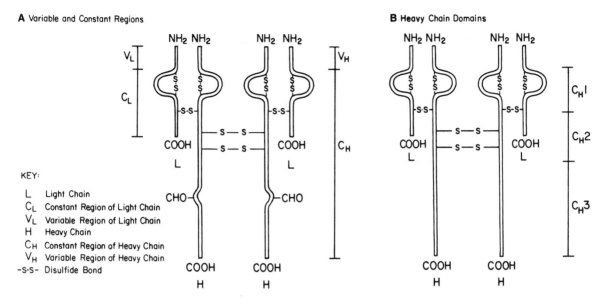

KEY:

L   Light Chain
C_L Constant Region of Light Chain
V_L Variable Region of Light Chain
H   Heavy Chain
C_H Constant Region of Heavy Chain
V_H Variable Region of Heavy Chain
-S-S- Disulfide Bond

FIGURE 8-2. *A*, The basic immunoglobulin structure is composed of two heavy and two light protein chains. Each chain has a variable and constant region. There are both intra- and interchain disulfide bonds. *B*, The heavy chain is composed of at least three constant domains. The specific number is cited in the text.

Pepsin cleavage of the molecule yields three different fragments. The two Fab fragments found with papain cleavage are held together by a disulfide bond and are called $F(ab')_2$. The pepsin cleavage produces two heavy chain fragments that are not joined together by a disulfide bond.[2,4]

Light Chains

There are two types of light chains kappa (κ) and lambda (λ). For any immunoglobulin molecule, only one type, κ or λ chains is present. For example, IgG may be either IgGκ or IgGλ, but it will never be

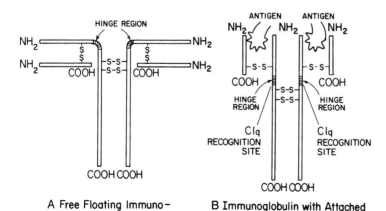

A Free Floating Immuno-
globulin (T-shape)

B Immunoglobulin with Attached
Antigen (Y-shape)

FIGURE 8-3. *A*, When the immunoglobulin is floating free in the plasma, it has a T shape. *B*, When attached to an antigen, the immunoglobulin changes from the T shape to the Y shape.

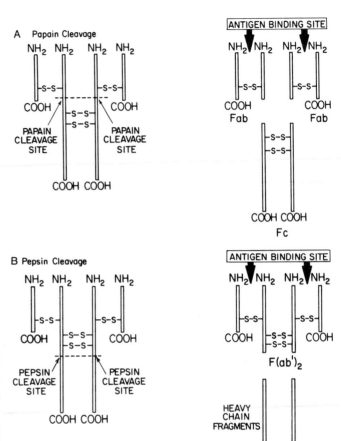

FIGURE 8-4. *A*, Papain cleaves the immunoglobulin molecule above the interchain disulfide bonds. Two different cleavage products are obtained: Fab, which has the ability to combine with the antigen, and Fc, which is crystallizable. Compared with the Fc, twice as many Fab fragments are formed. *B*, Pepsin cleaves the immunoglobulin below the interchain disulfide bond. Cleavage products are one F(ab')$_2$ and two heavy chain fragments.

IgGκλ. Both types of light chains have a molecular weight of approximately 23,000 d, though each is structurally different.[2] Even though there are structural differences between the two chains, some constraints are placed on structure variability. Both chains have amino acids threonine at position 5, glutamine at position 6, and glycine at position 16.[5] Approximately twice as many κ chains as λ chains are produced.[4]

Of the 214 amino acids in the κ chain, the variable region consists of the first 107 amino acids. Three hypervariable (HV) regions are found at amino acid residues 30 to 35, 50 to 55, and 95 to 100. Three allotypic variants are found in κ chains and are known as Km allotypes.[4]

The λ light chain consists of 213 to 216 amino acids. In some λ chains an amino acid is added or deleted from the normal sequence, although these differences are not considered allotypic variants. The variable and hypervariable regions of the λ chain occur at approximately the same amino acid positions as the κ chain; however, the addition or deletion of amino acids in the λ chain may slightly change these regions.[4]

Both the κ and λ chains have a cysteine molecule in the constant region that binds to a cysteine molecule on the heavy chain, forming the covalent disulfide bond. The cysteine molecule is the last amino acid of the κ chain and the penultimate (next to the last) amino acid of the λ chain. This disulfide bond linking the two chains creates the three-dimensional configuration that is essential for antibody and antigen interaction.[4]

In some diseases, such as multiple myeloma, free light chains are produced. These light chains do not polymerize with a heavy chain to form an immunoglobulin molecule but may form dimers through a disulfide bond with another light chain at the cysteine molecule that would normally bind to the heavy chain. A κ chain will associate with a second κ chain, and a λ chain will associate with a λ chain.[4] Free light chains or Bence-Jones protein have unique solubility properties. This protein precipitates at temperatures between 40° and 60°C and redissolves at 100°C.[6]

Heavy Chains

There are five major classes of immunoglobulins. Each class has a unique heavy chain that defines it: IgG has a gamma (γ) heavy chain, IgM has a mu (μ) heavy chain, IgA has an alpha (α) heavy chain, IgD has a delta (δ) heavy chain, and IgE has an epsilon (ϵ) heavy chain. All heavy chains consist of three or four constant domains and one variable domain. Each heavy chain is discussed when the Ig class is described.

Antibody Heterogeneity

Immunoglobulin variability may be divided into three types: isotypes, allotypes, and idiotypes (Table 8-1). Isotypes are the different heavy and light chains found in all healthy members of a species and are the classes, subclasses, and types. The constant domains of IgM, IgG (all subclasses), IgA, IgD, IgE, κ, and λ define the isotypes.[1]

Allotypes are genetic variation within the constant domains of a heavy or light chain. The alleles are inherited in a simple Mendelian pattern and ex-

pressed codominantly.[3] There are three allotypic markers for the κ chain (Km), two for α_2 heavy chain (A2m), and up to 25 for the heavy chain (Gm) class or subclass. Healthy individuals may not have all allotypes of a particular heavy or light chain.[1]

The idiotype is the variation within the variable region of an immunoglobulin molecule. Each immunoglobulin molecule from a single clone generally has a unique idiotype.[1] A portion of the idiotype may be an antigenic determinant, an idiotope, against which anti-idiotype antibodies are produced. It has been proposed that anti-idiotype antibodies have a role in the regulation of the immune response, either a positive or a negative effect.[7] Anti-idiotype antibodies have been used experimentally to detect antigen and antibody. Anti-idiotype antibodies also have a role in autoimmune disease, such as myasthenia gravis, Graves' disease, and insulin-resistant diabetes mellitis.

Additional Components of Immunoglobulins

J Chain

IgM and IgA classes are composed of more than one basic immunoglobulin unit held together by the J chain. The J chain is a small glycoprotein with a molecular weight of approximately 15,000 d that migrates electrophoretically in the prealbumin region. The J chain attaches via a disulfide bond near the carboxyl terminus of the heavy chains. Only one J chain is required for each IgM or IgA polymer. The J chain is believed to initiate polymerization.[4]

Secretory Component

The secretory component (SC) is a 70,000-d protein found on IgA and some IgM molecules in external secretions. Secretory IgA (or IgM) is released from the plasma cells located in mucosal tissue of the re-

Table 8-1: Antibody Heterogeneity

Type	Defines
Isotype	Heavy chain classes and subclasses (μ, μ_2; γ_1, γ_2, γ_3, γ_4; α_1, α_2; δ; ϵ)
	Light chain types (κ and λ)
	Healthy individuals have all isotypes
Allotype	Allelic variation of a class or light chain type (Gm, Am, and Km variants)
	Healthy individuals may express one or more of these
Idiotype	Variation in the variable region that is unique for each specificity of immunoglobulin

Immunoglobulin heterogeneity can be divided into three types: isotype, allotype, and idiotype. The heterogeneity occurs in different regions of the immunoglobulin molecule.

spiratory, gastrointestinal, and genitourinary tracts. The immunoglobulin diffuses toward the epithelial surface, where SC on the epithelial cell surface acts as a receptor for IgA. The IgA enters the epithelial cell and is transported across the cell in endocytic vesicles. The majority of secretory IgA released from the epithelial cells links the SC to the immunoglobulin via disulfide bonds. The SC attachment appears to be in the hinge region and other portions of the Fc region.[4] The function of the secretory component, in addition to facilitating IgA secretion, is to make the complex resistant to degradation by proteolytic enzymes present in secretions.[8]

Immunoglobulin Classes

IgG

The basic four-chain model of immunoglobulins is the basic structure of the immunoglobulin G (IgG) molecule. A γ chain is present in all IgG molecules.

Minor variation in heavy chains establishes the four IgG subclasses. The four subclasses of IgG vary in the amino acid sequence and the number of disulfide bonds between heavy chains. Gm allotypes define the variation in the γ chains in members of the same species. The carbohydrate content of IgG is 2.5% of its total molecular weight (Table 8-2). The IgG molecule has a sedimentation coefficient of 7S and a molecular weight of approximately 150,000 d. When serum is electrophoresed, the IgG migrates to the γ globulin region. The γ globulin region is a broad band because of the heterogeneity of IgG molecules. Each specific IgG molecule will have a slightly different charge and will migrate slightly differently. IgG, approximately 75% to 80% of all serum immunoglobulin, has a serum concentration ranging from 1000 to 1500 mg/dL. This concentration reflects the high rate of synthesis and the long half-life (low catabolic rate).

The variable region of the γ chain is the first 107 amino acids. Three hypervariable regions are located at nearly the same amino acid position as the hypervariable regions of the variable domain of the light chains: 30 to 35, 50 to 55, and 95 to 100. The constant region of the γ chain has three domains designated as CH_1, CH_2, and CH_3. CH_1 is adjacent to the variable region and encompasses amino acid residues 114 through 223. CH_2 is next, with amino acid residues 246 through 361; and CH_3 contains amino acid residues 362 through 496. Each heavy chain domain contains an intrachain disulfide bond and each constant domain has approximately 40% homology (same amino acid sequence) with the constant domain of the light chains. The hinge region of the γ chain (roughly between amino acid residues 220 and 241) is generally characterized by two interchain disulfide bonds linking the two heavy chains and has one disulfide bond linking one heavy and one light chain.[4]

IgG is the predominant antibody synthesized in the secondary antibody response. IgG is the exclusive antitoxin antibody. Both the intravascular and extravascular pools contain equal amounts of IgG. IgG is

Table 8-2: Properties of Immunoglobulins

Property	Immunoglobulin Class				
	IgG	IgM	IgA	IgD	IgE
Serum concentration (approximate in mg/dL)	1000–1500	100–125	200–250	3	0.01–0.05
Half-life (days)	21–23	5–6	5–6.5	2–8	1–5
Molecular weight (approximate in daltons)	150,000	900,000–1,000,000	150,000–350,000	180,000	190,000
Molecular formula	$\gamma_2\kappa_2$ or $\gamma_2\lambda_2$	serum $(\mu_2\kappa_2)_5 \cdot J$ or $(\mu_2\lambda_2)_5 \cdot J$	serum $\alpha_2\kappa_2$ or $\alpha_2\lambda_2$ secretory $(\alpha_2\kappa_2)_2 \cdot J \cdot SC$ or $(\alpha_2\lambda_2)_2 \cdot J \cdot SC$	$\delta_2\kappa_2$ or $\delta_2\lambda_2$	$\epsilon_2\kappa_2$ or $\epsilon_2\lambda_2$
Valence	2	5	2, 4	2	2
Activation of the classical pathway of complement	+	+++	–	–	–
Ability to cross the placenta	+	–	–	–	–
Subclasses	4	2	2	–	–

Immunoglobulins may be separated into five classes based on their molecular weight, valence, and half-life. The functions of each class differ as to the ability to activate the classical pathway of complement and to cross the placenta.

the only immunoglobulin class that can cross the placenta in humans. This allows maternal IgG to protect the fetus. If the mother is re-exposed to a microorganism, pre-existing specific IgG and newly synthesized specific IgG will protect the mother and fetus from infection by the microorganism. Since IgG has a relatively long half-life of 23 days, maternal antibodies present in the newborn at birth will continue to provide protection until the antibody is completely catabolized. Thus, maternal antibody provides the newborn with some protection for the first few months of life.

Most IgG activates the classical pathway of complement. The C1q recognition unit attaches to a receptor in the hinge region, and the pathway is activated when the C1q molecule attaches to two adjacent IgG molecules (see Chap. 5).

Each IgG subclass has a unique structure. Variations in the structure, function, and concentration are listed in Table 8-3. IgG1 is found in greatest serum concentration, approximately 900 mg/dL or 65% to 70% of the total IgG. IgG2 is approximately 25% of the total IgG with a serum concentration of 300 mg/dL. IgG3 is 4% to 7% of the total IgG and has

Table 8-3: Properties of IgG Subclasses

Property	Subclass of IgG			
	IgG1	IgG2	IgG3	IgG4
Serum concentration (approximate in mg/dL)	900	300	100	50
Activation of the classical pathway of complement	++	+	+++	−
Placental transfer	+	±	−	+
Reactivity with staphylococcal protein A (binds with the Fc portion of the molecule)	+	+	−	+
Gm allotypes	4	2	12	yes
Molecular weight (approximate in daltons)	146,000	146,000	170,000	146,000
Number of disulfide bonds linking heavy chains	2	4	15	2

IgG subclasses have varying concentrations in the serum with IgG1 > IgG2 > IgG3 > IgG4. Abilities to cross the placenta activate the classical pathway of complement and react with staphylococcal protein A are different in each subclass.

a concentration of 100 mg/dL. IgG4 is only 3% to 4% of the total IgG, with a concentration of approximately 50 mg/dL. The molecular weight, number of interchain disulfide bonds, and electrophoretic mobility also show variability. IgG1, IgG2, and IgG4 have a molecular weight of approximately 146,000 d, but IgG3 has a molecular weight of 170,000 d. The IgG3 heavy chain is 60,000 d compared with 52,000 d for the other subclass heavy chains.

IgG1 and IgG4 have two disulfide bonds between the heavy chains; but IgG2 has four and IgG3 has 15 interchain disulfide bonds. In addition to the greatest number of interchain disulfide bonds, IgG3 has the greatest number of Gm allotypes,[12] compared with IgG1 (4 Gm allotypes) and IgG2 and IgG4 (two Gm allotypes each). Under standard electrophoresis conditions, IgG2 and IgG4 migrate toward the anode, whereas IgG1 and IgG3 migrate toward the cathode. IgG3 has the shortest half-life, lowest synthesis rate, and highest catabolic rate of all the IgG subclasses.[1,2,4,5]

Macrophages have surface receptors for IgG1 and IgG3 that can bind to a site on the CH_3 domain of IgG1 and IgG3. This binding may lead to specific "arming" of the macrophage: first specific antibody binds to the macrophage Fc receptor, next antigen combines with the antibody, and finally antigen is phagocytized by the macrophage.[2]

Other variations between subclasses are noted. IgG3 does not cross the placenta, whereas IgG2 crosses the placenta poorly, compared with the other subclasses. IgG3 activates the classical pathway of complement very well, whereas IgG4 apparently fails to activate this pathway. The ranked order of IgG subclasses based on their ability to activate complement is IgG3 > IgG1 > IgG2.[1]

When exposed to an antigen, the antibody subclass response appears to be in the same proportion as the serum concentration. However, sometimes some antigens stimulate the production of a selected IgG subclass. For example, spontaneously occurring antibodies to coagulation factors are only subclass IgG4, whereas certain polysaccharides stimulate IgG2 subclass production.[5] Anti-DNA antibodies are primarily of IgG2 and IgG3 subclasses.

In some disorders the ability to synthesize IgG

subclasses is altered.[9-11] In recurrent sinopulmonary infections, some children were deficient in IgG2, some were deficient in IgG3, and a small percentage were deficient in both subclasses. The lack of IgG2 and/or IgG3 is an immune deficiency that allows repeated infections by *Streptococcus pneumoniae* and *Hemophilus influenzae*. An increase in IgG4 has been found in atopic allergy. It is speculated that IgG4 is a blocking antibody that is produced in response to an allergen. IgG4 binds to the same surface receptors on mast cells as IgE, preventing degranulation (see Chap. 27). The bond is weaker than that of IgE, though.[12]

IgM

Immunoglobulin M (IgM) is a pentamer with a molecular weight of 900,000 d; each of the five basic units has a molecular weight of 180,000 d. The J chain and the interchain disulfide bonds hold the molecule together (Fig. 8-5). Because IgM is so large, it has a sedimentation constant of 19S. Although it would appear that IgM could have a va-

lence of 10 (combines with 10 antigen molecules), in some experimental cases the IgM molecule could only bind with five molecules, probably due to steric hindrance.

IgM is 10% of the total serum immunoglobulin concentration or approximately 125 mg/dL. IgM migrates between the γ and α_2 regions during serum protein electrophoresis. The heavy chain, mu (μ) chain, has 576 amino acids and is composed of four constant domains and one variable domain.[4] Minor variation in the μ heavy chain establishes the two IgM subclasses. A secretory form of IgM has been found in body fluids, and its transport through the epithelial lining is the same as that for secretory IgA.

In an immune response, IgM is the first antibody produced in response to an antigen. IgM is the most common immunoglobulin found on the surface of B cells, though surface IgM is a monomer. When the immunoglobulin is found on the surface of the B cell, it is the antigen receptor. During B-cell maturation the μ chain is the first to be detected in the cytoplasm. IgM is the most efficient immunoglobulin

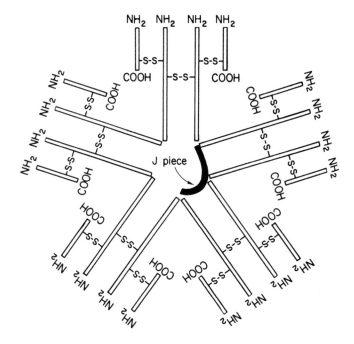

FIGURE 8-5. The IgM molecule is composed of five basic immunoglobulin units held together by the J piece at the carboxy terminus of the heavy chain.

class to activate the classical pathway of complement because only one molecule of IgM is required to activate this pathway.

IgA

Immunoglobulin A (IgA) exists as serum IgA and secretory IgA. The serum IgA molecule is a single basic immunoglobulin unit with a molecular weight of 160,000 d that migrates to the slow β or fast γ globulin regions. IgA differs from other immunoglobulin classes because of the α heavy chain. The α chain consists of 472 amino acids to include three constant domains. IgA has two subclasses. Subclass IgA1 has disulfide bonds linking the heavy and light chains, similar to those found in the basic immunoglobulin structure. No allotypes have been found in IgA1. IgA2, the second subclass of IgA, has no disulfide or other covalent bonds found between the heavy and light chains. Two allotypes (A2m1 and A2m2) are found in IgA2. The serum concentration of IgA is 15% to 20% of the total serum immunoglobulin concentration, with an approximate concentration of 250 mg/dL.

The second form of IgA, secretory IgA (sIgA), is found in the external body secretions. External body secretions include the colostrum and early milk, mucus (nasal, respiratory, bronchial, and intestinal), saliva, tears, prostatic fluid, and vaginal secretions.[2,8] sIgA has a molecular weight of 400,000 d, which reflects its composition: two basic immunoglobulin units with a J chain and the secretory component attached (Fig. 8-6). Secretory IgA and serum IgA are not in equilibrium with each other but are under separate control mechanisms.[2] Two supporting works provide evidence. Radiolabeled serum IgA does not appear as secretory IgA, and when IgA is administered to IgA-deficient patients, the serum IgA level increases but secretory IgA level does not.

The synthesis of secretory IgA molecules begins with the production of IgA monomers by plasma cells that are present in the mucosa. After the J chain is

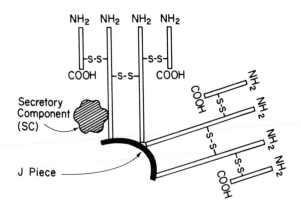

FIGURE 8-6. Secretory IgA is composed of two basic units held together by the J piece at the carboxy terminus of the heavy chain. In addition, there is a secretory component (SC) attached to the constant region of one heavy chain.

attached, the dimers are released from the plasma cell. The dimer is selectively transported across the mucosal epithelium by binding to the secretory component (SC) specific transport receptor found on the surface of the epithelial cell. The receptor–IgA dimer complex is endocytized, transported across the epithelial cell, and secreted into the mucosal secretions. SC is cleaved from the dimer before release into the secretions. Both sIgA and free SC are found in the mucosal secretions (Fig. 8-7).[8]

The function of serum IgA is unknown, though IgA may be important in antigen clearance and immune regulation. About 10% of the serum IgA is the dimeric form.[8] The functions of secretory IgA are numerous compared with serum IgA. Because of its unique association with the SC, the IgA dimer is resistant to proteolysis. sIgA does not activate the classical pathway of complement and appears to inhibit the complement-activating activity of IgG; however, IgA does activate the alternative pathway of complement. The inhibitory effect on IgG complement activation and the IgA activation of the alternative pathway may both provide protection and promote inflammation. Receptors for IgA have been found on inflammatory cells; IgA may help in the

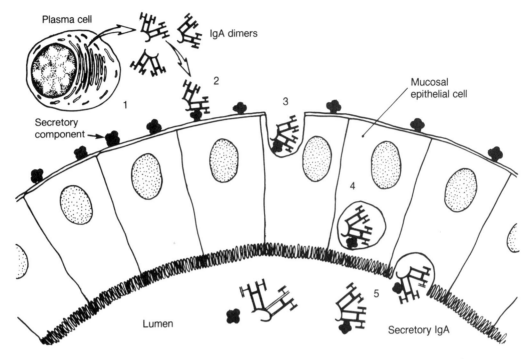

FIGURE 8-7. Step 1: The plasma cells secrete IgA dimers. Step 2: The IgA dimers bind to the secretory components (SC) located on the epithelial cell membrane. Step 3: The IgA–SC complex is endocytosed by the epithelial cell. Step 4: The endocytic vesicle moves through the epithelial cell to the cell membrane located on the lumen side. Step 5: The complexes are released into the lumen. The SC may be cleaved from the IgA dimer.

destruction of bacteria and other cellular pathogens by antibody-dependent cell-mediated cytotoxicity. sIgA can bind to some microorganisms, which may inhibit the ability of the microorganism to move or to bind to the mucosal wall, preventing colonization. Individuals who are IgA deficient have increased mucosal infections, atopy, and autoimmune diseases.[8]

IgD

IgD molecules have the same basic four-chain structure as the other immunoglobulin molecules. The heavy chain has a different sequence from the other classes and is the delta (δ) heavy chain. A single disulfide bond joins the δ heavy chains. Intact IgD has a molecular weight of 180,000 d, which suggests that the δ chain is composed of four constant domains. IgD migrates in the fast γ region in serum protein electrophoresis. The immunoglobulin can be degraded easily using proteolytic enzymes and heat. No subclasses or allotypes have been found.

The serum concentration of IgD is less than 1% of the total immunoglobulin or approximately 3 mg/dL. The relatively short half-life (2 to 3 days) and low synthesis rate (0.4 mg/kg/d) contribute to the low serum concentration.[4,8]

The exact function of IgD has not been determined; IgD has been reported to have antibody activity to insulin, penicillin, nuclear antigens, and thyroid antigen. IgD in association with IgM is found on the surface of B lymphocytes. One theory suggests that IgD is important in B-lymphocyte differentiation.[4,8]

IgE

Immunoglobulin E (IgE), first called reagin, is the immunoglobulin responsible for allergy. IgE has a molecular weight of approximately 190,000 d. The heavy chain, epsilon (ϵ), has four constant domains. The serum concentration of IgE is very low, about 0.004% of the total immunoglobulin. The effects of IgE are considerable and are discussed in Chapters 6 and 27. The Fc portion of IgE binds to receptors on mast cell. When an allergen binds to the hypervariable region of the IgE molecule, the mast cell releases mediators (i.e., histamine and leukotrienes), which are responsible for the symptoms observed in individuals with allergies.

Quantitation

Quantitation of serum immunoglobulin provides important information about humoral immunity. Some individuals may lack a class or subclass of immunoglobulin. For example, IgA deficiency is common and occurs with a frequency of 1 in 500 individuals. In some rare disorders, such as Bruton's agammaglobulinemia and severe combined immunodeficiency, no immunoglobulins are produced. In other diseases, such as multiple myeloma, an increase in a particular class and clone of immunoglobulin is present. Depending on which class is produced in excess, the β or γ globulin regions may be increased in protein electrophoresis. Another disorder in which immunoglobulins may be increased is acquired immunodeficiency syndrome (AIDS).

IgG and its subclasses, IgM, IgA, and IgD, may be quantitated using radial immunodiffusion or nephelometry. IgE quantitation requires more sensitive methods because the serum levels are very low. Total

serum IgE may be measured by radioimmunoassay or by enzyme immunoassay procedures.

References

1. Roitt IM, Brostoff J, Male DK: Immunology, p 5.1. London, Gower Medical Publishing, 1985
2. Goodman JW: Immunoglobulins I: Structure and function. In Stites DP, Stobo JD, Wells JV (eds): Basic and Clinical Immunology, 6th ed, p 27. Norwalk, Appleton and Lange, 1987
3. Roitt I: Essential immunology, 6th ed, p 31. Oxford, Blackwell Scientific Publications, 1988
4. Barrett JT: Textbook of immunology, 5th ed, p 103. St Louis, CV Mosby, 1988
5. Bloch KJ: Antibodies and their functions. In Benacerraf B, Unanue ER (eds): Textbook of Immunology, 2nd ed, p 31. Baltimore, Williams and Wilkins, 1984
6. Ricardo MJ, Tomar RH: Immunoglobulins and paraproteins. In Henry JB (ed): Clinical Diagnosis and Management by Laboratory Methods, 17th ed, p 860. Philadelphia, WB Saunders, 1984
7. Kennedy RC: Anti-idiotype antibodies: Prospects in clinical and laboratory medicine. Lab Manag 23:19, 1985
8. Ernst PB, Underdown BJ, Bienenstock J: Immunity in mucosal tissue. In Stites DP, Stobo JD, Wells JV (eds): Basic and Clinical Immunology, 6th ed, p 159. Norwalk, Appleton and Lange, 1987
9. Umetsu DT, Ambrosino DM, Quinti I, et al: Recurrent sinopulmonary infection and impaired antibody response to bacterial capsule polysaccharide antigen in children with selective IgG-subclass deficiency. N Engl J Med 313:1247, 1985
10. Lane P, MacLennan I: Impaired lung function in patients with IgA deficiency and low levels of IG2 or IgG3. N Engl J Med 314:924, 1986
11. Matter L, Wilhelm JA, Anghern W, et al: Selective antibody deficiency and recurrent pneumococcal bacteremia in a patient with Sjögren's syndrome, hyperimmunoglobulinemia G and deficiencies of IgG2 and IgG4. N Engl J Med 312:1039, 1985
12. Aalberse RC, van der Zee J, Vlug A: IgG4 antibodies in atopic allergy. Lab Manag 23:19, 1985

9

Nature of Antigens

Dorothy J. Fike

Antigens and Immunogens

Classically, an antigen was defined as any substance that induced an antibody response. Though the term *antigen* is still used, the more correct term is *immunogen*. An immunogen is a substance that causes a detectable immune response, whether the response be humoral (antibody), cellular, or both. Immunogenicity is the property of these substances to induce the immune response. Sometimes the immunogen elicits an allergic response and is known as an allergen. The term *antigen* now refers to the ability of a substance to combine with an antibody; therefore, when an immunogen combines with an antibody molecule, it is an antigen–antibody reaction rather than an immunogen–antibody reaction.[1,2]

Generally, an immunogen is a substance of high molecular weight, greater than 10,000 daltons, of which a small portion can combine with antibody. This portion of the immunogen molecule is the antigenic determinant, or epitope. It is thought that an immunogen must have at least two determinants per molecule to stimulate an antibody response. An epitope is approximately four to six amino acids or five to seven monosaccharides in length.[2]

For example, myoglobin, a muscle protein, has five different antigenic determinants on the molecule. Each antigenic determinant has a different amino acid sequence and is located in a different portion of the molecule. Different proteins will have the antigenic determinants located in other portions of the molecule (Fig. 9-1). Myoglobin antigenic determinants are adjacent amino acids, as shown in Fig. 9-2A. For other immunogens, the antigenic determinant is composed of amino acids or monosaccharides that are not in sequence but are in close proximity to each other because of the folding of the molecule (Fig. 9-2B).[3]

There are two major classes of immunogens: thymic-dependent immunogens and thymic-independent immunogens. The thymic-dependent antigens require the help of the T cells for the formation of antibody. Most immunogens are thymic dependent.

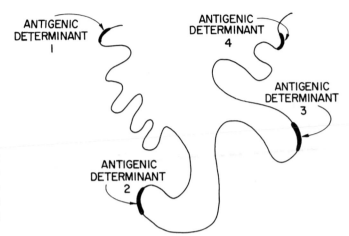

FIGURE 9-1. Antigenic determinants are most likely to be located at either the amino or carboxyl terminals of the molecule (antigenic determinants 1 and 4). Other antigenic determinants are located on exterior portions of the molecule (antigenic determinants 2 and 3).

Thymic-independent antigens stimulate antibody production without interacting with T cells. Structurally, thymic-independent antigens are composed of repeating units. Some bacterial polysaccharides are thymic-independent antigens. The response to thymic-independent antigens is of the IgM class, with little or no immunologic memory generated. Recently, some investigators found that some T-cell interaction was required for the production of antibody to T-cell independent antigens, suggesting that *thymus efficient*, rather than *thymus independent*, is a more appropriate term.[2]

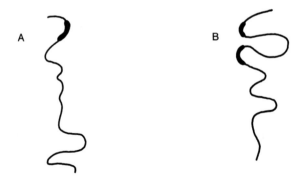

FIGURE 9-2. The antigenic determinant sequence may have the amino acids or sugars located next to each other in a linear sequence (A) or located next to each other because of folding of the molecule (B).

Factors Affecting Immunogenicity

Exactly what makes a substance immunogenic is unknown, but several characteristics of a molecule contribute to its immunogenicity. These characteristics are foreignness, molecular size, chemical composition and complexity, genetic composition of the host, and route and timing of administration of the immunogen (Table 9-1). All of these factors must be considered together when determining if there will be a response. One factor alone is not responsible for a response.[2]

An immunogen must somehow be recognized as "foreign" or "nonself." This important requirement encourages an immune response to a potentially harmful substance, rather than to substances of the individual. If a particular protein, such as C3, is removed from an individual and then injected into the same individual, there will be no response. If that same human C3 protein is injected into a rabbit, horse, or cow, there will be a response to the human C3 protein. The extent of the response depends on the degree of "foreignness" of the protein. Generally, the greater the phylogenic difference, the greater the immune response. The exact mechanism

Table 9-1: Factors Involved in Immunogenicity

Factor	Description
Foreignness	"Self" versus "nonself"; more unlike "self," more likely to have a response
Size	>10,000 d, best >100,000 d
Chemical composition and complexity	Proteins are best, complex carbohydrates are next, lipids and nucleic acids have a weak or no response
Genetic composition	HLA antigens are important to provide a "receptor" for the response to occur
Route, dose, and timing of administration	Variable; depends on the specific immunogen as to what the best response would be

There are several factors that cause a substance to be immunogenic. In some cases the more factors that contribute to immunogenicity, the better the response.

by which a host recognizes self immunogens versus nonself immunogens is not known.[2]

The molecular size of an immunogen necessary to provoke a response is unknown. Generally, molecules with a molecular weight of less than 10,000 d are poor immunogens, whereas complex substances with a molecular weight of more than 100,000 d are usually very immunogenic. Sometimes a substance with a molecular weight of less than 10,000 d may initiate an immune response by itself. Other low-molecular-weight substances require that a carrier protein be attached to induce a response. These substances are haptens; the mechanism of hapten induction of the immune response will be discussed later in this chapter.[1-3]

Chemical composition and complexity contribute to immunogenicity. Proteins and carbohydrates provide the best response. Lipids and nucleic acids are weak immunogens, though under certain circumstances, a response occurs. For example, in systemic lupus erythematosus, antibodies are found against nucleic acids and nuclear proteins.[1-3]

The immunogen molecule itself must be diverse, rather than being composed of a single amino acid or monosaccharide. In fact, the more complex the molecule is, the better the immunogen. Aromatic amino acids, such as tyrosine, provide more immunogenicity than nonaromatic amino acids.[2] The internal complexity also contributes to immunogenicity (Table 9-2). The primary, secondary, and tertiary structures of proteins define the internal complexity. Oligosaccharides, though sufficiently large, do not have internal complexity and are poor immunogens. Polysaccharides with extensive branching show

Table 9-2: Factors Involved in Internal Complexity

Factor	Comment
Primary structure	Oligosaccharides are poor immunogens, whereas polysaccharides, with their extensive branching, are good immunogens
Secondary structure	
Tertiary structure	
Hydrophilicity	Those portions of the antigens that contain hydrophilic portions are the antigenic determinants

The primary, secondary, and tertiary structure, as well as hydrophilicity, contribute to the internal complexity of an antigen.

more internal complexity and are good immunogens. Hydrophilicity, another factor in chemical composition and complexity, influences immunogenicity. Hydrophilic molecules are more immunogenic, and hydrophilic portions of immunogens are the antigenic determinants.[1]

Genetic composition of the individual contributes to the ability to respond to an immunogen. A particular polysaccharide will be immunogenic when injected in humans but will cause no immune response when it is injected into a guinea pig. To understand the genetic influence on responsiveness, intense research in the area of the major histocompatibility complex (MHC) antigens is ongoing. In humans if a particular MHC antigen is not present for an immunogen, there will be no response. It has been found that in 85% of the individuals expressing the HLA-A9 antigen, there was a high response to tetanus toxoid. In individuals with an HLA-B5 antigen, 71% had a low response to the tetanus toxoid.[4] The HLA-Dw2 and HLA-Dw3 have a general association with the atopic response. Specific allergy to cat dander is found more frequently in individuals who have the HLA-B7 or HLA-B8 antigen. Individuals with ragweed allergies have a higher frequency of the HLA-A2 and HLA-A28 antigen.[5] This ability to respond is inherited as an autosomal dominant trait.[2]

The last factor of immunogenicity is the route, dosage, and timing of immunogen administration. As with the other factors, the exact mechanisms by which route, dosage, and timing of immunogen exposure contribute to immune responsiveness are unclear. Generally, soluble immunogens injected intramuscularly or intravenously exhibit a better response than those same immunogens taken orally.[2] A notable exception is the polio vaccine, where a better response is found when the vaccine is administered orally, compared with the same dose administered intramuscularly.[6] Resistance to polio virus requires both intestinal and humoral immunity. Without intestinal immunity, some individuals may have a reservoir of the virus in the intestine and act as carriers.

The dose response may be partially dependent on the nature of immunogen processing: T-cell dependent or T-cell independent. Generally, a small dose of immunogen will produce little or no response. (Consult the section on immune tolerance in this chapter for a fuller discussion of dose response.)

Haptens

Haptens are low-molecular-weight substances (less than 10,000 d) that are not immunogenic but that can combine with an antibody. When a hapten combines with a carrier molecule, the complex is immunogenic. In the early 1900s Karl Landsteiner used haptens to study the specifity and cross-reactivity of antibodies and antigens. The carrier molecule, a protein, was immunogenic, whereas the hapten was not immunogenic when injected into a mouse. The hapten was covalently linked to the carrier molecule and the carrier-hapten complex was injected. Three antibodies were produced: one that combines with the hapten, one that combines with the carrier, and a

Table 9-3: Humoral Response With Hapten Injection

Injection	Humoral Response
Hapten alone	No antibodies produced
Carrier alone	Antibody to carrier produced
Hapten–carrier complex	Antibody to hapten produced Antibody to carrier produced Antibody to hapten–carrier junction produced
Free hapten and free carrier	Antibody to carrier produced

When haptens are injected into an animal, hapten antibody is only formed when the hapten is complexed to the carrier protein.

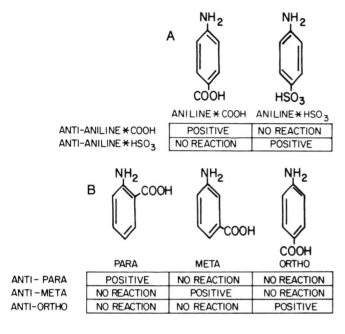

ANTI-ANILINE＊COOH	ANILINE＊COOH	ANILINE＊HSO₃
ANTI-ANILINE＊COOH	POSITIVE	NO REACTION
ANTI-ANILINE＊HSO₃	NO REACTION	POSITIVE

	PARA	META	ORTHO
ANTI-PARA	POSITIVE	NO REACTION	NO REACTION
ANTI-META	NO REACTION	POSITIVE	NO REACTION
ANTI-ORTHO	NO REACTION	NO REACTION	POSITIVE

FIGURE 9-3. Hapten antibody reactions are very specific. In (A) anti-aniline＊COOH reacts only with aniline＊COOH and not with aniline＊HSO₃, whereas anti-aniline＊HSO₃ reacts only with aniline＊HSO₃ and not with aniline＊COOH. In (B) aniline is substituted with -COOH in various positions; the antibody reacts only with the molecule that has the -COOH in the appropriate position (i.e., anti-*para*-aminobenzene carboxylate only reacts when the -COOH is in the *para* position).

third that combines with the hapten–carrier junction (Table 9-3). Each antibody is specific for the hapten, the carrier protein, or the hapten–carrier junction.[2]

In another experiment by Landsteiner, haptens similar in structure to the original hapten reacted with the original hapten antibody. (Fig. 9-3) In one experiment, aniline was monosubstituted in the ortho position with a carboxylic or sulfonic group. When specific antibody was produced against each immunogen, only the homologous antibody reacted. That is, aniline＊COOH reacted only with anti–aniline＊COOH and not with anti–aniline＊HSO₃, whereas aniline＊HSO₃ reacted only with anti–aniline＊HSO₃ and not with anti–aniline＊COOH. In a third experiment the aniline molecule was conjugated with a carboxylic group in the ortho, meta, and para positions. As in the previous experiment, the specific homologous antibody reacted with its specific immunogen. From these experiments, it was concluded that antibody reactivity is very specific and recognizes the three-dimensional structure of the antigen or hapten.[2]

Adjuvants

Adjuvants are agents that potentiate an immune response; they are not immunogens and cannot evoke a response alone. The most frequently observed response is an increase in the amount of specific immunoglobulin produced, although the activation of macrophages and cell-mediated immunity have also been observed.[1]

There are several types of adjuvants that act by slowing the release or escape of the immunogen from a particular region (Table 9-4). One type of adjuvant is the repository adjuvant, which includes aluminum and calcium salts. These salts combine with the immunogen to form an insoluble complex that slows the release of the immunogen from the subcutaneous or intramuscular site of injection. Because the repository adjuvant increases the size of the immunogen, phagocytosis is enhanced. Another type of adjuvant is the water-in-oil emulsifying agent. This type of adjuvant has had restricted use in humans. The emulsified adjuvants allow a slow release of immu-

Table 9-4: Adjuvants

  I. Insoluble complex, salts (aluminum and calcium)

     Aluminum hydroxide

     Aluminum potassium tartrate (alum)

     Calcium phosphate

  II. Slow release of antigen, oil in water

     Freund's incomplete, mineral oil

     Freund's complete, mineral oil with mycobacteria

 III. Increase in IgM production

     Lipopolysaccharide (LPS)

     Endotoxins

     Bordetella pertussis

 IV. Mobilizing T and B cells

     Bordetella pertussis

  V. Lysosomal release

     Vitamin A

     Beryllium salts

     Toxic forms of silica

     Quaternary forms of ammonium salts

Adjuvant action may be due to the formation of an insoluble complex, the slow release of antigen, an increase in IgM production, a mobilization of T and B cells, or lysosomal release. The agents that cause each of these actions are listed.

nogen from the oil droplets. Because there is a variety in droplet size, the droplets are degraded at different rates, resulting in the prolonged presence of immunogens. The oil droplets also aid in phagocytosis. Immunogens in oil droplets are more easily phagocytized than soluble immunogens.

Freund's adjuvant is the classic example of a water-in-oil adjuvant. Incomplete Freund's adjuvant is light mineral oil and an emulsifying agent. Freund's complete adjuvant contains light mineral oil, an emulsifying agent, and 0.5 mg/mL of killed mycobacteria. The mycobacteria induce granuloma formation at the site of injection. The granuloma further slows the release of the immunogen, because it is a physical barrier. Freund's complete adjuvant is not recommended for human use because the granuloma may be disfiguring.[7]

Lipopolysaccharides or endotoxins from gram-negative bacteria may also be used as adjuvants. These agents enhance the IgM response, though the exact mechanism for this increase of IgM is unknown. This adjuvant is not recommended for human use, because it induces a high fever.[7]

Bordetella pertussis is another adjuvant that increases the amount of IgM produced. In addition, *Bordetella* has a lymphocytosis-promoting factor that mobilizes T and B cells to the site of injection, thereby enhancing the immune reaction.[7]

Lysosomal enzyme release is another mechanism by which adjuvants may act. Vitamin A, beryllium salts, toxic forms of silica, and quaternary ammonium salts activate macrophages. These macrophages are stimulated to release lysosomal enzymes, which enhance the immune response.[7]

The ultimate effect of an adjuvant is to blend the primary and secondary (booster) responses together. Theoretically, this activity may be accomplished by (1) increasing the number of cells involved in the immune response, (2) providing more efficient processing of the immunogen, (3) prolonging the presence of immunogen, or (4) increasing the rate of synthesis and release of antibody.[7]

Immune Tolerance

Immune tolerance is the state of unresponsiveness to an immunogen in a host that normally responds. This response is restricted to a single antigen. Immune paralysis and immune nonresponsiveness are synonyms for immune tolerance.[7]

Several mechanisms may induce the state of tolerance (Table 9-5). One of the first mechanisms to be recognized was chimerism. Chimeras are fraternal

Table 9-5: Mechanisms of Immune Tolerance

Chimerism	T-cell tolerance
Fetal exposure (nonchimerism)	Clonal abortion
	Functional deletion
B-cell tolerance	T-cell suppression
Clonal abortion	
Clonal exhaustion	
Functional deletion	
Antibody-forming cell blockade	

Immune tolerance may be the results of chimerism, nonchimeric fetal exposure, B-cell tolerance, or T-cell tolerance. There are several factors that may cause either B-cell or T-cell tolerance.

twins that exchange tissue during fetal life; each twin can recognize the other twin's tissue antigens as "self." Consequently, no response is made to the foreign tissue.[8]

In addition to chimeras, exposure to the immunogen during fetal life will result in a state of unresponsiveness. Some immunogens that induce a state of tolerance are erythrocytes, bacteria, bovine serum albumin, and tissue cells.[8]

There may be both T- and B-cell tolerance. B-cell tolerance may be induced by clonal abortion, clonal exhaustion, functional deletion, and antibody-forming cell blockade (Fig. 9-4). Clonal abortion occurs when an immature B cell is exposed to a low concentration of antigen and the maturation of that B cell is arrested so that it may not respond to that antigen on subsequent exposure. Clonal exhaustion occurs when the B cell is repeatedly exposed to T-independent antigens. All mature B cells expressing the receptor for this antigen are already antibody-producing cells, so that no additional antigen binding and antibody production can occur.[8]

Functional deletion occurs when helper T cells are not present to help T-dependent antigens. Thus, B cells cannot mature into antibody-producing cells. Functional deletion occurs with T-independent antigens when the dose of the antigen is very high. There will be too few B cells that can respond to the large dose of antigen present. Antibody-forming cell blockade occurs when excess antigen binds to all the receptors and immunoglobulin secretion is inhibited. This last mechanism has a low ability to induce tolerance.[8]

T-cell tolerance may be induced by clonal abortion, functional deletion, and T-cell suppression (Fig. 9-5). Immature T cells may be clonally aborted, like immature B cells. When the immature T cell is exposed to low antigen concentration, its maturation is arrested, so that the T cell may not respond to that antigen on subsequent exposure. Functional deletion may occur when one T-cell subset becomes tolerant to an antigenic determinant and fails to stimulate a functional B cell to produce antibody. Cellular immunity may also be affected if the clone produces only a cellular immune response. T-cell suppression occurs when suppressor T cells actively suppress other T-cell subsets or B cells.[8]

B- and T-cell tolerance differ as to the time course, duration of tolerance, and dose of antigen required to tolerize the cells. T-dependent antigens may tolerize T cells found in the spleen and thymus within hours of challenge but require up to 4 days to tolerize adult splenic B cells. Bone marrow T cells may require up to 15 days to become tolerized to T-dependent antigens. T-independent antigens tolerize B cells more quickly than the 4 days required to tolerize the adult splenic B cells to T-dependent antigens.[8] Antigen persistence is a factor in tolerance. Immunogens that are continuously present maintain a state of tolerance. This may be due to constant exposure to the immunogen or a very slow catabolic rate. The tolerance has been found to be to a specific antigenic determinant, so that other antigens that have the same antigenic determinant will also be tolerized.[8]

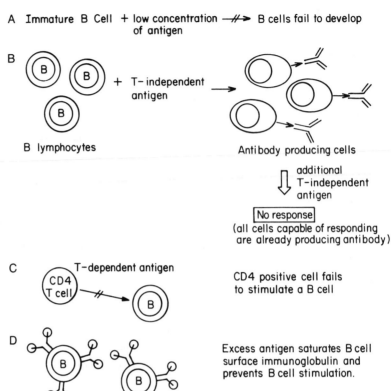

FIGURE 9-4. B-cell tolerance may be due to several mechanisms. (A) If an immature B cell is exposed to a low concentration of antigen, the B cells fail to develop. (B) If all the B cells have formed antibody-producing cells when the T-cell-independent (TI) antigen is again introduced into the animal, there will be no response, since all the cells are already producing antibody. (C) If a T-cell dependent (TD) antigen does not cause the CD4-positive cell to stimulate the B cell, the B cell will not become an antibody-producing cell. (D) Excess antigen prevents B-cell activation and antibody secretion.

The dose required to induce tolerance depends on the type of cells involved. B-cell tolerance requires a 100- to 1000-fold higher level of antigen than that required for T-cell tolerance. In some cases, low levels of immunogen will induce T suppressor cells to act and produce a state of tolerance. This type of tolerance is not completely effective.[8]

The duration of the state of tolerance depends on the mechanism by which tolerance was induced. Chimeras or fetal exposure may last throughout the entire life of the individual. When tolerance is due to clonal deletion, the tolerance remains until mature lymphocytes are regenerated from the stem cell.[8]

Self-tolerance is the ability of the body not to respond to autologous antigens. It appears that some B cells that recognize autologous antigens are pres-

ent normally in the individual but are inactive because of the lack of antigen recognition by T helper cells (functional deletion).[8]

Immunosuppression

Immunosuppression is the reduction of T- and B-lymphocyte and macrophage activity. This includes reduced phagocytic capacity by macrophages and reduced production of antibodies and lymphokines by lymphocytes. Use of immunosuppressive agents is usually not beneficial to normal individuals, but to those individuals who have autoimmune disorders, severe allergies unresponsive to other therapeutic

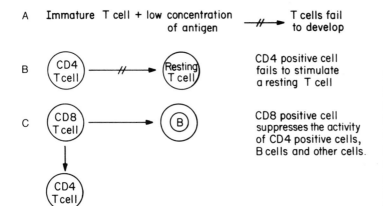

A   Immature T cell + low concentration of antigen →//→ T cells fail to develop

FIGURE 9-5. As with B-cell tolerance, T-cell tolerance may be due to several mechanisms. (A) If an immature T cell is exposed to a low concentration of antigen, it fails to develop into a mature T cell. (B) In some cases the CD4 (helper/inducer) cells are not activated and remain as resting T cells. Clonal expansion is prevented. (C) The CD8 (suppressor) cell inhibits the activity of the CD4-positive cells and B cells.

agents, or graft recipients, immunosuppressive therapy may be beneficial. Immunosuppression may be accomplished by many agents, which may be broadly categorized as physical, chemical, and biologic agents.

Physical agents include radiation and surgery. Radiation is an effective immunosuppressive agent if given within 4 days prior to antigen exposure. Radiation is less effective when given at the same time as the antigen and has little or no effect if the dose is given 4 days after antigen exposure. B cells are more sensitive to radiation than T cells. The reduction in the amount of antibody synthesized is temporary. The temporary reduction in antibody synthesis occurs because some cells are shielded from the radiation dose. Surgical removal of lymphoid organs such as lymph nodes, bone marrow, tonsils, appendix, spleen, Peyer's patches, and thymus will remove a concentrated area of lymphoid tissue. It is impossible to remove all lymphoid tissue, as well as all macrophages, since these cells are located in many areas. Thus, there is a reduction, not obliteration, of the immune response. If the thymus is removed shortly after birth, the immune response is reduced significantly. If the thymus is removed at a later time, there may only be a slight reduction in the immune response.[7]

Chemical agents include corticosteroids, purine and pyrimidine analogs, folic acid antagonists, alkyl-

ating agents, antibiotics, and cyclosporin A. Corticosteroids have two major effects on the lymphocytes: lymphocytolysis (both T and B cells) and inhibition of DNA, RNA, and protein synthesis by the lymphocyte. This last effect inhibits the production of antibodies and lymphokines. The corticosteroids also affect neutrophils and macrophages. Lysosomes are stabilized by the steroids so that the hydrolytic enzymes are not released and antigen processing is impaired. Oxidative metabolism is depressed, and phagocytic killing of bacteria by neutrophils is impaired. Monocyte, and sometimes neutrophil, chemotaxis is reduced by the steroids.[7]

Purine and pyrimidine analogs, including azathioprine and 6-mercaptopurine, inhibit the normal metabolism of the cell by using the analogs instead of the normal purine and pyrimidines. When these chemical agents are utilized instead of the natural purines and pyrimidines, a nonsense message results, and no protein is synthesized. These agents may also inhibit purine production from low-molecular-weight precursors. Folic acid antagonists, including methotrexate, inhibit DNA and protein synthesis. Cell division does not occur, and the primary response to an antigen is reduced. Alkylating agents, including cyclophosphamide, have an affinity for amino acids, sulfhydral groups, and other negatively charged molecules. DNA is affected by alkylating agents by breaking the strand. This results in impaired protein synthesis and cell division, and consequently, the primary and IgG responses to an antigen are impaired.[7]

Antibiotics and other miscellaneous agents have different effects on the immune system. Cyclosporin A, a fungal product, inhibits the effect of interleukin-2 on lymphocytes. Two enzymes, ribonuclease and asparaginase, have a suppressive effect on the immune system, though the exact mechanism is unknown.[7]

Biologic immunosuppression may be obtained using immunologic tolerance and antilymphocyte globulin (ALG) or antithymocyte globulin (ATG). Tolerance is used in experimental situations and has been previously discussed in this chapter. ALG is administered prior to, with, or after exposure to the antigen. There is generally a decrease in the number of circulating lymphocytes, with a cell loss in the lymph nodes and the white pulp of the spleen. The cell count returns to normal within 2 weeks of the last injection. With ATG there is a reduction in thymocytes, as shown by the decreased size of the thymus. The mode of action by ALG or ATG is the preferential elimination of the lymphocytes from the blood and other lymphoid centers. Both cellular immunity and immunoglobulin production are reduced.[7]

References

1. Barrett JT: Textbook of Immunology, 5th ed, p 29. St. Louis, CV Mosby, 1988

2. Goodman JW: Immunogenicity and antigenic specificity. In Stites DP, Stobo JD, Wells JV (eds): Basic and clinical immunology, 6th ed, p 20. Norwalk, Appleton and Lange, 1987

3. Hammarstrom S, Perlman P: Antigens. In Hanson LA, Widgzell H (eds): Immunology. Boston, Butterworth & Co, 1985

4. Sasazuki T, Kohno Y, Iwamoto I, et al: Association between an HLA haplotype and locus responsive to tetanus toxoid in man. Nature 272:359, 1978

5. Marsh DG, Meyers DA, Bias WB: Epidemiology and genetics of atopic allergy. N Engl J Med 305:1551, 1981

6. Benacerraf B, Unanue E: Textbook of Immunology, 2nd ed, p 12. Baltimore, Williams and Wilkins, 1984

7. Barrett JT: Textbook of Immunology, 5th ed, p 146. St. Louis, CV Mosby, 1988

8. Roitt I, Brostoff J, Male D: Immunology, p 12.1. London, Gower Medical Publishing, 1985

10

Antigen–Antibody Binding

Catherine Sheehan

When an antibody combines with its homologous antigen, an antigen–antibody complex or immune complex is produced. The reaction is reversible and depends on the chemical nature of each reactant. The specificity of the antibody is defined by the homologous antigen that stimulated the antibody production. When the three-dimensional structure and charge of the antibody are highly complementary for the antigen, the likelihood of binding is greater. This chapter will discuss the forces that bind an antigen to an antibody.

The Basis of Specificity

Since all antibody molecules are proteins, they are composed of amino acids. The protein structure dictates the idiotypic, allotypic, and isotypic variation of antibody molecules. There are four levels of protein structure:

1. *Primary:* Amino acids are joined by peptide bonds (Fig. 10-1).

2. *Secondary:* The conformation of the amino acid chain resulting from interchain hydrogen bonding (Fig. 10-2).

3. *Tertiary:* The folding of polypeptide chains through hydrophobic and hydrogen bonds.

4. *Quaternary:* The association of polypeptide subunits to form one protein (Fig. 10-3).[1]

The primary structure of antibody molecules, as defined by the genetic code, specifies the sequence of amino acids in a peptide chain. When amino acid sequences of different monoclonal immunoglobulins were studied, some portions of the amino acid sequence were remarkably constant, whereas other portions were variable. The similarity of amino acid sequence from one antibody molecule to another is homology. The constant domains of the heavy and light chains show little variability (or more homology). The constant domains of the heavy chain define the immunoglobulin class. Conversely, the variable

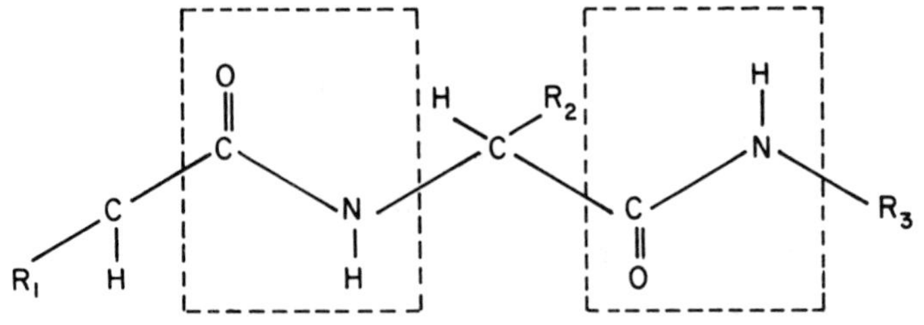

FIGURE 10-1. Primary structure of protein. The carboxy group of one amino acid joins the amino group of a second amino acid to create a peptide bond (indicated by ----). R = side chains of the amino acids.

domains of the heavy and light chains show more variability and less homology. Within variable domains, some amino acid positions are more frequently substituted than other amino acid positions; this is the hypervariable region. The hypervariable regions are believed to constitute the site of direct interaction with antigen.

The secondary structure of antibody molecules is the spatial arrangement of amino acids that results from the peptide bonds. This carbon-to-nitrogen linkage can result in an α-helix or β-pleated sheet formation. Immunoglobulins have the latter secondary structure almost exclusively.[2] The polypeptide chain can fold back on itself, creating parallel linear areas; the close proximity of these areas allows hydrogen bonding to stabilize the β-pleated structure.[3] The hinge region, a sequence rich in the amino acids proline and cysteine, does not display the same structure. The hinge region is thought to define the antibody subclass and to affect the flexibility of the

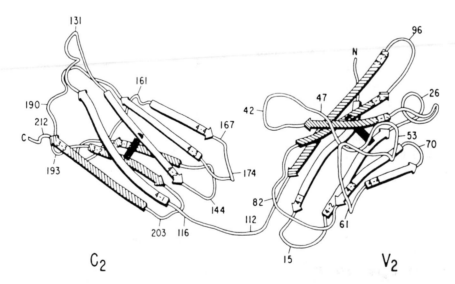

C_2 V_2

FIGURE 10-2. This schematic drawing of the constant (C) and variable (V) domains of a light chain illustrates the β-pleated structure. The striated arrows show a three-chain layer of β-pleated sheets; the white arrows show a four-chain layer. The intra-domain disulfide bonds are shown with a black bar. (From Edmunson AB, Ely KR, Abola EE, Schiffer M, Panagiotopoulos N. Rotational allomersim and divergent evolution of domains in immunoglobulin light chains. Biochemistry 14:3954, 1975. Copyright 1975 American Chemical Society.)

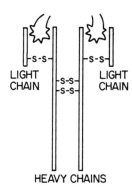

FIGURE 10-3. Quaternary structure of an immunoglobulin. The association of two heavy chains and two light chains forms a complete, biologically active molecule. Interchain disulfide bonds are shown by s-s.

molecule, its ability to bind complement, and its susceptibility to proteolytic enzymes.

The tertiary structure of immunoglobulin molecules results in its globular configuration. In the globular structure, hydrophilic areas are attracted to each other; likewise, hydrophobic areas complement each other. The hydrophilic areas generally are on the external surface of the molecule, and the hydrophobic areas are internal. The external hydrophilic areas promote immunoglobulin solubility in aqueous solutions. An exception to this internal–external arrangement is in the variable domain, where the hydrophilic area is more internal and interacts with the antigen. An intradomain disulfide bond in the middle stabilizes the peptide chain of the domain. The tertiary structure of the constant domains is responsible for the biologic functions specific for each immunoglobulin class.

The quaternary structure is the association of polypeptides, two heavy chains and two light chains for each basic immunoglobulin unit. Although each peptide chain contributes to primary, secondary, and tertiary structure, the quaternary structure is required for biologic activity. The spatial arrangement of the variable domains of the heavy and light chain defines the antigen-combining site of the antibody.

The antigen-combining capability of immunoglob-

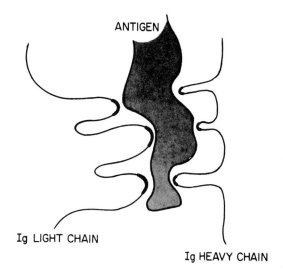

FIGURE 10-4. The hypervariable regions within the variable domains of the immunoglobulin (Ig) heavy chain and light chain form the antigen combining site. The darkened sections of the chains represent the hypervariable regions that interact with the antigen, which is the shaded area.

ulin molecules depends on all structural levels. The tertiary folding of heavy and light chains positions the hypervariable regions of each chain close together. As seen in Fig. 10-4, the quaternary structure brings the hypervariable region of one heavy chain in close proximity to the hypervariable region of one light chain.[4] Since the antigen interacts with the hypervariable regions, this is the antigen-combining site. Each immunoglobulin basic unit or monomer has two antigen-combining sites or a valence of 2. IgG, IgD, and IgE exist as monomers. Circulating IgM is a pentamer, with a valence of 10, whereas IgA most commonly is a monomer or dimer, with a valence of 2 or 4, respectively.

Forces Binding Antigen to Antibody

The union of an antibody with an epitope is reversible. The goodness of fit and the complementary nature of the two reactants determine the strength of this union. The forces include electrostatic force, hydrogen bonding, hydrophobic force, and Van der Waals force, as shown in Fig. 10-5.[5,6]

Electrostatic force is the attraction of a positively charged portion of a molecule (*e.g.*, the antibody) for a negatively charged portion of another molecule (*e.g.*, the antigen); the ionized state of the reactants influences the ability of each to combine. The pH and ionic strength of the environment greatly affect the ionic state of each molecule, the complementary nature of the charges, and the strength of attraction. The electrostatic force is inversely proportional to the square of the distance between the charges; therefore, the closer the two charged areas come, the greater the electrostatic force.

Hydrogen bonding is the attraction of two negatively charged atoms for hydrogen. This bond is weak, though common and numerous in antigen–antibody reactions. Since hydrogen bonding is an exothermic reaction, maximum binding occurs at lower temperatures, usually less than 37°C.[6] In laboratory procedures, hydrogen bonds are dissociated in the presence of 8 M urea or 6 M guanine, allowing polypeptide chains to be studied.

Hydrophobic force is related to the attraction between nonpolar groups. In an aqueous environment hydrophobic groups tend to associate and to reduce the total surface area exposed to water. The resulting lowered energy state provides the force of attraction. When an immune complex is sufficiently large, the complex excludes water, becomes insoluble, and precipitates.

Van der Waals force is a weak attractive force between the electron cloud of one atom and the nucleus of another atom. The force of attraction is inversely proportional to the seventh power of this distance: The closer the antigen comes to the antigen binding site, the stronger the force will be.

Antibody Affinity

Consistent with other chemical reactions, the law of mass action describes the relationship between an antibody molecule and a single binding site such as a hapten.[7,8] This reaction is reversible. In an aqueous solution, association of the hapten and antibody is related to the rate of diffusion of the two reactants

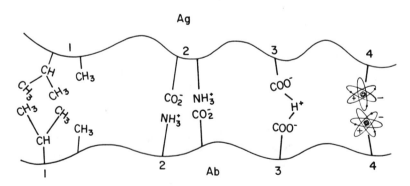

FIGURE 10-5. Forces of antigen–antibody binding. Site 1 shows the hydrophobic force, the complementary binding of a hydrophobic area of the antigen (Ag) with a hydrophobic area of the antibody (Ab). Site 2 shows the electrostatic force, the attraction of two charged areas. Site 3 shows hydrogen bonding in which two negatively charged groups attract hydrogen. Site 4 represents Van der Waals force, the weak attractive force between the electron cloud (−) of one atom and the nucleus (+) of another atom.

and to the probability that a collision will result in binding. For binding to occur during a collision, each reactant must have sufficient energy and a favorable orientation. Dissociation is related to the strength of the hapten–antibody bond; when this bond is strong, dissociation is low.

$$\text{Free Ab + free hapten} \underset{k_2}{\overset{k_1}{\rightleftharpoons}} \text{Ab–hapten complex}$$

At equilibrium, the rates of association and dissociation are constant, so that the amount of complex that forms equals the amount of complex that dissociates; therefore, the net change in the concentration of complex is zero. The ratio of these two rate constants is the affinity constant K_A and is specific for each antibody–hapten pair.

$$K_A = \frac{\text{Rate of association}}{\text{Rate of dissociation}} = \frac{k_1}{k_2}$$

In terms of concentration of reactants, the ratio of the concentration of the complex compared with the product of the concentrations of free antibody and free hapten is called the affinity constant.

$$K_A = \frac{[\text{Ab-hapten complex}]}{[\text{Free Ab}] [\text{Free hapten}]}$$

The more tightly an antibody and hapten bind, the greater the concentration of antibody–hapten complex that will exist at equilibrium. A high-affinity antibody is highly complementary for the hapten and does not dissociate easily from it (Fig. 10-6).

Here is another way to describe the affinity constant: When the concentration of free antibody

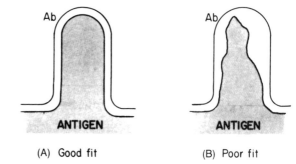

(A) Good fit   (B) Poor fit

FIGURE 10-6. The goodness of fit between the immunoglobulin molecule and an antigenic determinant determines the affinity. The shaded area in (A) represents an epitope that is highly complementary for the antibody; hence, there is a good fit, or high affinity. (B) The poor fit between the antibody and the epitope results in lower affinity.

equals the concentration of antibody complexed to the hapten, then 50% of the antibody is bound to the hapten. In the preceding equation, an equal concentration of free and complexed antibody will allow these two terms to be eliminated.

$$K_A = \frac{[\text{Ab-hapten complex}]}{[\text{Free Ab}] [\text{Free hapten}]} = \frac{1}{[\text{Free hapten}]}$$

Thus, the affinity constant will be the reciprocal of the concentration of free hapten when half of the total antibody is free. The affinity constant is expressed as liters per mole or molarity^{-1}. The smaller the hapten concentration that saturates half of the total antibody, the greater the affinity of the antibody for the hapten: The antibody is highly complementary for the hapten, there is a good fit, and the antibody does not easily release the hapten. For example, if the affinity constant for an antibody and hapten pair is 1×10^{10} L/mole, then the concentration of hapten needed to bind 50% of the antibody is 1×10^{-10} moles/L. This is an example of an antibody with high affinity for the hapten.

Avidity

The preceding discussion concerning antibody affinity is based on the interaction of a single epitope or a monovalent hapten with the combining site of an antibody. However, most naturally occurring antigens and antibodies are polyvalent, and in a naturally occurring immune response, a mixture of antibodies with different specificities, affinities, and valences is synthesized. Avidity describes the tendency for multiple antibodies and multivalent antigens to combine and is the cumulative binding strength of all antibody–epitope pairs. Thus, avidity is related to the specific affinity constants of each antibody–epitope pair, yet avidity is greater than the sum of affinity constants. Avidity is the bonus effect and is the product of affinity constants. For dissociation to occur, multiple bonds must be broken simultaneously (Fig. 10-7).[5,9]

Specificity and Cross-reactivity

The specificity of an antibody is defined by the antigen that induced antibody production. In other words, the antibody reacts with the homologous antigen so that the antibody is specific for the antigen. Ideally, an antibody would react with only one antigen, but this is not always the case. The interaction of an antibody with an antigen that is structurally similar, but not identical, to the homologous antigen is a cross-reaction. The greater the similarity between the cross-reacting antigen and the homologous antigen, the stronger the bond between the antibody and the cross-reacting antigen. So there is a continuum of potential reactions of an antibody with various antigens, from the strong binding with the homologous antigen, to weak binding with a similar antigen, to no binding with a dissimilar antigen (Fig. 10-8).

Heterophile Antibodies

A heterophile antibody is an antibody produced in response to a foreign antigen that also reacts with an antigen from a phylogenetically different species. That is, the antibody recognizes an antigen that is similar to the stimulating antigen but is found in another species. For example, an infection with group A streptococcal bacteria stimulates an antibody response to the epitopes of the organism. One antibody produced reacts with the organism and with

FIGURE 10-7. The combined forces of multiple-antigen combining sites and multiple-antibody combining sites result in avidity. A multivalent antigen (⊶) combines with a divalent antibody (O——O). In (A) there is only one antibody present and low avidity. In (B) the same multivalent antigen combines with several different antibodies, increasing avidity.

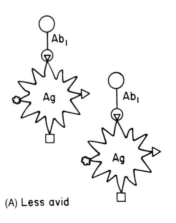

(A) Less avid

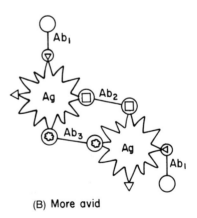

(B) More avid

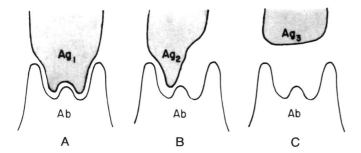

FIGURE 10-8. (*A*) The homologous antigen (Ag₁) stimulates the production of the antibody (Ab) and reacts with the antibody. (*B*) The same antibody reacts with another structurally similar antigen (Ag₂), showing cross-reactivity. (*C*) The same antibody cannot react with the dissimilar antigen (Ag₃).

a structurally similar antigen, human myocardium, and results in the damage associated with rheumatic fever.

The prototype heterophile antibody is associated with infectious mononucleosis. This disease results from Epstein-Barr virus infection that stimulates the immune system to produce many antibodies that react with epitopes of the virus. One of these antibodies, the heterophile antibody, cross-reacts with an epitope on the surface of sheep red blood cells. Thus, by measuring the heterophile antibody reaction with sheep red blood cells, there is indirect evidence of a recent Epstein-Barr virus infection.

Other heterophile antibodies are used to detect serologically a variety of recent infections. For example, antibodies produced in response to several rickettsial organisms can react with antigens of *Proteus vulgaris*. Therefore, one laboratory test strategy is to measure the antibodies that react with *Proteus* antigens and to interpret the titers in light of clinical indications of rickettsial infection. A second example is the cross-reactivity of the cold agglutinin produced in response to *Mycoplasma pneumoniae* infection. This antibody presumably reacts with the organism and reacts with the I antigen on adult human red blood cells. When the titer of cold agglutinin is sufficient, it suggests a recent *Mycoplasma* infection.

Given the wide variety and complexity of antigens in nature, it is not surprising that cross-reactivity between similar antigens and an antibody is seen. In clinical immunology, well-characterized cross-reactions are used to identify antibodies associated with a recent infection or with damage to the host. Further examples and explanations will be presented in the clinical immunology section.

Conclusion

The sequence of amino acids, as defined by the genetic code, determines the inherent properties and functions of all protein, including antibody molecules. For full biologic activity of antibody, all four levels of protein structure must be intact and unmodified. When the hypervariable regions within the variable domains of heavy and light chains are in close proximity, the antigen-combining site is created. The reversible association of antigen and antibody occurs through hydrogen bonding and electrostatic, Van der Waals, and hydrophobic forces. Affinity relates the strength of an antibody–hapten or antibody–epitope bond, whereas avidity relates the overall binding between multivalent antibodies and antigens. Antibody specificity is defined by the antigen that induced the production of that antibody; the opposite of specificity is cross-reactivity in which a second, structurally similar antigen can bind to the antibody. Heterophile antibodies are cross-reacting antibodies that react with antigens from different species.

References

1. Danishefsky I: Biochemistry for medical sciences, p 24. Boston, Little Brown and Company, 1980
2. Jeske DJ, Capra JD: Immunoglobulins: Structure

and function. In Paul WE (ed): Fundamental Immunology, p 131. New York, Raven Press, 1984

3. Edmunson AB, Ely KR, Abola EE, et al: Rotational allomerism and divergent evolution of domains in immunoglobulin light chains. Biochemistry 14:3953, 1975

4. Goodman JW: Immunoglobulins I: Structure and function. In Stites DP, Stobo JD, Well JV (eds): Basic and Clinical Immunology, 6th ed, p 27. Norwalk, Appleton and Lange, 1987

5. Roitt IM: Essential Immunology, 6th ed. Oxford, Blackwell Scientific Publications, 1988

6. Howard PL: Principles of antibody elution. Transfusion 21:477, 1981

7. Berzofsky JA, Berkower IJ: Antigen-antibody interaction. In Paul WE (ed): Fundamental Immunology, p 595. New York, Raven Press, 1984

8. Steward MW, Steensgaard J: Antibody affinity: Thermodynamic aspects and biological significance, p 1. Boca Raton, CRC Press, Inc., 1983

9. Eisen HN: Immunology, 2nd ed, p 298. New York, Harper & Row, 1980

CHAPTER **11**

Precipitation

Dorothy J. Fike

The reaction between soluble antigen and soluble antibody results in a precipitation reaction. Maximal precipitation occurs when the concentrations of antigen and antibody are in the zone of equivalence (Fig. 11-1). When the concentration of antigen is greater than that of the antibody, the amount of precipitate observed may be diminished or absent; this is postzone. The same observation, diminished or absent precipitate, also occurs when the antibody concentration is greater than the antigen; this is prozone.

The precipitate development requires that each antigen have at least two antigenic determinants per molecule. When bivalent antibody combines with the bivalent antigen, the antigen may become cross-linked and form a lattice (Fig. 11-2). The lattice forms when the antibody molecule combines with two different antigen molecules. A second antibody molecule combines with the second antigenic determinant on one of the antigen molecules and a third antigen molecule so that a complex is formed. Repeated so many times, the complex continues to grow

until it is sufficiently large to become insoluble and to precipitate. If the antigen is monovalent, no lattice will be formed and a different methodology must be used to detect the antigen or antibody. The reaction time may be hours or days, depending on the type of precipitation reaction that is employed. Consistent with all antigen–antibody reactions, precipitation reactions can occur using polyclonal or monoclonal antibodies.

Types of Reactions

Many different types of precipitation test systems (Table 11-1) can be used in the clinical laboratory. Each system can detect antigens or antibodies, depending on what is desired. Moreover, each system has different sources of error that must be remembered when performing a particular laboratory procedure. In every case, the lattice must form in the

123

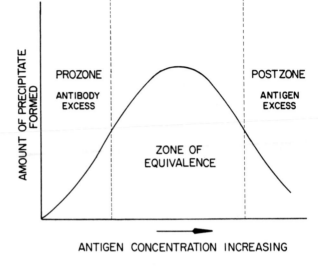

FIGURE 11-1. The precipitation curve shows the maximal amount of precipitation in the zone of equivalence. This reaction is obtained using several tubes, each with the same concentration of antibody. The tubes have an increasing amount of antigen added.

zone of equivalence to visualize the antigen–antibody reaction. In general, precipitation techniques are not as sensitive as other techniques.

Fluid Phase Precipitation

One of the first precipitation reactions was the passive diffusion of fluid phase antigen and antibody. This double diffusion method in a capillary tube layers an antigen solution over an antibody solution. Both the antigen and antibody will diffuse toward each other; when antibody recognizes antigen, precipitate forms at the interface. The amount of precipitate is proportional to the concentration of both the antigen and antibody. In Figure 11-3, (A) and (B) show precipitation of antigen–antibody complexes; (B) shows more precipitate than (A). In (C) no precipitate is formed. This procedure may be used to detect either unknown antigen or unknown antibody.

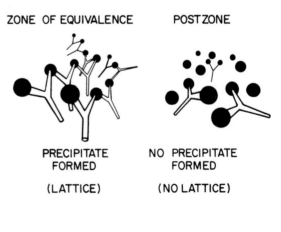

FIGURE 11-2. The amount of precipitation in each of the zones of the precipitation curve is determined by the amount of lattice formed. In prozone, little or no precipitate is formed; antibody excess prevents cross-linking of antigen molecules. In the zone of equivalence, precipitate is formed because the lattice is large and insoluble. In postzone, little or no precipitate is formed, since lattice formation does not occur in antigen excess.

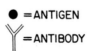

Table 11-1: Types of Precipitation Reactions

PASSIVE

Fluid

    Double diffusion

    Capillary tube precipitation

Gel

    Double diffusion Ouchterlony

    Single diffusion radial immunodiffusion (RID)

ELECTROPHORESIS

Countercurrent immunoelectrophoresis (CIEP)

Immunoelectrophoresis (IEP)

Immunofixation electrophoresis (IFE)

Rocket technique (Laurell)

Precipitation reactions may be done by passive diffusion in fluids or gels or by electrophoresis.

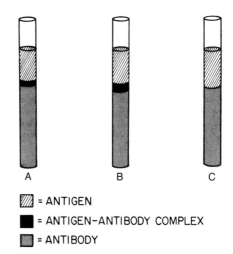

= ANTIGEN

= ANTIGEN–ANTIBODY COMPLEX

= ANTIBODY

FIGURE 11-3. The antigen and antibody solutions are placed on top of each other in a capillary tube. After diffusion the antigen and antibody precipitate in the zone of equivalence. In samples A and B some precipitate is formed at the interface, with B having more than A. In sample C there is no precipitate.

If an antigen is to be detected, a fixed amount of antibody is placed in the capillary tube; the greater the amount of precipitate formed, the greater the concentration of antigen. C-reactive protein (CRP), an acute phase protein, is an antigen that can be detected with this method.[1,2] In Fig. 11-3, if the antiserum contained CRP antibody, example B had more CRP than example A. The lack of sensitivity and the extensive time required to obtain results in double diffusion favor newer methodologies to detect CRP. If this procedure is used to detect antibody, a known amount of antigen is used.

Precipitation Reactions in Gel

Other passive diffusion methods use gel as a solid medium. Gels are semisolid media that allow soluble antigen and/or antibody to diffuse through the pores until the antigen and antibody reach the optimal concentration for lattice formation. The size of the molecule determines the rate at which it diffuses through the gel. In general, smaller molecules move through the gel faster than larger molecules. If there is a mixture of antigens and/or antibodies, there may be several precipitin lines, since each antigen and the corresponding antibody will form a lattice in its zone of equivalence.[2] Besides the molecular weight of the antigen, other factors that affect the diffusion rate are temperature, gel viscosity and hydration, and interactions between the gel matrix and the reactants.[3]

Double Diffusion

One gel diffusion method, the Ouchterlony technique, is a double-diffusion method in which both antigen and antibody diffuse. Antigen is placed in one well and antibody in another; diffusion occurs,

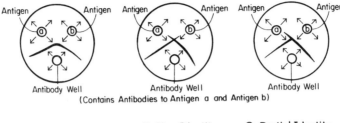

FIGURE 11-4. (A) Antigens a and b are identical. Where the lines of precipitate come together on the plate, a smooth curve is formed. (B) Antigens a and b are not the same. In the area on the plate where the two antigens may react with antibody, the lines of precipitate will cross through each other. (C) Antigens a and b are similar but not completely identical. Where the lines of precipitate join, the line is not completely smooth. The spur points to the antigen that is dissimilar.

and where the two meet in the gel, a line of precipitation is formed. If multiple wells of antigen are used opposite an antibody well on the same plate, several patterns of reactivity may be observed (Fig. 11-4). In Figure 11-4(A), if antigen a is the same as antigen b, the reaction of each with the antibody will be the same. The result is a solid, continuous, smooth line of identity between the antigen wells and the antibody well. If antigen a is different from antigen b and both react with the antibody as shown in (B), the precipitin lines cross and a double spur is formed. This line of precipitate is known as a line of nonidentity. The double spur is formed, since both antigens and antibodies are diffusing in all directions. Each antigen–antibody lattice forms its own distinct precipitin line; the two lines cross where each antigen–antibody complex is in its own zone of equivalence. If antigen a and antigen b have some common elements, a single spur will be formed. This is known as the line of partial identity, as seen in Figure 11-4(C). If antigen a and antigen b share some of the same amino acids or sugars in a particular sequence, the antibody can react with both antigens. The spur is formed when the antibody reacts with the more simple antigen to form a precipitin line; additional antibodies react with the more complex (or "true") antigen as it mi-

grates through this line. In Figure 11-4(C) the "spur" points to the well containing antigen b, although in other test systems the "spur" may point to antigen a. The spur always points to the more simple antigen.[1]

Some problems that may occur with the Ouchterlony technique are irregular patterns due to overfill-

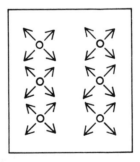
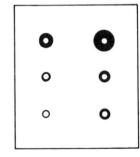

A Diffusion Pathway   B Ending Pattern

FIGURE 11-5. (A) The antigen is placed in the well; it diffuses into the agar in all directions. (B) The area around the well where precipitation occurs is the area of the zone of equivalence between the antigen and antibody. The diameter of the area of precipitation (including the well diameter) is measured to determine the concentration of antigen.

ing of wells, irregular well punching, or nonlevel incubation.[3] Other problems may include gel drying and overheating. If inadequate time for diffusion has been allowed, band intensity may be weakened. Antigen or antibody degradation may occur because of bacterial or fungal contamination. Considering the lattice theory, antigen or antibody excess may yield false negative results. This may be partially overcome by using several concentrations of both antigens and antibodies, so that the combination will be in the zone of equivalence.

Radial Immunodiffusion

A commonly used gel precipitation technique is that of radial immunodiffusion (RID) (Fig. 11-5). In this technique antiserum is added to the liquified gel, which is poured into a plate and allowed to solidify by cooling to room temperature. The antiserum should be monospecific, highly specific, and of excellent precipitating ability. The antigen solution is added to wells cut into the agar. The antigen diffuses in all directions from the well, and precipitation occurs in a ring surrounding the well in the zone of equivalence. The time required for the diffusion depends on the size of the antigen being measured, larger molecules diffuse more slowly and require more time for full diffusion and maximum precipitin ring formation.

There are two standard reading measurement times—the Fahey, or kinetic diffusion, method[4] and the Mancini, or endpoint diffusion, method.[5] In the Fahey, or kinetic diffusion, method, the diameter of the precipitin rings is measured at 18 hours. The logarithm of the concentration of the standards is proportional to the diameter of the precipitin ring. Using semilogarithmic paper, the y-axis is the analyte concentration and the x-axis is the diameter of the ring (including well diameter). The standards used are generally a high concentration, a normal concentration, and a low concentration. If these three points do not fall in a straight line, then a line is drawn point to point. The analyte concentration of

the patient and control sera may be read from the graph.[2] Figure 11-6 is an example of a kinetic diffusion graph.

In the endpoint method the antigen is allowed to diffuse fully to achieve maximal precipitation. The time needed varies, depending on the molecular weight of the protein being measured. For example, IgG quantitation requires a 48-hour incubation, whereas IgM requires a 72-hour incubation. The longer incubation time required for IgM is due to its large molecular weight. Using linear graph paper, the concentration of the antigen is plotted on the y-axis and the diameter squared of the precipitin ring is plotted on the x-axis. The relationship between the concentration of the standards and the square of the diameter of the precipitin rings is the line of best fit (Fig. 11-7). The concentration of the unknown sera is read from this graph. Patient values can only be obtained if the precipitin ring diameter is within the values obtained for the reference sera. If the diameter of the precipitin ring of the patient sample is greater than that of the highest reference serum, the line should not be extended to obtain the patient concentration, since linearity above the reference line cannot be guaranteed. It is recommended that the serum be diluted with normal saline and the assay repeated. The result obtained should be multiplied by the dilution factor. If the diameter of the precipitin ring of the patient sample is below the lowest reference standard, the results should be reported as less than the standard value or the sample should be assayed on a "low-level" plate.

This single-diffusion method may be used for the quantitation of immunoglobulins and other serum proteins, including complement components. In this particular procedure antiserum is always in the gel, so if immunoglobulins are quantitated, the immunoglobulin is the antigen.

Sources of error include over- or underfilling the wells, spilling the patient's serum on the gel, nicking the side of the well when filling, and improper incu-

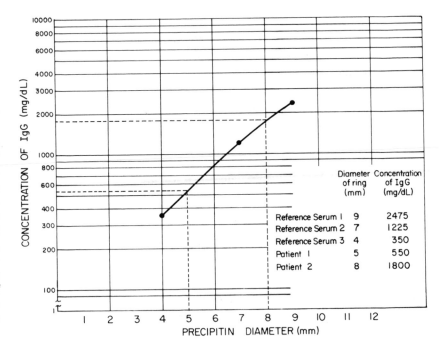

FIGURE 11-6. In the kinetic diffusion method, the diameter of the ring is plotted versus the concentration on semilogarithmic graph paper. Values of high, normal, and low reference samples are plotted, and the points are connected. Concentrations of unknown samples may be determined using this graph. For example, if the patient sample has a diameter of 5 mm, the sample contains 550 mg/dL of IgG. If the patient sample has a diameter of 8 mm, the sample contains 1800 mg/dL.

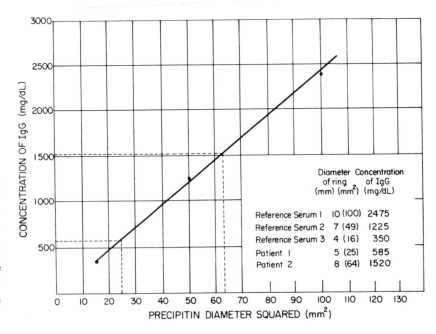

FIGURE 11-7. In the endpoint method, the square of the diameter of the ring is plotted against the concentration of antigen on linear graph paper. Values of high, normal, and low reference samples are plotted and the line of best fit is drawn. Concentrations of unknown samples may be determined using this graph. For example, if the patient sample has a diameter of 5 mm, the sample contains 585 mg/dL. If the patient sample has a diameter of 8 mm, the sample contains 1520 mg/dL of IgG.

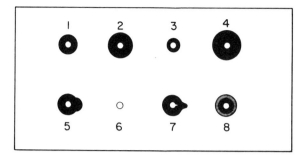

FIGURE 11-8. Ring patterns on a RID plate should be equal around the well. In this figure, wells 1 through 4 are normal. Well 5 has more precipitate on one side, which indicates that some of the sample spilled on the gel. There is no precipitate around well 6, which indicates that the well was not filled or was underfilled or that the sample contained little or no analyte. Well 7 has an irregular shape on one side, which indicates that the well was nicked during filling. Well 8 is an example of double precipitin rings.

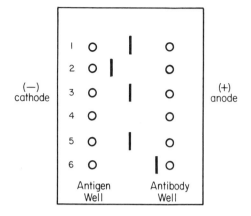

FIGURE 11-9. In countercurrent electrophoresis, antigen and antibody wells are placed opposite each other. In this figure, unknown antigen is detected using known antibody. The plate is electrophoresed and a precipitin line is formed at the zone of equivalence, which may not always be midway between the two wells. Samples 1, 3, and 5 have antigen present and in equal concentration to the known antibody. Sample 2 has antigen present, but in less concentration compared to the antibody concentration. Sample 4 has no antigen present. Sample 6 has antigen present in a higher concentration than that of the antibody.

bation time and temperature. These will all lead to inaccurate quantitation requiring the sample to be reassayed (Fig. 11-8).

Countercurrent Immunoelectrophoresis

A third precipitin reaction in gel is the technique of countercurrent immunoelectrophoresis (CIEP). Gel is poured onto a plate and cooled. Two columns of wells are created; antigen is placed in one well and the antibody is placed in the other well. The plate is placed in an electric field, causing migration of the antigen and antibody based on the charge of each. At pH 8.6 the antigen will migrate toward the anode, and the antibody toward the cathode. At equivalence, precipitation occurs (Fig. 11-9). The electric current shortens the time required to produce precipitation of antigen–antibody complexes. This qualitative procedure is used to detect autoantibodies, antibodies to infectious agents, and certain microbial antigens.[3,6]

This method can be semiquantitative by using serial dilutions. If a particular antigen is serially diluted and the concentration of antibody is kept constant, as the concentration of antigen increases the precipitin line moves closer to the antibody well. If the concentration of antibody is serially diluted and the concentration of antigen is constant, higher concentrations of antibody will move the precipitin line toward the antigen well.

Sources of error are related either to electrophoresis or to precipitation. One electrophoresis error is the reversal of the wells so that the current is applied in the wrong direction. Other problems associated with the electrophoresis technique are improper pH of the buffer and insufficient electrophoresis time. There will be no or reduced precipitation if there is no lattice formed in prozone or postzone. Also, if the wells are not parallel, the reaction might not occur.

(text continues on page 132)

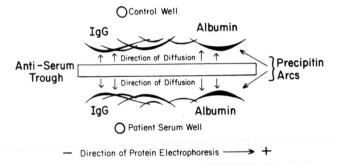

FIGURE 11-10. The first step required to form precipitin arcs in immunoelectrophoresis is to separate proteins in patient and control sera. The proteins migrate to the same area as in routine protein electrophoresis (Fig. 8-1). The second step requires total anti-human serum, which contains specific antibodies to different serum proteins, to be added to the trough and allowed to diffuse through the gel. Wherever the patient or control sera and each specific antibody in the total anti-human serum are in the zone of equivalence, a precipitin arc is formed. The relative serum protein concentration determines the size of the arc. For example, the anti-albumin in the trough diffuses toward the albumin in the patient or control serum. Where the two meet, the precipitin arc forms. Because more albumin is present than IgG in normal serum, the size of the arc for albumin is larger than that for IgG.

FIGURE 11-11. In some cases more information may be obtained from serum immunoelectrophoresis by using monospecific antibodies. In each case, the sample is placed in the well and electrophoresed; monospecific antiserum is placed in the trough. (A) This is an example of normal patient serum compared to the control serum. The two patterns are identical. Since κ and λ chains are found on all heavy chains, the arc formed with κ and λ antisera will be in all regions where IgG, IgM, IgA, and IgD are found. (B) This is an example of a patient with an IgMκ paraprotein. Note the increase in the precipitin arcs of the patient serum with anti-μ and anti-κ antiserum when compared to the precipitin arcs of the control.

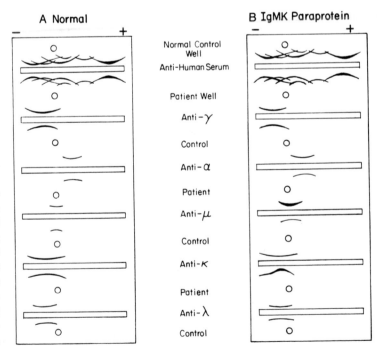

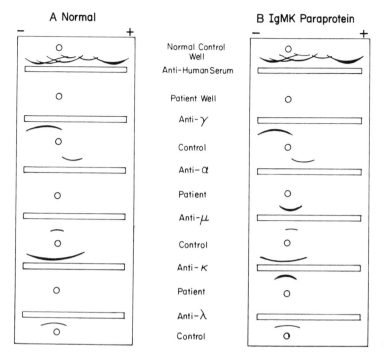

A Normal

B IgMK Paraprotein

Normal Control
Well

Anti-Human Serum

Patient Well

Anti-γ

Control

Anti-α

Patient

Anti-μ

Control

Anti-κ

Patient

Anti-λ

Control

FIGURE 11-12. Urine immunoelectrophoresis from the same two patients whose sera were evaluated in Figure 11-11 are shown here. (A) Normally urine contains little protein; therefore, no precipitin arcs are formed. The control used in this procedure is normal human serum. (B) The patient urine has increased μ and κ precipitin arcs compared to the control. This is consistent with the serum findings in Figure 11-11. No other arcs are formed because no other urine proteins are present in detectable quantities.

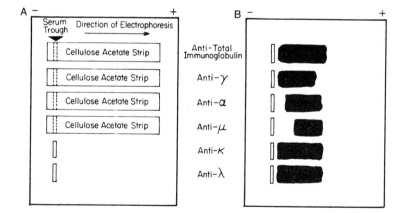

FIGURE 11-13. (A) After gel electrophoresis of serum, urine, or cerebrospinal fluid, cellulose acetate strips impregnated with antiserum are placed on the gel. No bubbles should be between the strip and the gel so that the antiserum can completely diffuse into the gel. (B) After incubation to allow for the diffusion, the cellulose acetate strips are removed and the precipitin bands are stained. As with other electrophoresis procedures, the stained area identifies the location of the specific protein as it would be found on routine protein electrophoresis. Since κ and λ light chains are usually associated with all heavy chain classes, the anti-κ and anti-λ reactions will occur in all regions where immunoglobulin has been electrophoresed.

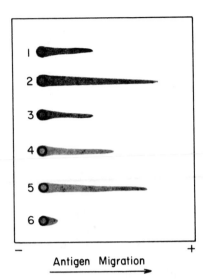

FIGURE 11-14. In the Laurell rocket technique, the agar contains a specific antiserum. The samples are electrophoresed. The area where the antigen and antibody are in the zone of equivalence will show precipitation. The rocket area may be quantitated. Sample 2 has the highest concentration of antigen; sample 6 has the least amount.

Immunoelectrophoresis

Immunoelectrophoresis (IEP) is another gel electrophoretic technique commonly performed in the clinical immunology laboratory. This qualitative procedure is used to identify monoclonal proteins, including free κ and λ chains. This procedure utilizes both electrophoresis and double diffusion (Fig. 11-10). Patient serum is placed in a well and electrophoresed. The movement of the serum proteins is similar to protein electrophoresis, with albumin migrating toward the anode and the immunoglobulins migrating to the α, β, and γ globulin regions.[2,7] Anti–human serum is placed in the trough, and the antiserum and the separated patient's proteins diffuse toward each other.

Precipitin arcs form at the zone of equivalence between the antigen and specific antisera. Anti–total

human serum is a mixture of antibodies against all serum proteins and will produce many precipitin arcs. If a monospecific antiserum is placed in the trough, then only one arc will be formed if that particular serum component is present. The plate may be stained and photographed. The precipitation patterns of identity, nonidentity, and partial identity are observed. A normal control serum is performed simultaneously, so that the two may be compared.

This procedure is relatively insensitive to the antigen and antibody ratios, so it has been used for the detection of free light chain proteins.[3] It can also be used as a screening procedure to detect immunoglobulin classes (Fig. 11-11). Since the size of the arc is an indication of the amount of immunoglobulin pres-

Table 11-2: Test Procedures Using Precipitation Techniques

Test	Method
C-reactive protein	Capillary tube precipitation

Immunoglobulin quantitation
  IgG, total and subclasses
  IgA
  IgM
  IgD
	RID

Complement proteins
  C3
  C4
	RID

Microbial antigens	CIEP
Monoclonal proteins (Serum, urine, and cerebrospinal fluid)	IEP and IFE

Several procedures can use precipitation reactions for the detection of antigens. These reactions may be qualitative, semi-quantitative or quantitative. Refer to the text for specific information.

ent, the procedure is semiquantitative.[3,7] The shape and position of precipitin arcs can provide clues as to the monoclonality of a protein.

Some problems associated with this procedure include prolonged diffusion that will result in artifacts, especially at the anode and cathode. Marked antibody excess may result in multiple concentric arcs that could be mistaken for multiple antigen reactions.

IEP may also be used to identify urine proteins. Urine is placed in the well and electrophoresed, troughs are filled with antisera, and diffusion occurs. Free light chain and intact immunoglobulin molecules can be characterized (Fig. 11-12).

Immunofixation

Immunofixation electrophoresis (IFE) is another gel electrophoretic technique useful in the clinical laboratory. Serum, urine, or cerebrospinal fluid (CSF) are electrophoresed, followed by the application of antisera. A cellulose acetate strip impregnated with antiserum is placed over the separated proteins (Fig.

Table 11-3: Advantages and Disadvantages of Precipitation Techniques

Technique	Advantages	Disadvantages
Capillary tube precipitation	Easy to set up	Insensitive
		Reaction time long
		Semiquantitative
Radial immunodiffusion (RID)	Sensitive	Reaction time long (kinetic: 18 hrs; endpoint: 48 hrs)
	Quantitative	Can only detect one antigen per plate
Double diffusion (Ouchterlony)	Can detect similarities among antigens	Semiquantitative
		Reaction time long
Counter immunoelectrophoresis (CIEP)	More rapid reaction than other tests	Semiquantitative
Immunoelectrophoresis (IEP)	Sensitive	Semiquantitative
	Less problem with antigen/ antibody ratio	
Immunofixation electrophoresis (IFE)	Sensitive	Semiquantitative
	Can detect genetic variations among antigens	Antigen/antibody ratio is important
Rocket Technique (Laurell)	Rapid reaction time	Can only detect one antigen per plate
	Quantitative	

Each type of precipitation reaction has advantages and disadvantages. The requirements for detection of a specific antigen will determine which type of precipitation reaction may be used.

11-13). Diffusion of the antiserum into the gel occurs rapidly, resulting in precipitation of antigen–antibody complexes. The resolution of IFE is greater than that in IEP. Compared with IEP, the IFE technique is more sensitive to the antigen and antibody ratios. In many instances, serum dilution or antiserum dilution is necessary to produce the precipitin reaction. Urine and CSF must be concentrated to be in the zone of equivalence; typically, urine is concentrated 25 times and CSF is concentrated 50 to 100 times. If there are air bubbles, when the cellulose acetate is applied to the gel, diffusion cannot occur at these points, and a precipitation reaction may be missed.[3]

Rocket Technique

Another electrophoretic precipitation technique, used primarily in research laboratories, is the rocket or Laurell technique.[7] This technique is used to quantitate antigens other than immunoglobulins. Antiserum is incorporated into the agar. The unknown antigen is placed in the well and electrophoresed. As the antigen migrates through the gel, it combines with antibody. Precipitation occurs along the lateral boundaries and resembles a rocket (Fig. 11-14). The total distance of antigen migration and precipitation is directly proportional to the antigen concentration.[7]

As previously discussed, a variety of procedures may be used in the clinical and research laboratories using precipitation techniques. The specific methodology used depends on the concentration of the antigen and whether quantitation is necessary. Table 11-2 summarizes some of these tests and which procedure may be used for each. Table 11-3 summarizes the advantages and disadvantages of each procedure.

References

1. Barrett JT: Textbook of Immunology, 5th ed, p 292. St Louis, CV Mosby, 1988
2. Stansfield WD: Serology and Immunology: A clinical approach, p 135. New York, Macmillan, 1981
3. Johnson AM: Immunoprecipitation in gels. In Rose NR, Friedman H, Fahey JL (eds): Manual of Clinical Immunology, 3rd ed, p 14. Washington, DC, American Society for Microbiology, 1986
4. Fahey JL, McKelvey EM: Quantitative determination of serum immunoglobulins in antibody-agar plates. J Immunol 94:84, 1965
5. Mancini G, Carbonara AO, Heremans JF: Immunochemical quantitation of antigens by single radial diffusion. Immunochemistry 2:235, 1965
6. Roitt I: Essential Immunology, 6th ed, p 69. Oxford, Blackwell Scientific Publications, 1988
7. Stites DP, Rodgers RPC: Clinical laboratory methods for detection of antigens and antibodies. In Stites DP, Stobo JD, Wells JV (eds): Basic and Clinical Immunology, 6th ed, p 241. Norwalk, Appleton and Lange, 1987

CHAPTER 12

Agglutination and Agglutination Inhibition

Dorothy J. Fike

General Considerations

Agglutination is the cross-linking of a particulate or insoluble antigen and the corresponding antibody; this is observed as clumping. If the particles are red cells, the reaction is hemagglutination. If latex particles are the insoluble particle, the reaction is latex agglutination. Antigens that participate in agglutination reactions may be referred to as agglutinogens, whereas antibody may be known as an agglutinin. As in precipitation, this serologic reaction results when antigen and antibody molecules complex and form a lattice (Fig. 12-1).

Excess antibody or antigen in agglutination reactions behave similarly to prozone and postzone of the precipitation curve, which may also be referred to as the agglutination curve (see Fig. 11-1). For lattice formation to occur, the antigen must have at least two antigenic determinants.[1] Lattice formation is more rapid in agglutination than in precipitation, minutes or hours compared with hours or days. Because there is an insoluble particle in the agglutination reaction, fewer antigen–antibody complexes are required for the reaction to be visible. Agglutination and precipitation are compared in Table 12-1.

The class of antibody also plays a role in the agglutination reaction. IgM class molecules agglutinate particles very readily since their large size, five basic immunoglobulin units, allows the attachment of up to five antigens. IgG class molecules are poor agglutinins.[2] In some cases, altering incubation conditions allows IgG class molecules to produce good agglutination. Because IgG molecules require special conditions in agglutination reactions, they were mistakenly referred to as incomplete antibodies. This is a misnomer, since IgG molecules are structurally and functionally complete.[3]

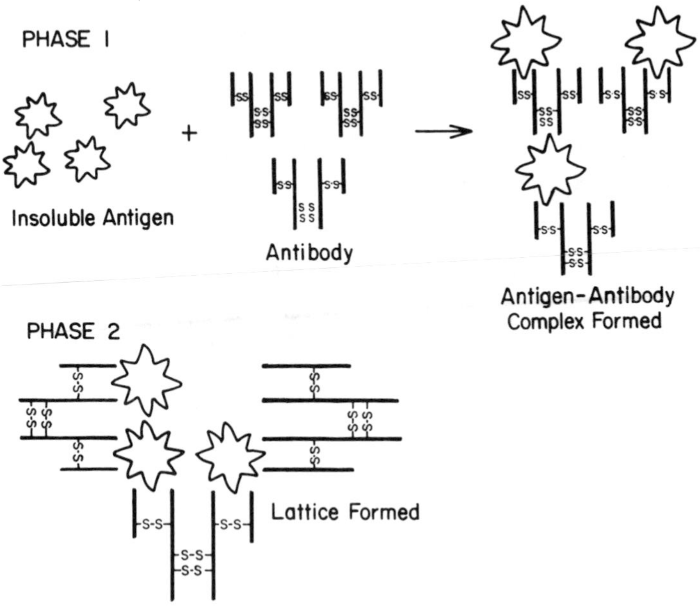

FIGURE 12-1. Agglutination reactions result in lattice formation. The lattice formation occurs in two phases. Phase 1 is the attachment of the antibody molecule to the insoluble antigen and the formation of individual antigen–antibody complexes. Phase 2 is the formation of the lattice.

Phases of Agglutination

Agglutination requires two phases: (1) specific binding of antigen and antibody and (2) lattice formation (Fig. 12-1). Although this reaction is faster than that of precipitation, one major disadvantage of agglutination reactions is that often the results are qualitative. In qualitative test procedures, the presence of an antigen or antibody is detected, but the amount of antigen or antibody is not determined. In some test

Table 12-1: Comparison of Agglutination and Precipitation Reactions

Agglutination	Precipitation
Insoluble or particulate antigen	Soluble antigen
Antigen must have at least two antigenic determinants	Antigen must have at least two antigenic determinants
Antigen excess results in a postzone reaction	Antigen excess results in a postzone reaction
Antibody excess results in a prozone reaction	Antibody excess results in a prozone reaction
Reaction time: minutes to hours	Reaction time: hours to days
Test results: qualitative or semiquantitative	Test results: qualitative, semiquantitative, or quantitative

This table is a comparison between agglutination and precipitation reactions. Both types of reactions have lattice formation, so that the number of antigenic determinants, prozone reaction, and postzone reaction influence lattice formation. The antigen, reaction time, and test results for each are different.

procedures the results are semiquantitative when a titration is performed. The results give the relative concentration of antigen or antibody present in the sample. If it is necessary to know the specific quantity of the antigen or antibody, other methods must be used. In many instances, though, only a rough estimate of the concentration is sufficient. For example, it may be necessary to know if a particular organism is present (qualitative) or to know if a recent infection has occurred (semiquantitative). In these cases the agglutination procedure is adequate.

Agglutination procedures may be performed as slide, tube, or microtiter techniques. Figure 12-2 represents the appearance of agglutination in each system.[1] In slide test procedures, the antigen–antibody reaction occurs on a glass or paper slide. Reaction time for the slide procedures is short, with most procedures requiring slide rotation for 2 to 3 minutes at room temperature. The maximum time required for a slide test procedure is the Rapid Plasma Reagin test, which requires slide rotation for 8 minutes. Tube test reactions generally require a longer incubation pe-

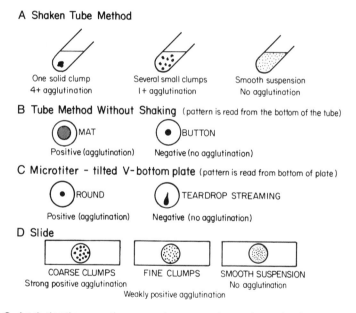

FIGURE 12-2. Agglutination reaction procedures may be performed using test tubes, microtiter plates, or slides. The reaction patterns for each are shown. (A) Test tubes may be shaken and the amount of agglutination observed. In some reactions the antigen–antibody lattice formation results in one solid clump, a 4+ reaction. In other reactions, more than one clump results when the tube is shaken. If there are many small clumps, this is a 1+ reaction. A negative reaction is a completely smooth suspension of the particles or cells. (B) In some procedures, the tube is not shaken and the pattern of reactivity is read from the bottom of the tube. If a mat is formed, agglutination has occurred. If there is a button, no agglutination has occurred. (C) When a V-bottom microtiter plate is tilted, a round pattern indicates the presence of agglutination; a tear drop shape indicates that no agglutination has occurred. (D) Coarse clumps in a slide procedure indicate strong positive agglutination. Fine clumps occur in a weak agglutination, and a smooth suspension of antigen indicates that no agglutination has occurred.

riod and may be incubated at 4°C, room temperature, or 37°C. The incubation time ranges from 15 minutes to overnight. Microtiter techniques are generally adaptations of tube test procedures. The major advantage of microtiter techniques is that less patient sample and fewer reagents are required for the assay. Most slide procedures are qualitative, whereas the tube test or microtiter assays are semiquantitative.

Classification of Agglutination Reactions

Direct Agglutination

There are three major types of agglutination reactions: direct, viral hemagglutination, and passive (indirect).[4] Direct agglutination uses antigens found naturally on the surface of cells such as red blood cells or bacteria. Human red cell antigens (blood groups) are very diverse, with more than 400 antigens that have been defined. ABO and Rh systems are the most important red blood cell antigens. ABO antigens are found on all cells in the body, not just on red cells. If the individual lacks a particular ABO antigen, antibodies against that antigen will develop through exposure to natural antigens sharing a similar structure to the human antigen (see Table 2-4). The detection of these antigens and the corresponding antibodies is important in blood and tissue transplantation. The Rh(D) antigen is important, since it is highly antigenic and the antibody can cause hemolytic disease of the newborn.

Red blood cells may be used to detect antibodies to infectious agents. One serologic test, the cold agglutinin test, uses adult human red blood cells to detect antibodies against *Mycoplasma pneumoniae*. Following a recent infection, antibodies to the *M. pneumoniae* will react with the I antigen found on human red cells.

Another direct hemagglutination test uses the antigens found on horse, sheep, or beef red blood cells to detect heterophile antibodies in human serum. Heterophile antibodies are produced in response to one antigen yet can react with a second antigen from a phylogenetically different species. In infectious mononucleosis and serum sickness, heterophile antibodies are detectable.

Bacterial natural antigens have been used to demonstrate a recent infection by measuring the titer of antibody against a specific species of bacteria. Evidence of a recent infection is indicated by a diagnostic titer or a rising antibody titer. A diagnostic titer is the minimum concentration of antibody in one specimen that is significant; through clinical evidence and observation, when this titer is achieved, there has been a recent infection. Demonstrating a fourfold increase in antibody titer between acute and convalescent specimens also suggests antigenic stimulation by a recent infection.

Febrile agglutinins are antibodies produced in response to bacterial infections in which fever is a prominent feature. The Widal test uses *Salmonella* bacteria to detect antibodies in typhoid and paratyphoid fevers. In this test procedure, antibodies to both H antigens (flagellar antigens) and O antigens (somatic antigens found in the cell wall) are detected. The Weil–Felix reaction has been used to detect antibodies in rickettsial diseases, such as Rocky Mountain spotted fever. Rickettsial antibodies cross-react with and agglutinate subspecies of *Proteus vulgaris*. Other febrile agglutinins are detected following infection with *Brucella*, *Francisella*, and *Bordetella*. Since these direct agglutination tests lack sensitivity and specificity, other procedures are recommended to provide serologic evidence of a recent infection.[1,3,5]

Viral Hemagglutination

Viral hemagglutination, a natural phenomenon, occurs when a virus, such as the rubella or influenza virus, agglutinates red blood cells by binding to receptors on the red blood cell surface. Most commonly, viral hemagglutination inhibition tests are used to detect the presence of patient antibody. In this reaction, antibody inhibits the virus from agglutinating the red blood cells.[3]

Passive and Reverse Passive Agglutination

A third major type of agglutination reaction is passive agglutination in which the antigen is attached to a particulate "carrier." Passive agglutination is also referred to as indirect agglutination. In this chapter indirect procedures will be used to refer to an indirect antiglobulin procedure, and passive agglutination will refer to the use of a carrier particle coated with antigen. Antibody may also be attached to a particulate "carrier," and this technique is reverse passive agglutination.

Carriers currently used in clinical laboratory tests are charcoal, latex particles, gelatin particles, and red blood cells. Some antigens, such as lipopolysaccharide, endotoxin, DNA, and penicillin, attach to the red cell membrane spontaneously. Other antigens, especially proteins, only adsorb onto red cells after the cells have been treated to increase the cell membrane reactivity. Most often, red cells are treated with tannic acid, so that additional protein will adhere to the surface of the cell. Antigens adsorbed onto the surface of the red cell membrane must not be released during the antigen–antibody reaction. Generally, this problem has been evaluated and is controlled by the manufacturer.[1]

Latex particles and charcoal are inert substances that must have a minimum size for agglutination reactions. This is controlled in the manufacturing process. Latex is a polystyrene polymer sphere 0.81 μm in diameter. Polystyrene is an inert colloid with a negative charge that adsorbs protein. Because different proteins adsorb onto latex particles in varying degrees, optimal coating of the particle is necessary to yield maximal agglutination. Charcoal is inert carbon onto which protein may adsorb.[1] The only test in the clinical laboratory that utilizes carbon particles is the rapid plasma reagin test.

Passive agglutination procedures can be used to detect the nontreponemal antibody in syphilis, rheumatoid factor, rubella antibody, and thyroglobulin antibody. As in direct agglutination, the test format may be slide, tube, or microtiter techniques. Each specific test procedure depends on the carrier that will best adsorb the antigen and whether the procedure is quantitative or qualitative. These tests are summarized in Table 12-2.

Latex particles and red cells may also be used to detect antigen in the reverse passive agglutination procedure. Antibody is attached to the particle, and agglutination occurs when specific antigen is present. C-reactive protein (CRP) is commonly detected by the reverse passive latex agglutination method. The high levels of CRP produced during acute inflammation make postzone a serious source of error.

Sources of error in passive or reverse passive techniques include those stated for direct agglutination, prozone and postzone reactions, and cross-reactivity. In addition, false negative results may be obtained if test reagents are not at the appropriate pH, if the antigen or antibody is released from the carrier, or if the red cells are fragile. It is important for the carrier to bind a high concentration of antigen or antibody, so that maximal agglutination is observed. For this reason different carriers are used.

Antiglobulin Techniques

Sometimes an agglutination reaction must be enhanced to visualize the reaction. Since red cells have a net negative charge, they repel each other. IgG molecules are small and cannot link one antigen-binding site on one cell with another antigen-binding site on a second red cell. No lattice is formed, and the reaction is not visible. To overcome this spatial defi-

Table 12-2: Tests Using Agglutination or Agglutination Inhibition Techniques

Test	Detecting Antigen or Antibody	Insoluble Particle	Type of Technique
Rapid plasma reagin (syphilis)	Antibody	Charcoal with lecithin–cardiolipin attached	Agglutination (passive)
Cold agglutinin (primary atypical pneumonia)	Antibody	Human group O red cells (natural I antigen on red cells)	Agglutination (direct)
Febrile agglutinins	Antibody	Bacteria (natural antigens)	Agglutination (direct)
Widal		*Salmonella typhi* and *paratyphoid*	
Weil–Felix (*Rickettsia*)		*Proteus vulgaris*	
Francisella		*Francisella tularensis*	
Brucella		*Brucella abortus*	
Infectious mononucleosis (heterophile)	Antibody	Sheep, horse, or beef red cells (natural heterophile antigens)	Agglutination (direct)
Rheumatoid factor	Antibody	Latex particle with human IgG attached	Agglutination (passive)
Rubella	Antibody	Tanned red cells with rubella antigen attached	Agglutination (passive)
Thyroglobulin	Antibody	Red cells with thyroglobulin attached	Agglutination (passive)
C-reactive protein	Antigen	Latex particle with anti-CRP attached	Reverse passive agglutination
Pregnancy	Antigen	Latex or red cells with hCG attached	Agglutination or hemagglutination inhibition

Tests in the laboratory that utilize the agglutination principle may be direct, passive, or reverse passive. In direct procedures the antigen may be human, sheep, or beef red cells or different species of bacteria. In passive and reverse passive the antigen or antibody may be attached to red cells, latex, charcoal, or another particle. In agglutination inhibition the procedures may utilize natural antigens or latex particles with antigen attached.

ciency, anti–human IgG may be used to detect the presence of antibodies coating a red cell. This is known as the antiglobulin technique. Usually the antiglobulin reagent is prepared in rabbits by injecting purified human γ chains; following an immune re-sponse, rabbit anti–human IgG is harvested (Fig. 12-3). An anti–human immunoglobulin reagent may also be used in fluorescence immunoassays, radioimmunoassays, and enzyme immunoassays. In some situations, IgA-sensitized red cells are suspected.

A   Specific heavy chain injected
    into an animal

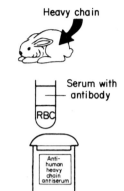

Heavy chain

B   After an immune response,
    specific antibody is produced.
    The animal is bled to harvest
    the antibody.

Serum with
antibody

RBC

C   After purification,
    specific antiserum is available
    for diagnostic testing.

Anti-
human
heavy
chain
antiserum

FIGURE 12-3. (A) Anti–human globulin is prepared by injecting the IgG heavy chain (γ chain) into a rabbit or other animal. (B) After the immune response, a specific antibody is produced, and the animal is bled to obtain it. (C) After purification the specific antibody may be used for diagnostic procedures.

Using an anti-IgA (α-chain-specific) serum to detect cell-bound IgA may be possible in the future.

Two specific procedures use anti–human globulin: direct and indirect. In the direct anti–human globulin test, the antigen–antibody reaction has occurred *in vivo*, whereas the indirect antiglobulin technique requires an *in vitro* incubation. In both procedures the red cells are washed with isotonic saline after antibody has bound to the red cells to remove any un-

bound antibody. The anti–human immunoglobulin reagent is added and will bind to the human immunoglobulin on the surface of the red cell to form a lattice; agglutination will be observed (Fig. 12-4).

Direct Antiglobulin Technique

The direct antiglobulin technique is performed when an *in vivo* attachment of a red cell antibody to the individual's red cells has occurred. The *in vivo* attachment of antibody occurs in four disease states or conditions: hemolytic disease of the newborn, autoimmune hemolytic anemia, hemolytic transfusion reactions, and drugs binding to the red cell membrane. In any of these conditions, premature red cell destruction results in anemia. In hemolytic disease of the newborn (HDN), maternal IgG anti–red cell antibodies cross the placenta; and if the specific antigen is on the fetal red cells, the cells will be destroyed. Several red cell antibodies, such as anti-D, anti-A, and anti-B, cause HDN. In autoimmune hemolytic anemia, the individual produces antibodies to autologous red cells. Generally, in hemolytic transfusion reactions, the patient has produced antibodies to previously transfused red cell antigens. When the antigen is encountered again, antibody attaches to the cells. In drug reactions the drug attaches to the red cell membrane; antibodies to the drug may attach and initiate the destruction of the red cell.

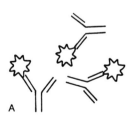

A

Antibody-coated antigen
without visible agglutination

(No lattice formation)

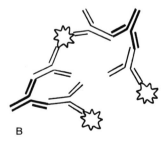

B

Anti-human globulin is added
which reacts with the antibody
on the antigen.

Visible agglutination occurs.

(Lattice formation)

FIGURE 12-4. (A) In some agglutination reactions the antigen–antibody complex will not form a lattice. (B) When anti–human globulin (AHG) is added, the AHG will react with the antibody on the surface of the particle and form a lattice. Agglutination will be observed.

Indirect Antiglobulin Technique

The indirect antiglobulin procedure is performed to detect red cell antigens, to detect red cell antibodies, or to determine compatibility. In these procedures, the red cells are incubated *in vitro* with serum to allow the antibody to bind to the antigen. After an incubation period of 10 to 60 minutes at 37°C, the red cells are washed with isotonic saline to remove any unbound antibody; anti–human immunoglobulin is added. If antigen–antibody binding occurred during incubation, agglutination will be observed after anti-human immunoglobulin is added.

Agglutination Inhibition Reaction

Sometimes the direct or passive agglutination procedure is not appropriate to detect the presence of an antigen. In these cases a two-step agglutination inhibition procedure may be used (Fig. 12-5). If red cells are used, the procedure is known as hemagglutination inhibition, and if latex particles are used, it is latex agglutination inhibition. In the first step, soluble antigen in the patient's sample is incubated with known antibody reagent. If the soluble antigen is present, the two will react, though the reaction is not visible. In the second step of the procedure, the particulate antigen, either a natural antigen or a red cell or latex particle with an antigen attached, is added. If the antigen was present in the patient sample, there is no free antibody to attach to the particulate antigen. This means that agglutination was inhibited and is a positive test result. If there was no antigen in the patient sample, antibody is available to agglutinate the particulate antigen and is a negative test result. Agglutination inhibition is used to detect human chorionic gonadotropin (hCG) in serum or

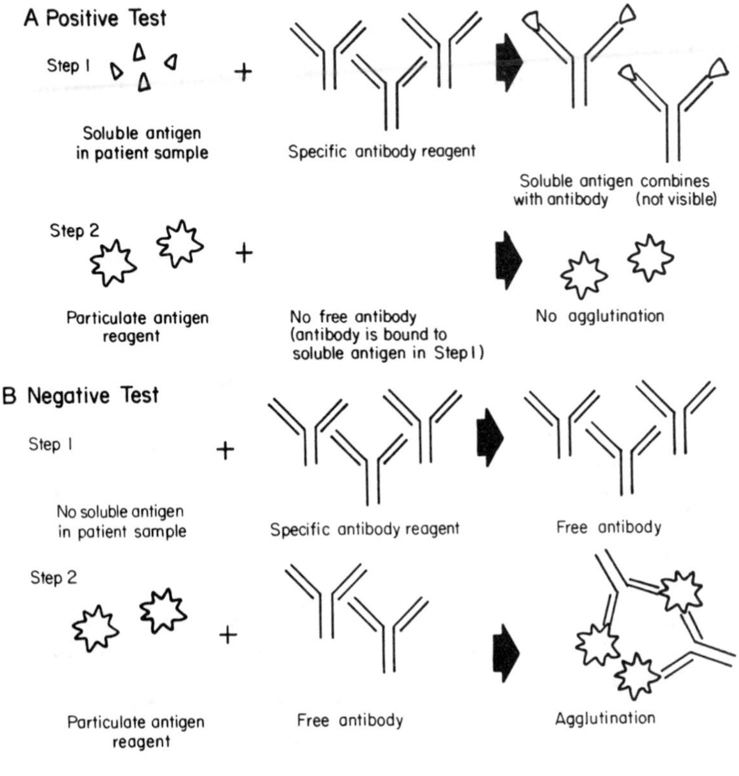

A Positive Test

Step 1

Soluble antigen in patient sample   +   Specific antibody reagent   Soluble antigen combines with antibody (not visible)

Step 2

Particulate antigen reagent   +   No free antibody (antibody is bound to soluble antigen in Step 1)   No agglutination

B Negative Test

Step 1

No soluble antigen in patient sample   +   Specific antibody reagent   Free antibody

Step 2

Particulate antigen reagent   +   Free antibody   Agglutination

FIGURE 12-5. (*A*) In a positive test for agglutination inhibition, soluble antigen in the patient sample combines with the specific antibody reagent in step 1 to form soluble antigen–antibody complexes that are not visible. In step 2, when particulate antigen reagent is added, there is no free antibody to react, so no agglutination occurs. (*B*) In a negative test, there is no antigen in the patient sample to react with the specific antibody reagent in step 1. In step 2, when particulate antigen reagent is added, the antibody from step 1 is free to react with the particulate antigen reagent to form a lattice. Agglutination will be observed.

urine and the presence of soluble A, B, and H substances in body fluids.

Slide tests to detect hCG are based on the principle of agglutination inhibition or hemagglutination inhibition. The hCG is adsorbed onto latex particles or red cells. In the first step, antibody to the β chain of the hCG is added to patient urine. If the urine contains hCG, there will be antigen–antibody attachment but no lattice is formed. In the second step, the carrier hCG is added. If hCG is present in the urine, agglutination will be inhibited because the antibody is bound in step 1. (No agglutination indicates a positive test result). If there is no hCG present in the urine, the anti-hCG will be able to bind to the hCG carrier and agglutination will be observed. (Agglutination indicates a negative test result.)

Detection of the soluble red cell antigens may be performed in the case of rape or other crimes. Eighty percent of the white population secretes A, B, or H substances in such body fluids as urine, saliva, and semen. In step 1, the body fluid is incubated with known anti-A, anti-B, or anti-H antibodies. In step 2, red cells with the corresponding antigen are added. If the soluble substance is present in the body fluid, agglutination is inhibited in step 2. If there is no soluble substance present, agglutination will be observed after the addition of the red cell antigens.

Sources of error in agglutination inhibition reactions include prozone and postzone reactions (false positive result), addition of the reagents in the incorrect order (false negative result), outdated or inactive reagents (false positive result), and incorrect incubation (false positive result). It is important that controls be used to identify sources of error, especially those caused by the reagent failure.

References

1. Nicols WS, Nakamura RM: Agglutination and agglutination inhibition. In Rose NR, Friedman H, Fahey JL (eds): Manual of Clinical Laboratory Immunology, 3rd ed, p 49. Washington, DC, American Society for Microbiology, 1986

2. Barrett JT: Textbook of Immunology, 5th ed, p 313. St. Louis, CV Mosby, 1988

3. Stansfield WD: Serology and Immunology: A Clinical Approach, p 168. New York, Macmillan, 1981

4. Stites DP, Rodgers MPC: Clinical laboratory methods for detection of antigens and antibodies. In Stites DP, Stobo JD, Wells JV (eds): Basic and Clinical Immunology, 6th ed, p 275. Norwalk, Appleton and Lange, 1987

5. Bryant NJ: Laboratory Immunology and Serology, 2nd ed, p 171. Philadelphia, WB Saunders, 1986

CHAPTER 13

Assays Involving Complement

Dorothy J. Fike

The complement system is a complex series of events that can lead to cell lysis. The components, pathways, control mechanisms, and deficiencies are discussed in Chapter 5. This chapter will discuss assays that measure complement proteins and pathway activity and assays that use complement as a reagent.

Evaluation of Complement

Complement components in patient serum can be quantitated immunologically when the component reacts with monospecific antiserum. The functional ability of the complement cascade can be measured by lysing red blood cells. Some complement components—C1q, C3, C4, and C5—are extremely labile, so that proper sample handling is critical. Prolonged exposure to heat will decrease complement activity and will produce different fragments of complement components. To preserve complement activity, blood should clot for 1 hour at room temperature, and the serum should be removed and stored at $-70°C$ in small aliquots.[1,2]

Functional Assays

The CH_{50} assay tests the functional capability of serum complement components of the classical pathway to lyse sheep red blood cells (SRBC) when these cells are coated with rabbit anti–sheep red blood cell antibody. When the antibody-coated (sensitized) SRBC are incubated with patient serum, the classical pathway of complement is activated and hemolysis results. If a complement component is absent, the CH_{50} level will be zero; if one or more components of the classical pathway are decreased, the CH_{50} will be decreased. The initial serum dilution of 1:50 or 1:60, depending on the specific method used, is serially

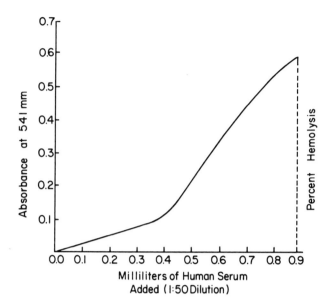

FIGURE 13-1. The CH_{50} absorbance curve. The absorbance of the hemolysis of various concentrations of a 1:50 serum dilution is read at 541 nm.

diluted.[1,2] A fixed volume of optimally sensitized SRBC is added to each serum dilution. After incubation, the mixture is centrifuged and the degree of hemolysis is quantitated by measuring the absorbance of the supernatant at 541 nm.

A typical sigmoid curve obtained can be seen in Figure 13-1. Since these results do not yield a straight line, the CH_{50} titer may be obtained graphically by plotting the reciprocal of the serum dilution versus the percent lysis on semilog graph paper or by using the von Krogh transformation (Fig. 13-2). The von Krogh transformation is a graphic representation of the log of milliliters of serum versus the log of $Y/(1 - Y)$, where Y is the percent hemolysis. When $Y/(1 - Y) = 1$, 50% of the SRBC are hemolyzed. The reciprocal of the corresponding volume of serum when $Y/(1 - Y)$ is the CH_{50} unit. The reference range of CH_{50} units varies with the method used in the laboratory. If the method described by Mayer is used, the reference range is 25 to 50 U/mL; but if the method of Kent and Fife is used, the reference range is 125 to 300 U/mL. Variation in these methods and reference ranges is due to the quantity of SRBC used, the concentration of SRBC, and the total vol-

ume of the test solution. The method of Mayer uses 1.0 mL of 5% SRBC suspension in a total volume of 7.5 mL, whereas the method of Kent and Fife uses 0.6 mL of a 1% SRBC suspension in a total volume of 1.5 mL. Regardless of the method used, each laboratory performing this test should establish its own reference range.[1]

The CH_{50} assay is a labor-intensive, demanding procedure subject to many interferences. Some SRBC are more fragile than others, resulting in spontaneous hemolysis that is unrelated to the complement activity. The affinity of the rabbit antibody varies from lot to lot and from one manufacturer to another; this affects the amount of antibody that binds to the SRBC. Also, the process of sensitizing SRBC with antibody results in cells with differing amounts of antibody coating the SRBC. Specimen collection and storage are an important potential source of error. To detect as many sources of error as possible, it is critical to test a control serum with a known CH_{50} value every time the assay is performed and to reproduce the accepted value of the known serum control.[1,2]

A second assay, the CH_{100} assay, can be used to

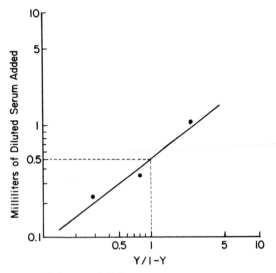

Y = **Corrected O.D.** (Correct with O.D. of tube with 100% lysis)

FIGURE 13-2. Since the CH_{50} cannot be calculated from the absorbance curve, a Von Krogh transformation must be plotted. Y is the corrected optical density as corrected with the optical density of the tube with 100% lysis.

assess the function of the classical pathway of complement. In this diffusion assay, sensitized SRBC are mixed with agar, and serum is placed in a well and allowed to diffuse. The complement in the serum will hemolyze the cells, producing a clear zone around the well. The diameter of the zone of hemolysis is measured and is proportional to the complement activity.[3]

The activity of the alternative or properdin pathway of complement may be measured by modifying the CH_{50} procedure. Rabbit red blood cells are capable of initiating the alternative complement pathway. When they replace the sensitized SRBC in the traditional CH_{50} assay, the degree of hemolysis indicates the functional ability of the alternative pathway. Antibody and C1q are not required for activation of this pathway.[1]

Complement Component Assays

All assays that measure individual specific complement components require specific antisera to react with the complement protein. Methodologies include radial immunodiffusion (RID), nephelometry, radioimmunoassay, and latex agglutination photometric immunoassay. Sample collection and handling are extremely important. Care must be taken to prevent activation of the complement cascade prior to the assay. In some cases, plasma is used instead of serum to assure that the classical pathway of complement is not activated during the coagulation of the blood.

All complement components (except Factor D) and two inhibitor proteins (C1 inhibitor and C3b inactivator) may be measured by RID. The agar gel contains the specific antibody for the complement protein to be measured. Patient serum or plasma is placed in the well and diffuses in all directions, producing a concentric precipitin ring. The reference range for some complement components is listed in Table 13-1.[4,5] Some investigators believe that all laboratories should establish their own reference range, since the variation between normal populations in

Table 13-1: Reference Range of Some Complement Components

Component	Reference Range
C1q	11–21 mg/dL
C3	80–180 mg/dL
C4	15–50 mg/dL
C5	7–17 mg/dL
Properdin	1.0–2.0 mg/dL
Factor B	17.5–27.5 mg/dL

different geographic areas is great.[1] The reference range for each complement component should reflect the normal mean of the area population. Commercial kits are available to measure the concentrations of C3, C4, and Factor B, the three complement components most commonly measured. Improper handling of the specimen may result in elevated values of C3 and C4. These two components are heat labile and are split into smaller fragments that diffuse faster than intact molecules. The antibody in the agar reacts with these fragments and produces a larger diameter of precipitation, thus falsely elevating the results.

Other methods to detect specific complement proteins are nephelometry, to detect all components of complement (including Factor D); latex agglutination photometric immunoassay, to detect C3 and C4; and radioimmunoassay, to detect C3a, C4a, and C5a. The assays to detect anaphylatoxin peptides are currently for research use only.

Complement Components in Disease

The most frequent observation in disease is an increase in C3 and C4 as well as the total hemolytic activity. C3 and C4 are acute phase reactants and will be increased during acute inflammation. This increase is associated with diseases listed in Table 13-2. In rheumatoid arthritis, systemic erythematosus and other rheumatic diseases, complement is increased in the acute phase of the disease and may be decreased when the disease process is consuming or activating complement *in vivo*. Other conditions in which complement levels are increased in an acute phase response are myocardial infarction, viral hepatitis, diabetes, and pregnancy. The increases are generally not more than twofold, which is less than the dramatic hundredfold increase of C-reactive protein.[1,7]

Table 13-2: Some Diseases Associated With Increased Complement Levels

AUTOIMMUNE DISORDERS	OTHER
Rheumatoid arthritis	Gout
Ulcerative colitis	Obstructive jaundice
Diabetes mellitus	Thyroiditis
Systemic lupus erythematosus	Acute myocardial infarction
	Pregnancy
	Oral contraceptives
INFECTIVE DISORDERS	
Acute rheumatic fever	
Typhoid fever	
Acute viral hepatitis	

Some diseases are associated with increased complement levels, including some autoimmune and infective disorders. Other conditions may also lead to an increase in complement levels.

In some diseases there is a decrease in the CH_{50} value, which may be due to a congenital component deficiency, *in vivo* consumption by antigen–antibody complexes, decreased synthesis of one or more components, increased catabolism of the components, or presence of an inhibitor (Table 13-3). Though the CH_{50} test assesses the overall function of the pathway, it is less sensitive than the immunologically based specific component assays. The immunologic measurement of individual components better reflects changes in the serum concentration. Slight decreases in the CH_{50} value have been associated with a reduction of up to 50% in the C1, C2, or C3 levels.[7]

Complement deficiencies are rare; however, they provide a means to study and understand the function of the component. In general, deficiency of a specific component causes an autoimmune disease,

Table 13-3: Some Diseases Associated With Decreased CH$_{50}$ Levels

AUTOIMMUNE DISEASES

Systemic lupus erythematosus with glomerulonephritis

Myasthenia gravis

IMMUNE DEFICIENCY DISORDERS

Severe combined immunodeficiency

Hereditary angioedema (C1INH deficiency)

Hereditary C2 deficiency

INFECTIVE DISORDERS

Acute glomerulonephritis

Infected ventriculoarterial shunts

Infective hepatitis with arthritis

OTHER

Disseminated intravascular coagulation (DIC)

Paroxysmal cold hemoglobinuria

Allograft rejection

Diseases associated with decreased CH$_{50}$ levels may be found in autoimmune disorders, immune deficiency disorders, and infective disorders. Besides these disorders, other conditions may lead to the decrease in CH$_{50}$ levels.

increased infections, or both. Most important, a deficiency of C1 inhibitor (C1INH) causes hereditary angioedema.[2,7] These individuals have repeated, potentially life-threatening episodes of edema, especially of the skin, upper respiratory tract, and gastrointestinal tract.[1]

Decreased serum levels of complement components, other than a deficiency, may be due to hypo-synthesis. Many complement components are synthesized in the liver, so that in severe liver disease, complement production is decreased. Likewise, in protein calorie malnutrition, such as that seen in anorexia nervosa, complement production is decreased.[1]

Hypercatabolism is associated with diseases that have circulating immune complexes, such as systemic lupus erythematosus, acute glomerulonephritis, malaria, rheumatoid arthritis, and pneumococcal infections. Both C3 and C4 are decreased because the classical pathway is activated by immune complexes. C4 levels may be reduced first, followed by a decrease in C3 levels; this pattern occurs most frequently in systemic lupus erythematosus. In systemic lupus erythematosus, complement component levels are decreased when immune complex–mediated renal disease is prominent, whereas in rheumatoid arthritis, the component levels are decreased when immune complex–mediated vasculitis is present. The serum levels of C3 and C4 may also be normal or increased in rheumatoid arthritis, but the synovial fluid level is decreased (Table 13-4).[1,2,4]

Decreased levels of C3 are also found in diseases that activate the alternative pathway of complement, such as membranoproliferative glomerulonephritis, paroxysmal nocturnal hemoglobinuria, and circulating endotoxin. The C4 levels are normal, since this component is not activated in the alternative pathway. Some diseases can activate both cascades, thereby decreasing both C3 and C4. To distinguish activation of the classical and alternative pathways from activation of the classical pathway only, Factor B should be measured. Factor B will be decreased if the alternative pathway is activated and will be normal if only the classical pathway is activated.[1,2,4]

Two conditions deserve special consideration of the complement levels. In disseminated intravascular coagulation, the decreased concentration of C3 is due to the catabolism of C3 by enzymes involved in clot fibrinolysis. The C4 levels are unaffected. Sepsis, trauma, surgery, and neoplasms may cause dissemi-

Table 13-4: Diseases Associated With Decreased Levels of Complement Components

Disease	C3 Level	C4 Level
CLASSICAL PATHWAY ACTIVATION WITH CIRCULATING IMMUNE COMPLEXES	D	D
Systemic lupus erythematosus		
Glomerulonephritis		
Rheumatoid arthritis		
Pneumococcal infections		
Malaria		
ALTERNATIVE PATHWAY ACTIVATION OF C3	D	N
Membranoproliferative glomerulonephritis		
Paroxysmal nocturnal hemoglobinuria		
Circulating endotoxins		
OVERT IMMUNOLOGIC ACTIVATION: BOTH PATHWAYS ACTIVATED	D	D
TISSUE INJURY: C3 CLEAVAGE BY PROTEOLYTIC ENZYMES	D	N
Disseminated intravascular coagulation		
HEREDITARY ANGIOEDEMA (C1 INHIBITOR DEFICIENCY)	N	D

A decrease in C3 and C4 may be found in certain diseases. This may be associated with the classical pathway activation, alternative pathway activation, or both. N indicates that the level of the component is normal; D indicates a decreased concentration.

nated intravascular coagulation. A deficiency of C1 inhibitor (C1INH), either inherited or acquired, may cause a decrease in the C4 concentration.[1,4] In normal individuals, once the classical cascade is activated, activated C1 cleaves C4 into C4a and C4b until activated C1 is inactivated by the regulatory protein, C1INH. A deficiency of C1INH prevents inactivation of C1. In the inherited form of C1INH deficiency, the concentration of C4 is low even when the patient is asymptomatic and may become undetectable during an acute episode. The acquired form of C1INH deficiency may develop in lymphoid malignancies and autoimmune disease when the regulatory protein is consumed or destroyed. In either inherited or acquired C1INH, the C3 levels are normal.

Complement Fixation

In the complement fixation technique the test system and indicator system compete for the binding of complement. If complement is bound (fixed) by the antigen–antibody complex formed in the test system, complement will not be available to react in the indicator system. If no antigen–antibody complex is formed in the test system, complement will be available to bind to the antigen–antibody complex in the indicator system. The complement fixation techniques can be useful in viral, rickettsial, and fungal serology. Some diseases that may be diagnosed by complement fixation are Rocky Mountain spotted fever, *Herpes simplex* infection, and influenza. Prior to the development of radioimmunoassays and enzyme immunoassays, complement fixation procedures were the most sensitive available.

Before performing this technique, the complement present in the patient sample must be inactivated by heating at 56°C for 30 minutes. This critical step ensures that only the fresh guinea pig complement is available to participate in the complement fixation test.

A Identification of Unknown Antigen

Step 1   Patient sample + Known antibody + Guinea pig complement
(antigen)
→ incubate

Step 2   Add sheep red blood cells coated with hemolysin
→ incubate

Step 3   Read for hemolysis

B Identification of Unknown Antibody

Step 1   Patient sample + Known antigen + Guinea pig complement
(antibody)
→ incubate

Step 2   Add sheep red blood cells coated with hemolysin
→ incubate

Step 3   Read for hemolysis

FIGURE 13-3. (*A*) Complement fixation procedures may be used to detect the presence of unknown antigen in patient serum. In step 1 a known antibody is incubated with the patient sample. (*B*) Unknown antibody may also be detected. In step 1 a known antigen is incubated with the patient sample. For both techniques, steps 2 and 3 are identical.

The complement fixation technique may be used to detect an unknown antigen or an unknown antibody in the patient sample. As seen in Figure 13-3, the procedure for antibody detection requires two steps. The first step, the test system, is the incubation of the test antigen with patient serum or control serum with fresh guinea pig complement. If the serum contains the homologous antibody, it will bind to the test antigen. Complement will then bind to the antigen–antibody complex. The second step is the incubation of the test mixture with the indicator system, sensitized sheep red blood cells (SRBC). The extent of hemolysis is measured. To prepare sensitized SRBC, the SRBC are incubated with an anti–sheep red blood cell antibody that causes hemolysis of the red cell in the presence of complement. This antibody is referred to as hemolysin or amboceptor.

If there is no hemolysis, the serum contains the antibody. As shown in Figure 13-4*A*, an antigen–

A Positive Reaction

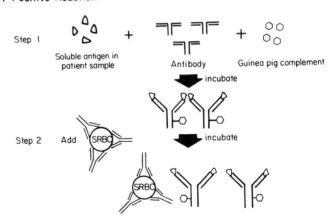

Step 1   Soluble antigen in patient sample   +   Antibody   +   Guinea pig complement
→ incubate

Step 2   Add SRBC
→ incubate

Step 3   No hemolysis

FIGURE 13-4. (*A*) A positive result is shown. An antigen–antibody reaction has occurred in step 1 and guinea pig complement binds to this complex. There is no free complement to bind with the anti–sheep red cell antibody in step 2. No hemolysis will be observed. (*B*) and (*C*) There is no antigen (*B*) or antibody (*C*) present in the patient sample. There is no antigen–antibody complex formed in step 1, so complement is free to bind with the anti–sheep red blood cell antibody added in step 2. Hemolysis will occur.

B Negative Reaction for Unknown Antigen

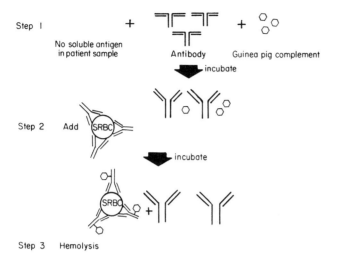

Step 1

No soluble antigen in patient sample

Antibody

Guinea pig complement

incubate

Step 2   Add   SRBC

incubate

Step 3   Hemolysis

C Negative Reaction for Unknown Antibody

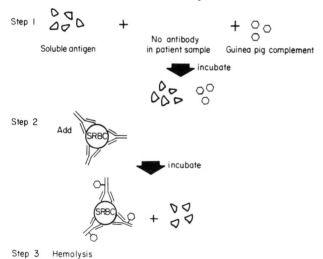

Step 1

Soluble antigen

No antibody in patient sample

Guinea pig complement

incubate

Step 2   Add   SRBC

incubate

Step 3   Hemolysis

Figure 13-4 (*continued*)

antibody complex is formed in the test system (step 1) and guinea pig complement is activated. In this step the complex formation and complement activation are not visible. The indicator step is used to detect unreacted complement. In this case there is no unreacted complement and no hemolysis occurs.

If hemolysis is observed, the serum does not contain the antibody. As shown in Figure 13-4*B*, no serum antibody is present, so no antigen–antibody complex is formed. Therefore, the guinea pig complement is not fixed. When the sensitized SRBC are added, complement is available to react with the sensitized SRBC. The complement cascade is activated, resulting in visible hemolysis.

The complement fixation test can be modified to detect antigen in the patient sample, as shown in

Figure 13-4C. In this case a known antibody would be used in the test system to complex with the antigen to be detected. The indicator system is the same as that described earlier. No hemolysis indicates the presence of the antigen, and hemolysis indicates the absence of the antigen.

Some reagents are tested prior to the complement fixation procedure and are additionally controlled during the complement fixation test. The SRBC are washed prior to use, and the supernatant from the second wash is examined for visible hemolysis. If hemolysis is present, the cells are fragile and should be discarded. A new lot of cells should be washed and used. Prior to sensitization of the SRBC, the hemolysin is titered to determine the optimal concentration of antibody. Complement is also titered prior to use; generally, a 1:400 dilution is sufficient to produce adequate hemolysis. The antigen or antibody reagent is also titered to obtain its optimal concentration to use in the test system.

The complement fixation technique is a titration procedure with many controls. In the clinical laboratory the procedure is usually performed in a microtiter tray, as shown in Figure 13-5. Controls to be run include a known positive serum, a known nega-tive serum, antigen control, patient serum control, cell control, and complement control. These controls are used to detect the instability of complement, the variability of sheep red blood cells, the immunochemical variation of hemolysin, and the narrow optimal range of diluent components.[8]

In the complement fixation assay both positive and negative serum controls are titered in parallel with the patient serum, and the titer produced must be within the acceptable limit. If the titer is unacceptable, the results of the patient are invalid. The cell control is a mixture of sensitized SRBC and buffer incubated under test conditions. To be acceptable, no hemolysis should be seen. Hemolysis would invalidate the complement fixation assay and is most likely due to fragile cells. The complement or hemolytic control contains all reagents except the patient serum. It is used to indicate the ability of the complement to function by lysing the sensitized SRBC. Total hemolysis is expected.[8]

The serum control is the test system (without the test antigen) and the indicator system. It is a check on the ability of the patient serum to bind complement nonspecifically or to inhibit complement activity in the absence of the test antigen. It should show

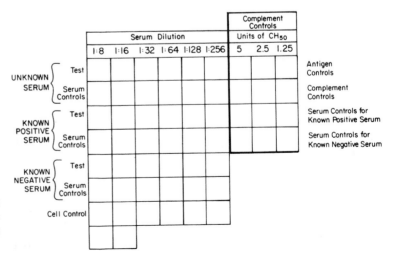

FIGURE 13-5. The complement fixation technique is performed using a microtiter plate. Serum dilutions are performed on the unknown sample, known positive serum, and known negative serum. Cell controls, complement controls, and antigen controls are also performed.

hemolysis. When it does not, it is anticomplementary; the complement appears to be neutralized by the patient serum.

The antigen control is the test system without the patient serum and the indicator system. It is used to determine if the test antigen can nonspecifically bind complement or to inhibit the complement activity. It should show hemolysis. If it shows no or little hemolysis, it is anticomplementary; the complement appears to be neutralized by the test antigen.

False positive reactions occur if the serum control or antigen control are anticomplementary, if the complement is inactive, if the antigen of antibody is not added to the test system, or if the patient serum is too concentrated. A summary of the sources of error is presented in Table 13-5.

False negatives may occur if the sheep cells are fragile, if the SRBC are mechanically damaged, or if the patient serum is incompletely heat inactivated prior to testing. In the latter situation more comple-

ment will be present: the patient's complement plus the guinea pig complement. The extra complement may react with the sensitized SRBC, thus causing a falsely negative result. If the patient serum is too dilute, a false negative may occur.

Conclusion

Complement components and functional activity can be measured in patient samples; decreased levels are an indication of *in vivo* activation, *in vitro* activation during coagulation, or a component deficiency. Specific assays are used to pinpoint the pathway or component that is decreased in activity or concentration. CH_{50} and CH_{100} assays are functional assays to evaluate the ability of the classical pathway to lyse sensitized sheep red blood cells. When rabbit red blood cells are used in the modified CH_{50} assay, it evaluates the ability of the alternative pathway to be activated. Individual components are quantitated by immunologic methods.

Complement can be used as a reagent in the complement fixation technique. Most often, patient serum antibody reacts with a known antigen, forming a complex that is capable of fixing guinea pig complement. When the indicator (sensitized sheep red blood cells) is added, unreacted complement can lyse the sensitized sheep red blood cells. This sensitive assay has largely been replaced by other assays that have comparable or better sensitivity but are easier to perform.

Table 13-5: Sources of Error in Complement Fixation Tests

FALSE POSITIVE (NO OR DECREASED LYSIS)

Inactive complement

Patient serum insufficiently diluted

Anti–complementary components in patient serum

Anti–complementary antigen

FALSE NEGATIVE

Fragile sheep red cells

Failure to heat-inactivate the serum

Failure to add antigen or antibody

Patient serum diluted too much

Sources of error may yield either false positive or false negative reactions.

References

1. Ruddy S: Complement. In Rose NR, Friedman H, Fahey JL (eds): Manual of Clinical Laboratory Immunology, 3rd ed, p 175. Washington, DC, American Society for Microbiology, 1986

2. Gaither TA, Frank MM: Complement. In Henry JB (ed): Clinical Diagnosis and Management by Laboratory Methods, 17th ed, p 879. Philadelphia, WB Saunders, 1984

3. Lint TF: Laboratory detection of complement activation and complement deficiencies. Am J Med Technol 48:743, 1982

4. Luskin AT, Tobin MC: Alterations of complement components in disease. Am J Med Technol 48:749, 1982

5. Satoh P, Yonker TC, Kane DP, et al: Measurement of anaphylatoxins: An index for activation of complement cascade. BioTechniques 1:90, 1983

6. Stites DP, Rodgers RPC: Clinical methods for detection of antigens and antibodies. In Stites DP, Stobo JD, Wells JV (eds): Basic and Clinical Immunology, 6th ed, p 277. Norwalk, Appleton and Lange, 1987

7. Frank MM: Complement in the pathophysiology of human disease. N Engl J Med 316:1525, 1987

8. Palmer DF, Whaley SD: Complement fixation test. In Rose NR, Friedman H, Fahey JL (eds): Manual of Clinical Laboratory Immunology, 3rd ed, p 57. Washington, DC, American Society for Microbiology, 1986

CHAPTER 14

Immunofluorescence

Catherine Sheehan
Ann C. Albers

Immunofluorescence combines immunologic methods and histochemical methods to demonstrate the presence of an antigen or an antibody in tissue, in serum, or on an organism. There are two types of fluorescent antibody techniques, the direct and indirect. In the direct method the homologous antibody is conjugated (labeled or tagged) with a fluorochrome (fluorescent dye) and the labeled antibody is allowed to react with a test antigen. In the indirect method, the test antigen is allowed to react with unlabeled antibody, and subsequently the antigen–antibody complex is layered with conjugated antiglobulin that is species specific. The fluorescent antigen–antibody (or antigen–antibody–antibody) complex is rendered fluorescent when the specimen is illuminated with excitation light, which, when it strikes the fluorochrome, produces light emission of a longer wavelength (in the visible spectrum).

The immunofluorescence assay is both sensitive and reliable. Minute concentrations of antibodies and of soluble protein antigens can be detected. Soluble protein antigens or antibodies can be detected in concentrations of 10^{-4}/mL.[1] Moreover, insoluble antigens in tissues can be tested for directly by using immunofluorescence.

Fluorescence

Molecules capable of absorbing electromagnetic radiation or light energy become excited, altering the electron configuration of that molecule. The absorbed energy is dissipated, usually in the form of heat; however, some molecules emit a photon of light as it reverts to the stable ground state. This is luminescence.[2,3]

There are two types of luminescence, fluorescence and phosphorescence. In fluorescence the length of time between excitation and emission of light energy is short ($\leq 10^{-8}$ seconds). In phosphorescence the

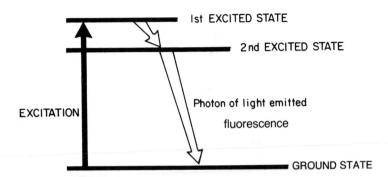

FIGURE 14-1. The movement of an electron that produces fluorescence.

length of time is longer ($>10^{-4}$ seconds). The light energy is emitted in all directions, regardless of the direction of the excitation light.

Fluorescence occurs when a molecule absorbs light energy, causing an electron to move from a stable ground state to an excited state by moving the electron from one orbital to another. Some energy will be lost as heat as the electron shifts to a second excited state, one with lesser energy. Finally, as the electron returns to its original orbital, the ground state, a photon of light is emitted. This is fluorescence (Fig. 14-1). The amount of energy emitted is always less than the amount of excitation energy; hence, the wavelength of the emitted light is always longer than the wavelength of the excitation light (Fig. 14-2).

Though a fluorescent label may be called a fluorochrome, fluorophore, or fluor, in immunofluorescence, the term *fluorochrome* is used. In general, the fluorochrome is attached to a specific antibody to be used in an immunofluorescence assay. The fluorochrome labels the antibody reagent so that the presence of the antibody reagent can be visualized. When an antibody is labeled or conjugated with a fluorochrome, it is called a conjugate. The most commonly used fluorochromes are fluorescein, rhodamine, acridine, and phycoerythrin.

Methods

Two major types of immunofluorescence methods are commonly performed in clinical immunology: the

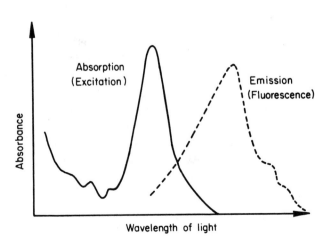

FIGURE 14-2. Absorption and emission spectra of a fluorescent compound.

direct immunofluorescence (DIF) and indirect immunofluorescence (IIF). DIF is used to detect an antigen that is part of the tissue, cell, or microorganism. IIF is used to detect circulating antibody in a patient sample.

Direct Immunofluorescence

The antigen (tissue biopsy, bacterial suspension, or cell suspension) is fixed onto a microscope slide. A conjugate specific for the antigen is overlaid onto the antigen. The labeled antibody will bind to the antigen. Excess conjugated antiserum is washed off. A coverslip is mounted onto the slide with buffered glycerol, and the preparation is examined for specific fluorescence using a fluorescence microscope. This method is used to detect organisms (viral, fungal, or parasitic) in host tissue, to detect lymphocyte surface markers, and to detect immune complexes in tissue biopsies (most commonly in skin and kidney biopsies) (Fig. 14-3).

Indirect Immunofluorescence

Indirect immunofluorescence is a two-stage test. In the first stage unlabeled antibody from a patient sample reacts with an antigen fixed onto a slide. This antigen expresses known epitopes and may be called the substrate. After washing away the unreacted protein in the patient sample, the antigen–antibody complex (antigen in the substrate and antibody from the patient sample) is exposed to a labeled antiglobulin serum. The slide is washed to remove excess conjugate, a coverslip is mounted with buffered glycerol, and the preparation is viewed for a specific pattern of fluorescence using a fluorescent microscope. A specific, known antigen (or substrate) is used to capture an antibody from a patient sample that is visualized by a fluorochrome-labeled antibody. This method is used to detect serum antibody to bacterial organisms and to autologous tissue antigens (Fig. 14-4).

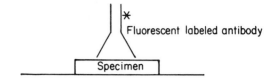

FIGURE 14-3. Schematic of direct immunofluorescence.

Fluorochromes

Fluorochromes are organic dyes that fluoresce when exposed to short-wavelength light energy. Each has an excitation spectrum in which there is one wavelength that optimally excites the fluorochrome. The emission spectrum of each fluorochrome identifies the wavelength at which maximum fluorescence is emitted. To assure that the optimal excitation wavelength interacts with the fluorochrome and that the optimal emission wavelength is viewed, filters are employed in the fluorescence microscope. The filters must be matched for the fluorochrome used.

Fluorescein is the most commonly used of the fluorochromes in immunofluorescence (Fig. 14-5). To increase its ability to label antibody molecules, the more reactive fluorescein derivative, fluorescein isothiocyanate (FITC), is used. The molar fluorescein-to-protein ratio (F/P ratio) is an indication of the relative number of fluorescein molecules per antibody molecule. This molar ratio compares to a weight ratio by a factor of approximately 0.6 (*i.e.,* a molar ratio of 5 will have substantially more activity

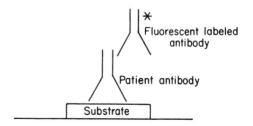

FIGURE 14-4. Schematic of indirect immunofluorescence.

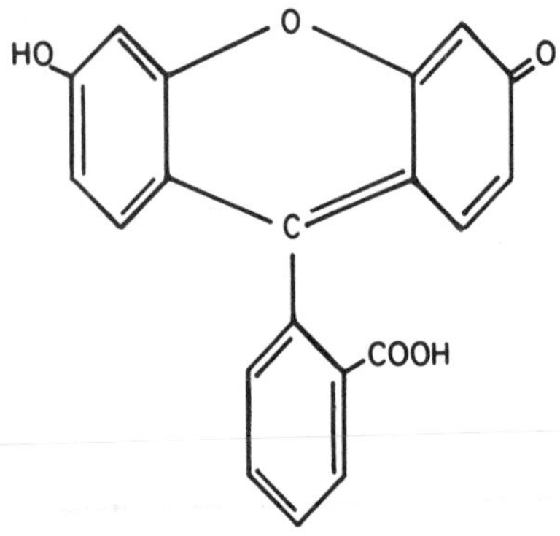

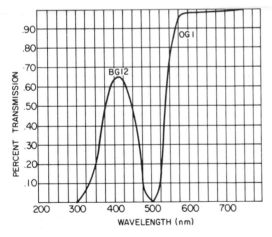

FIGURE 14-5. Structure of fluorescein.

than a weight ratio of 5). In IIF the molar ratio should be between 1 and 6, although the usual ratio is between 2 and 4.[1,4,5] If this ratio is too high, the conjugate will bind nonspecifically to the tissue or substrate, causing nonspecific fluorescence that may be difficult or impossible to distinguish from the desired specific fluorescence. If the ratio is too low,

FIGURE 14-6. An example of a filter system that can be used with fluorescein. The BG 12 filter is the excitation filter, which allows the optimal excitation wavelength (490–495 nm) to be transmitted to the specimen. The OG 1 filter is the barrier filter, which can transmit the emission wavelength of fluorescein (520 nm) and does not transmit the excitation wavelength.

specific staining will be diminished, causing decreased antibody titers or false negative results.

The conjugated antibody must contain sufficient antibody to ensure acceptable sensitivity. In DIF the conjugate should contain approximately 100 to 200 μg antibody/mL. In IIF the concentration of conjugate should be 25 to 50 μg antibody/mL.[1]

Fluorescence Microscope

A fluorescence microscope creates a darkfield and then, using special components, produces the proper conditions for separating excitation and emission wavelengths. The special components are the light source, the excitation filter, and the barrier filter.

Light sources for fluorescence microscopes must emit light rich in the wavelength necessary for excitation of the fluorochrome. The two common light sources are tungsten halogen lamp and mercury vapor arc lamp. The tungsten halogen lamp produces a continuous spectrum, has a short life-span (about 30 hours), maintains its intensity until it burns out, and can be used in a standard lamp housing. The mercury vapor arc lamp produces a discrete spectrum, has a long life-span (about 200 hours), loses intensity with the lamp age, and requires a special protective lamp housing. When the fluorochrome is fluorescein, the mercury vapor arc lamp produces a more intense light emission at 577 nm compared with the tungsten halogen lamp, thereby producing stronger fluorescence.

The excitation or primary filter is placed between the light source and the specimen and allows the wavelength of light that can be absorbed by the fluorochrome to reach the specimen and removes undesired wavelengths of light. The barrier or secondary filter is placed between the specimen and the ocular lens. It allows the light emitted from the specimen to pass through the filter while preventing undesired wavelengths from passing. Most commonly, these filters are glass (Fig. 14-6).

There are two configurations for fluorescence microscopes: transmitted light microscope and epifluorescence microscope. In the transmitted light fluorescence microscope, the light travels from the light source through the excitation filter through a dark-field condenser through the specimen. The light emitted from the specimen passes through the barrier filter to the ocular lens to be viewed by the observer. Because the light beam is transmitted from below and then passes through the specimen, some of the light is diffused, thereby decreasing the fluorescence (Fig. 14-7).

The epifluorescence microscope, described by Ploem in 1967, employs vertical illumination and a dichroic mirror. In this system light travels from the light source through the excitation filter and is reflected by the dichroic mirror at a 45° angle to pass through the objective (which serves as the condenser) to the surface of the specimen. The fluorescence emitted from the specimen enters the objective and passes through the dichroic mirror and the barrier filter to the ocular lens. The dichroic mirror is an interference filter that allows specific wavelengths of light to be reflected (the excitation light) and other

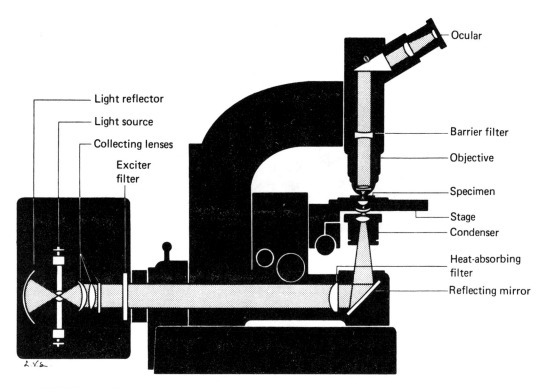

FIGURE 14-7. Fluorescence microscope with transmitted light. Light beam is generated by a mercury vapor lamp, reflected by a concave mirror, and projected through collecting lenses to the exciter filter, which emits a fluorescent light beam. A reflecting mirror directs the beam from underneath the stage, through the condenser into the specimen. A barrier filter removes wavelengths other than those emitted from the fluorescent compound in the specimen, and the fluorescent pattern is viewed through magnification provided by the objective and ocular lenses. (Reproduced with permission from Stites DP, Stobo JD, Wells JV: Basic and Clinical Immunology, 6th ed. Copyright Appleton and Lange, 1987.)

wavelengths of light to be transmitted (the emitted light). Because the excitation light is passed down through the objective and stops on the specimen, a darkfield is created. Also, since the excitation light travels down, it does not interfere when the specimen is viewed; thus, the fluorescence is more distinct. The filter systems are easily changed, so that viewing more than one fluorochrome is a simple change. Epi-illumination may be combined with transmitted light from brightfield or phase contrast microscopes (Fig. 14-8).

The objectives in fluorescence microscopy must be nonfluorescent and should have the highest numerical aperture (N.A.) possible. The higher the N.A. of an objective lens, the greater the light-gathering capability of the objective; therefore, the fluorescence is brighter. The immersion oil must be nonfluorescing.

In immunofluorescence the mounting medium must be water-soluble. When the fluorochrome is fluorescein, most often buffered glycerol is used (nine parts glycerol to one part of 0.2 M carbonate

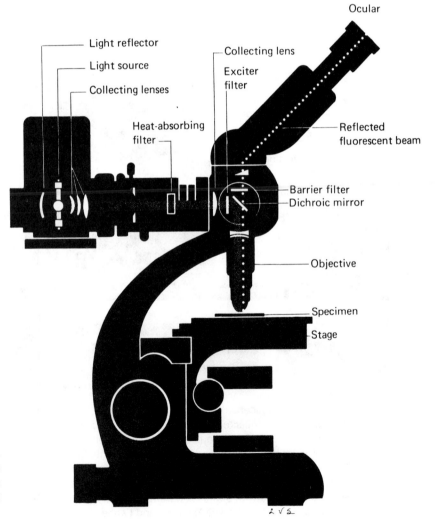

FIGURE 14-8. Fluorescence microscope with epi-illumination. The light beam is directed through the exciter filter and down onto the specimen. A dichroic mirror allows passage of selected wavelengths in one direction but not another. After reaching the specimen, the light is reflected through the dichroic mirror and emitted fluorescent light is visualized at the ocular. (Reproduced with permission from Stites DP, Stobo JD, Wells JV: Basic and Clinical Immunology, 6th ed. Copyright Appleton and Lange, 1987.)

buffer, pH 9.0).[6] The pH should be above 8 to enhance fluorescence and retard fading on exposure to ultraviolet light.[7] Stored buffered glycerol mounting medium may absorb CO_2, resulting in a decrease in pH.

Standardization

Types of Fluorescence

Specific staining (both desired and undesired) is the result of an immunologic reaction between the conjugate and the antigen. Undesired specific staining may be due to a cross-reaction with a heterologous antigen or an impure antibody preparation. Nonspecific staining is a nonimmunologic interaction of the conjugate with the antigen. This may be due to the presence of free (unconjugated) fluorochrome or of labeled serum protein other than immunoglobulin (such as globulin), or it may result when the specimen dries out during the staining procedure. Nonspecific staining can be decreased or eliminated by appropriate dilution of the conjugate and by control of the reaction time and temperatures.

Autofluorescence is the natural fluorescence of tissue or substrate. The color of autofluorescence depends on the filter system used and ranges from blue to blue-green to yellow to red. Proper filter selection allows sufficient contrast between autofluorescence and specific fluorescence. Autofluorescence is increased by formalin fixation, embedding in paraffin, and long storage time.

Optimal Conjugate Dilution

To determine the proper dilution of conjugated antiserum to be used in a particular IIF test, a chessboard titration must be performed. For this titration, slides containing the appropriate substrate are incubated with serial dilutions of a known positive control serum and are then tested with a serial dilution of the conjugate. The performance of conjugate will be constant for several conjugate dilutions for a specific control serum dilution (the plateau titer) and is related to the F/P ratio. One twofold dilution less than the highest conjugate dilution (plateau endpoint) to generate this constant fluorescence is the optimal dilution of conjugate to be used in the assay.

Control Serum

Positive control serum and negative control serum must be run in every IIF assay and should produce the proper specific fluorescence pattern. In antinuclear antibody testing, a World Health Organization 66/233 Reference Preparation provides a standard preparation to which a fluorescent pattern and intensity can be referenced for the homogeneous pattern.

References

1. Kwapinski G: The Methodology of Investigative and Clinical Immunology, p 245. Malabar, Robert E. Krieger Publishing Co., 1982
2. Huth JA: Fluorometry and fluorescence polarization. In Hicks MR, Haven MC, Schenken JR, et al (eds): Laboratory Instrumentation, 3rd ed, p 87. Philadelphia, JB Lippincott, 1987
3. Skoog DA, West DM: Fundamentals of Analytical Chemistry, 2nd ed, p 638. New York, Holt, Rinehart and Winston, 1969
4. Cavallaro JJ, Palmer DF, Bigazzi PE: Immunofluorescence Detection of Autoimmune Diseases, p 128. Atlanta, US Dept Health Education and Welfare, 1976
5. Nakamura RM, Tucker ES: Antibody as reagent. In Henry JB (ed): Clinical Diagnosis and Management by Laboratory Methods, 17th ed, p 908. Philadelphia, WB Saunders, 1984
6. Batty I: Standardization of reagents and methodology in immunology. In Rose NR, Friedman H, Fahey JL (eds): Manual of Clinical Laboratory Immunology, 3rd ed, p 957. Washington, DC, American Society for Microbiology, 1986
7. Narin RC: Standardization in immunofluorescence. Clin Exp Immunol 3:465, 1968

CHAPTER 15

Ligand Assays

Catherine Sheehan

The term *ligand*, derived from the Latin term *ligare*, meaning "to bind," refers to any substance that will complex to another molecule. In practical terms, the ligand is the substance to be measured in a ligand assay. The ligand could be an antigen combining with an antibody, a hormone with a transport protein, or a drug with an antibody. In a ligand assay one reactant is labeled so that the amount of binding can be monitored. Assays are named according to the attached label: Radioimmunoassay uses a radiolabel, enzyme immunoassay uses an enzyme label, chemiluminescent assay uses a light-emitting label, and fluorescence immunoassay uses a fluorescent label. The various methods use either monoclonal antibodies, polyclonal antibodies, or binding proteins to capture the ligand, and they can be qualitative or quantitative. Reactions may be designed to occur in the soluble or solid phase. Some methods require a step to separate the free labeled reactant from the bound labeled reactant; other methods do not. These vari-

ables in methodology contribute to diversity of assays currently performed in the clinical laboratory.

This chapter introduces the concepts of ligand assay, defines terminology, describes available methods, discusses commonly used labels, and cites examples of assays.

General Considerations

A ligand is a substance that combines with a specific binding reagent. The general reaction can be summarized as

Ligand + binding reagent $\rightleftharpoons$

ligand–binding reagent complex

To measure the amount of complex that is formed, either the ligand or the binding reagent must be labeled. The earliest assays used a labeled ligand known as the tracer. Examples of ligands are hormones (T_4, cortisol, thyroid stimulating hormone, human chorionic gonadotropin), drugs (digoxin, theophylline, gentamycin), autoantigens (DNA, thyroglobulin), infectious agents (hepatitis B surface antigen, chlamydia), antibodies (directed against rubella, human immunodeficiency virus), and tumor markers (alpha fetoprotein, carcinoembryonic antigen).

Binding reagents must have a specific configuration to bind to a ligand. These reagents can be receptors, binding proteins, or antibodies, as listed in Table 15-1. If the binding reagent is a receptor, the test is a receptor assay. Receptors may be located in the nucleus or cytoplasm or on the surface membrane of cells. For example, one receptor assay uses labeled progesterone to identify cytoplasmic receptors for progesterone in tumor cells, whereas another assay uses corpus luteum membrane receptors to quantitate human chorionic gonadotropin.

The second type of binding reagent is binding protein. These are naturally occurring transport proteins. Examples include transcortin (a binding protein for cortisol), sex hormone binding globulin (for testosterone and estrogen), and thyroid binding globulin (for T_3 and T_4).

The third and most commonly used binding reagent is an antibody; when used as the binding reagent, the test is an immunoassay. The ability to produce polyclonal or monoclonal antibodies commercially, each with a well-defined specificity and affinity, has expanded the number and diversity of analytes quantitated by immunoassay.

The amount of ligand that binds to the binding reagent is related to the capacity and affinity of the binding reagent. The capacity of the binding reagent is the number of available binding sites. The affinity of the binding reagent is the strength of binding with the ligand and equals the sum of the forces of attraction between the ligand and binding reagent. These forces include hydrogen binding, ionic forces, and Van der Waal's forces. (For further discussion of these forces, consult Chapter 10.) At equilibrium, the rate of the forward reaction (k_1) equals the rate of the reverse reaction (k_2), so that the proportion of free and bound ligand is constant.

$$\textbf{Free} \text{ ligand} + \text{binding reagent} \underset{k_2}{\overset{k_1}{\rightleftharpoons}} \textbf{Bound} \text{ ligand}$$
$$\text{(L)} \qquad\qquad \text{(BR)} \qquad\qquad \text{(L-BR)}$$

Table 15-1: Types of Ligand Assays

Assay	Binding Reagent	Typical K_A (in L/mole)	Examples
Receptor	Receptor	10^8–10^{11}	Human chorionic gonadotropin Progesterone receptors Estrogen receptors
Protein binding	Binding proteins	10^7–10^8	T_3, T_4 Cortisol Testosterone Estrogen
Immunoassay	Antibody	10^9–10^{11}	Rubella virus Rubella antibody Human chorionic gonadotropin

This binding obeys the law of mass action and can be expressed mathematically as:

$$\frac{[\text{L-BR}]}{[\text{L}][\text{BR}]} = \frac{k_1}{k_2} = K_a = \text{affinity constant}$$

K_a is the affinity or equilibrium constant and represents the reciprocal of free ligand concentration when 50% of the binding sites of the binding reagent are occupied. The affinity constant is expressed in L/mole or moles/L^{-1}. The greater the affinity of the ligand for the binding protein, the smaller the concentration of ligand required to achieve 50% saturation. For example, if the affinity constant of binding reagent A is 3×10^{11} L/mole, it means that a ligand concentration of 3×10^{-11} moles/L is needed to occupy half of the binding sites, and if the affinity constant of binding reagent B is 3×10^9 L/mole, a ligand concentration of 3×10^{-9} moles/L would saturate 50% of the available binding sites. The affinity of binding reagent A for the ligand is 100 times greater than the affinity of binding reagent B for the ligand. Typically, the affinity constants for antibodies used in radioimmunoassay procedures range from 10^9 to 10^{11} L/mole, whereas the affinity constants for binding proteins in radioligand assays range from 10^7 to 10^8 L/mole and the affinity constants for receptors range from 10^8 to 10^{11} L/mole.[1,2]

Classification of Methods

Ligand assays can be classified as heterogeneous or homogeneous. A heterogeneous assay requires the separation of the free label from the bound label before quantitating the bound label. The design of homogeneous assays does not require a separation step prior to quantitating the label. Types of heterogeneous assays are the competitive assay, sandwich assay to detect antigen, and sandwich assay to detect antibody. Examples of homogeneous ligand assays are enzyme multiplied immunoassay technique (EMIT™, Syva Corporation) and fluorescence polarization immunoassay (Table 15-2).

Heterogeneous Methods

Competitive Binding Assays

In competitive binding assays, labeled and unlabeled ligand compete for a limited number of binding sites on the binding reagent. When the binding reagent is a binding protein, the assay is a competitive protein binding assay, whereas in the more common radioimmunoassay, the radiolabeled antigen (Ag*) competes with an unlabeled antigen (Ag) for the combining sites of the specific antibody (Ab).

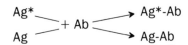

Table 15-2: Classification of Ligand Assays

HETEROGENEOUS (REQUIRES SEPARATION)
Competitive
Sandwich assay to detect antigen (antigen capture)
Sandwich assay to detect antibody (antibody capture)
HOMOGENEOUS (DOES NOT REQUIRE SEPARATION)
Enzyme-multiplied immunoassay techniques
Fluorescence polarization immunoassay

A relatively small, yet constant, number of Ab combining sites is available to combine with a relatively large, constant amount of Ag* (tracer); when Ag is added, it will displace or prevent the tracer from binding. The displacement of the tracer will be proportional to the amount of Ag present. Consider the example in Table 15-3. The amount of tracer and antibody are constant, and the amount of tracer exceeds the antibody binding sites. The only variable in the test system is the amount of unlabeled antigen. The greater the concentration of unlabeled antigen,

the greater the concentration of free tracer or the greater the percentage of free tracer.

By using different concentrations of standards (known concentrations of unlabeled antigen) in an assay, a dose response or standard curve is established. As the concentration of unlabeled Ag increases, the concentration of tracer that binds to the Ab decreases. The amount of either free tracer or bound tracer can be measured. In the example presented in Table 15-3, if the amount of unlabeled antigen is 0, maximum tracer will combine with the

Table 15-3: Competitive Binding Assay Example:

$$Ag \quad + \quad Ag^* \quad + \quad Ab \quad \rightarrow \quad AgAb \quad + \quad Ag^*Ab \quad + \quad Ag^*$$

Concentration of Reactants			Concentration of Products		
Ag	Ag*	Ab	AgAb	Ag*Ab	Ag*
0	200	100	0	100	100
50	200	100	20	80	120
100	200	100	34	66	134
200	200	100	50	50	150
400	200	100	66	34	166

Sample Calculations

Dose of [Ag]	%B	B/F
0	$\dfrac{100}{200} = 50$	$\dfrac{100}{100} = 1$
50	$\dfrac{80}{200} = 40$	$\dfrac{80}{120} = .67$
100	$\dfrac{66}{200} = 33$	$\dfrac{66}{134} = .49$
200	$\dfrac{50}{200} = 25$	$\dfrac{50}{150} = .33$
400	$\dfrac{34}{200} = 17$	$\dfrac{34}{166} = .20$

antibody. When the amount of unlabeled antigen is the same as the tracer, each will bind equally to the antibody. Several graphic representations, shown in Figure 15-1, can be used to relate the dose of known unlabeled antigen (standard) to the measurable tracer. When a patient sample is assayed, the unlabeled antigen in the patient sample competes with the tracer, and the amount of bound tracer is measured. When compared with the dose response curve, the concentration of the unlabeled antigen is assigned.

To determine the amount of free or bound tracer, competitive binding assays require that free tracer be separated from bound tracer. Separation techniques are discussed later in this chapter.

A representative protocol for simultaneous incubation of tracer and unlabeled antigen is summarized here. A schematic is shown in Figure 15-2.

1. Pipet serum (control, standard, or patient sample) into test tubes.

2. Pipet tracer into each tube.

3. Pipet binding reagent into each tube.

4. Incubate to allow binding to occur.

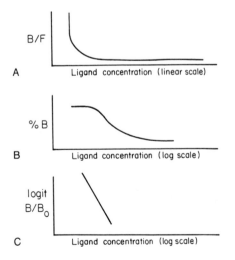

FIGURE 15-1. Dose-related curves in competitive immunoassay. B = bound counts per minute; F = free counts per minute; B_0 = maximum binding.

5. Separate free tracer from bound tracer.

6. Measure the amount of bound tracer.

Sandwich Assay to Detect Antigen

The sandwich assay to detect antigen, also known as the antigen capture assay, requires the binding reagent, usually an antibody, to be immobilized. The inert surface to which the antibody is attached is the solid phase. When the unlabeled antigen is added, it binds to the immobilized antibody. To quantitate the amount of bound antigen, a labeled antibody is then added that combines with the antigen. The amount of labeled antibody is measured and is directly proportional to the amount of bound antigen. Specific sandwich assays are named according to the binding reagent and label used. For example, immunoradiometric assays use an antibody that is radiolabeled, and immunoenzymetric assays use an enzyme-labeled antibody.

A representative protocol for an immunometric assay is presented in Figure 15-3 and is summarized here.

1. Pipet serum (control, standard, or patient sample) into test tubes.

2. If tube is not coated with the antibody, add the antibody-coated solid phase.

3. Incubate to allow the antigen to bind to the solid-phase antibody.

4. Wash to remove unbound serum components.

5. Add labeled antibody; incubate.

6. Wash to remove unbound labeled antibody.

7. Measure the bound antibody.

Sandwich Assay to Detect Antibody

The antibody capture assay is a variation of the sandwich assay. In the sandwich assay to detect antibody, the ligand or antigen is attached to the solid phase. A serum containing an unknown amount of specific antibody is added, and the antibody is captured by the solid-phase antigen. To identify the amount of specific antibody bound to the antigen, a

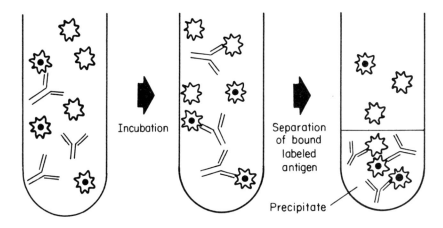

FIGURE 15-2. Competitive immunoassay. During simultaneous incubation labeled antigen (⬡) and unlabeled antigen (✪) compete for the antibody binding sites (≼). The bound label in the precipitate is measured.

labeled anti–human globulin is added. The amount of bound labeled antibody measured is directly proportional to the amount of specific antibody present. This assay can be modified to determine the immunoglobulin class of the specific antibody present in serum. For example, if the labeled antibody were monospecific (such as a rabbit anti–human IgM [μ-chain specific]), it would detect and quantitate only human IgM captured by the solid-phase specific antigen.

A sample protocol to detect antibody is summarized here. A schematic is presented in Figure 15-4.

1. Pipet serum (control, standard, or patient sample) into the test tubes.

2. If the antigen is not bound to the tube, add the antigen-coated solid phase.

3. Incubate to allow the specific antibody to bind to the solid-phase antigen.

4. Wash to remove unbound serum components.

5. Add the labeled anti–human globulin; incubate.

6. Wash to remove unbound labeled antibody.

7. Measure the bound labeled antibody.

Homogeneous Assay

Homogeneous immunoassays do not require separating free from bound labeled antibody or antigen.

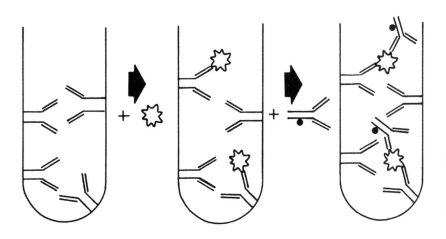

FIGURE 15-3. Sandwich assay to detect antigen. In sequential incubation, first unlabeled antigen (✪) binds to immobilized antibody followed by incubation with labeled antibody (≼). The bound label is measured.

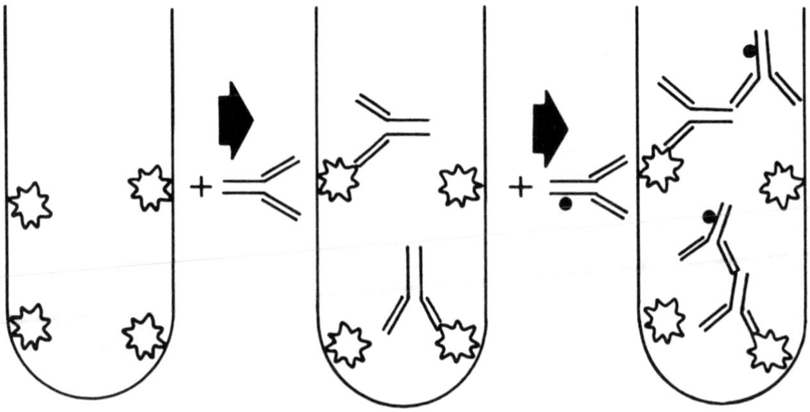

FIGURE 15-4. Sandwich assay to detect antibody. Unlabeled antibody (≼) is incubated with immobilized antigen (✿). In a second step, labeled anti–human globulin (≼) is added. The bound label is measured.

These assays are designed so that bound label selectively separates from the free label or so that the label is active only when it is free. One of the earliest homogeneous assays was an enzyme immunoassay named enzyme multiplied immunoassay technique (EMIT™) and is currently produced by Syva Corporation.[3] As shown in Figure 15-5, the reactants in the test system include an enzyme-labeled ligand (in this example, a drug), an antibody directed against the ligand, and the substrate. The enzyme is catalytically active when the labeled ligand is free (not bound to the antibody). It is thought that when the antibody combines with the labeled ligand, the antibody sterically inhibits the enzyme. The conformational changes that occur during antigen–antibody interaction inhibit the enzyme activity. The unlabeled ligand

(from the control, standard, or patient sample) competes with the labeled ligand for the antibody binding sites; as the concentration of unlabeled ligand increases, it prevents enzyme-labeled ligand from binding to the antibody. Therefore, more labeled ligand is free, and the enzymatic activity is greater.

A second homogeneous immunoassay, enzyme immunochromatography, is quantitative and does not require instrumentation.[4] A dry paper strip with immobilized antibody is immersed in a solution of unlabeled ligand and an enzyme-labeled ligand; the liquid migrates up the strip by capillary action. As the labeled and unlabeled ligand migrate, they compete and bind to the immobilized antibody. A finite amount of labeled and unlabeled antigen mixture is absorbed. The migration distance of the labeled li-

FIGURE 15-5. Enzyme-multiplied immunoassay technique. (A) Without unlabeled drug, the enzyme-labeled drug (drug-E) binds maximally to the antibody (Ab). In the Ab-drug-E complex, the enzyme is inactive. Only free enzyme-labeled drug is enzymatically active. (B) In the test system, the unlabeled drug in a patient sample competes with the labeled drug, thereby increasing the amount of free enzyme-labeled drug.

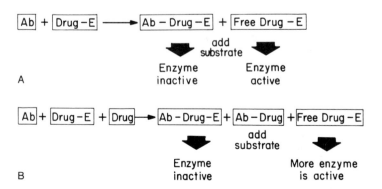

gand is visualized when the strip reacts with a substrate reagent and develops a colored reaction product. Comparing the migration distance of the sample with the calibrator allows the concentration of the unlabeled ligand to be assigned.

Separation Techniques

In heterogeneous ligand assays, separation of bound from free tracer or bound from free labeled antibody is accomplished by several different techniques. Ideally, there should be a clean and total separation of the free tracer and the bound tracer; likewise, if the antibody is labeled, free and bound labeled antibody must be separated. Separation techniques—adsorption, nonimmune precipitation, immune precipitation, and use of solid phase—are summarized in Table 15-4.[5]

Adsorption techniques use particles to trap the free ligand.[1] Most commonly, a mixture of charcoal and cross-linked dextran is used. Charcoal is porous and readily combines with small molecules to remove them from solution; dextran prevents nonspecific protein binding to the charcoal. The size of the dextran influences the size of the molecule that can be absorbed; the lower the molecular weight of dextran used, the smaller the molecular weight of free ligand that can be adsorbed. Other adsorbents include silica, ion exchange resin, and sephadex. After adsorption and centrifugation, the free tracer is found in the precipitate.

Nonimmune precipitation refers to precipitation of protein-bound ligand. Most nonimmune precipitation methods alter the solubility of the protein in the complex, thus causing the complex to precipitate. Compounds such as ammonium sulfate, sodium sulfate, polyethylene glycol, and ethanol precipitate protein nonspecifically; free protein and protein–ligand complexes will precipitate. Ammonium sulfate and sodium sulfate "salt out" protein and protein–ligand complexes. Ethanol denatures the protein and protein–ligand complexes, causing precipitation. Polyethylene glycol precipitates larger protein molecules with or without the ligand attached. All of these precipitants are nonspecific, precipitating all

Table 15-4: Characteristics of Separation Techniques

Separation Technique	Example	Action
Adsorption	Charcoal and dextran Silica Ion exchange resin Sephadex	Traps the free tracer
Nonimmune (chemical) precipitation	Ethanol Ammonium sulfate Sodium sulfate Polyethylene glycol	Denatures all protein, including the bound tracer
Immune precipitation	Second antibody	Antibody recognizes the species of primary antibody and forms an insoluble complex
Solid phase	Polystyrene (paddles, stars, beads, tubes, microtiter wells) Membranes (nylon, nitrocellulose, polymers)	Either the analyte or the antibody is immobilized on an inert physical surface

protein that is present. To facilitate separation of the precipitate, centrifugation is used. Ideally, all protein-bound labeled ligand will be in the precipitate, leaving free tracer in the supernatant; thus, complete separation occurs.

A soluble antigen–antibody complex can be precipitated by a second antibody that recognizes the antibody molecule of the soluble complex. The result is an antigen–antibody–antibody complex that is insoluble and will precipitate. Centrifugation is again used to aid in the separation. This immune precipitation method is also known as the double-antibody or second-antibody method. For example, in a growth hormone assay, the primary or antigen-specific antibody produced in a rabbit recognizes growth hormone. The second antibody, produced in a sheep or goat, would recognize rabbit antibody. Labeled antigen–antibody complexes, unlabeled antigen–antibody complexes, and free primary antibodies are precipitated by the second antibody. This separation method is more specific than nonimmune precipitation because only the primary antibody is precipitated.

Solid-phase immobilization of antibody or antigen provides a method to separate free from bound labeled reactant without centrifugation. The solid-phase support may be, but is not limited to, tubes, paddles, stars, beads, discs, paper, membranes, or microtiter wells. In the sandwich assay to detect antigen, antibody is immobilized on the solid phase, whereas in the sandwich assay to detect antibody, the antigen is immobilized. The immobilized antigen or antibody may be covalently or noncovalently bound to the solid-phase support; covalent linkage prevents spontaneous release of the immobilized antigen or antibody. Immunoassays using solid-phase separation are easier to perform, require less manipulation, and require less time to perform than other immunoassays. However, relatively large amounts of antibody or antigen are required to coat the solid-phase surfaces, and consistent coverage of the solid phase is difficult to achieve. Solid-phase assays are

more expensive to produce and require greater technical skill to perform to minimize intra-assay and interassay variability.

Recently, solid-phase technology using membranes as the solid support medium have been developed. The membranes are thin, porous material, such as nitrocellulose, nylon, or other polymers. Protein can bind to membranes whereas liquid can pass through membranes. These immunoassays are simple and rapid to perform. For example, one approach is to immobilize an antibody to human chorionic gonadotropin (hCG) to a nylon membrane that is attached to an absorbent material.[6] The absorbent material draws fluid, such as urine or serum, through the membrane so that hCG can be captured by the specific antibody bound to the membrane. Subsequently, the antibody-bound hCG can react with an enzyme-labeled antibody and substrate to produce a visible color. The porous nature of membranes increases the surface area to which the protein can bind. The more protein (such as the capture antibody or capture antigen) that binds to the membranous solid phase, the greater the potential sensitivity of the assay. Compared with other forms of solid phase, membranes offer more surface area for protein binding, thus improving sensitivity. By reducing the nonspecific binding of protein to the membrane, the specificity of the assay is enhanced. The versatility of configurations using membranes is great: It can be used as the bottom of a microtiter plate, as a dipstick, or in a flow-through chamber.

Using membranes as the solid phase is increasingly popular. Refinement of the general format uses microsphere particles trapped in discrete areas.[7] One scheme, ICON™ (Hybritech, Inc.), creates three zones of specifically treated particles: In the assay zone the particles are coated with antiserum specific for the assay; in the negative control zone the particles are coated with nonimmune antibody; and in the positive control zone the particles are coated with an immune complex specific for the assay. The patient sample (serum or urine) passes through the membrane, and the analyte attaches to the specific antibody in the assay zone. Next, a conjugated antibody passes through the membrane, which fixes to the specific immune complex formed in the assay zone or the positive control zone. Following color development, a positive reaction is noted when the assay and positive zones are colored.

Characteristics of Labels

Radioactive Labels

Radioactive labels are atoms with unstable nuclei that spontaneously emit radiation.[8] The emission is known as radioactive decay and is independent of chemical or physical parameters, such as temperature, pressure, or concentration. Three forms of radiation can be emitted: alpha, beta, and gamma. Alpha particles are the nuclei of helium atoms consisting of two protons and two neutrons. They are positively charged, large particles from heavy radioactive nuclides. These particles are of little clinical laboratory significance.

Beta particles are emitted from the nucleus of the atom and can be negatively charged electrons, called negatrons, or positively charged electrons, called positrons. A specific spectrum of energy levels is associated with each beta-emitting radionuclide. Most commonly, these radionuclides are used in research.

Gamma emission is a portion of the electromagnetic radiation spectrum. Gamma rays have very short wavelengths originating from unstable nuclei; the properties of gamma rays are similar to those of x-rays and light waves. Radionuclides emitting gamma rays are the most common radiolabel used in the clinical laboratory.

As a radionuclide releases its energy and becomes more stable, it disintegrates or decays, releasing energy. The standardized unit of radioactivity is the becquerel (Bq), which is equal to one disintegration per second. The traditional unit is the curie (Ci), which equals 3.7×10^{10} Bq; 1 μCi equals 37 kBq. The half-life of the radionuclide is the time needed for 50% of the radionuclide to decay and to become more stable. The longer the half-life, the more slowly it decays, thereby increasing the length of time it can be measured. For those radioactive substances used in diagnostic tests, it is preferable that the emission have an appropriate energy level and that the long half-life be relatively long; ^{125}I satisfies these requirements and is the most commonly used gamma-emitting radionuclide in the clinical laboratory.

Gamma-emitting nuclides are detected using a crystal scintillation detector. The energy released during decay excites a fluor, such as thallium-activated sodium iodide. The excited fluor releases a photon of visible light, which is amplified and detected by a photomultiplier tube where the light energy is translated into electrical energy. Detectable decay of the radionuclide is expressed as counts per minute.

In ligand assays, one reactant is radiolabeled; in competitive assays, the ligand is labeled (the tracer); and in immunoradiometric assays, the antibody is labeled. The radiolabel must allow the tracer to be fully functional; the tracer must compete equally with the unlabeled ligand for binding sites on the binding reagent, and the tracer must not be damaged in the process of labeling. When the antibody is radiolabeled, the antigen-combining site must remain biologically active.

Enzyme Labels

Enzymes may be used to label the ligand or antibody. Enzyme immunoassay (EIA) is the generic term to describe any assay in which the label is an enzyme and the binding reagent is an antibody.[9,10] Heterogeneous EIA requires the separation of free from bound labeled reactants. An EIA method in which the separation technique is a solid phase is termed enzyme-linked immunosorbent assay (ELISA). The enzymes most often used to label the antibody in ELISA techniques include horseradish peroxidase, glucose oxidase, glucose-6-phosphate dehydrogenase, and alkaline phosphatase. The enzyme label chemically converts a substrate into a product, which is then quantitated by measuring its absorbance, its fluorescence, or its ability to modify another chemical reaction. A typical reaction uses horseradish peroxidase–labeled antibody (Ab-HRP) and the substrate, a peroxide, to generate the product, oxygen; this reaction is coupled to a second reaction to produce a colored product. The oxygen oxidizes a reduced chromogen (reduced orthophenylenediamine [OPD]), producing a colored compound (oxidized OPD), which is measured.

$$Ab\text{-}HRP + peroxide \rightarrow Ab\text{-}HRP + O_2$$

$$O_2 + reduced\ OPD \rightarrow oxidized\ OPD + H_2O$$

Fluorescent Labels

Fluorescent labels are specific compounds that absorb electromagnetic radiation of one wavelength and emit electromagnetic radiation of a longer wavelength. The fluorescence of biologic compounds occurs between 10^{-9} and 2×10^{-8} seconds. Generally, the emitted light is measured at a 90° angle from the path of excitation light. The difference between the excitation wavelength and emission wavelength, called Stokes shift, usually ranges between 20 and 80 nm for most fluorochromes. Some fluorescence immunoassays simply substitute a fluorescent label for an enzyme label and quantitate the fluorescence.[11] Another approach, time-resolved fluorescence immunoassay, requires a highly efficient fluorescent label.[12,13] When this fluorescent label is

excited by electromagnetic radiation, it fluoresces approximately 1000 times more slowly than the natural background fluorescence. This delay allows measurement of the fluorescent label without interference from other fluorescing compounds in the system. In addition, the label used in time-resolved fluorescence immunoassay has a long Stokes shift that facilitates separating the emission wavelength (to be measured) from the excitation wavelength. The resulting assay is highly sensitive, is time-resolved, and has little background fluorescence. One commercially available label that satisfies these requirements is europium chelate. Assays are either competitive or immunometric methods, using polyclonal or monoclonal antibodies.

Fluorescence polarization immunoassay (FPIA) is another assay that uses a fluorescent label.[14,15] This homogeneous immunoassay utilizes polarized light to excite the fluorescent label. Polarized light consists of parallel light waves oriented in one plane and is created when light passes through special filters. When polarized light is used to excite a fluorescent label, the emitted light could be polarized or depolarized, depending on the size of the fluorescent label. Large molecules, such as those created when the fluorescent label binds to an antibody, randomly rotate slowly and emit polarized light parallel to the excitation polarized light. Small molecules, such as free fluorescent-labeled hapten, rotate more rapidly and emit light in many directions, thus producing depolarized light. The polarized light is measured at a 90° angle compared with the path of the excitation light. In one FPIA, a fluorescent label is bound to a small ligand, a hapten; following excitation with polarized light, the free labeled ligand will emit mostly depolarized light and little polarized light. In a competitive assay, as shown in Figure 15-6, fluorescent-labeled hapten (tracer) and unlabeled hapten (in the patient sample) compete for limited antibody sites. When no unlabeled hapten is present, the tracer binds maximally to the antibody, creating large complexes that rotate slowly and demonstrate a high level of polarization. When hapten is present, it competes with the tracer for the antibody sites; thus, as the hapten concentration increases, more tracer is displaced and is free. The free tracer rotates rapidly and demonstrates reduced fluorescence polarization. The degree of tracer displacement is inversely related to the amount of unlabeled hapten present.

Luminescent Labels

Luminescent labels emit a photon of light that is measured by a luminometer. If a chemical reaction is involved, the light is called chemiluminescence, and if a biologic system is involved, it is called bioluminescence.[16] The energy generated in these reactions must directly excite at least one reactant to emit a photon of light or transfer energy to a secondary reaction capable of emitting light. The two popular systems for luminescent immunoassays utilize luminol or luciferase.

Luminol is a cyclic diacylhydrazide that emits light energy under alkaline conditions in the presence of a catalyst or co-oxidant. Because peroxidase can serve as the catalyst, assays may use this enzyme as the label; the chemiluminogenic substrate, luminol, will produce light that is directly proportional to the amount of peroxidase present.

$$\text{Cyclic diacylhydrazine} + 2H_2O_2 + OH^- \xrightarrow{\text{peroxidase}}$$

$$\text{open diacylhydrazine} + N_2 + 3H_2O + \text{photon of light}$$

Luciferase is an enzyme from bacteria or fireflies that releases light energy and requires cofactors, such as NADH or ATP. When the light-emitting reaction is coupled with a reaction producing the required cofactor, the light is proportional to the rate-limiting cofactor. Examples of luminescence using luciferase are diagrammed as follows:

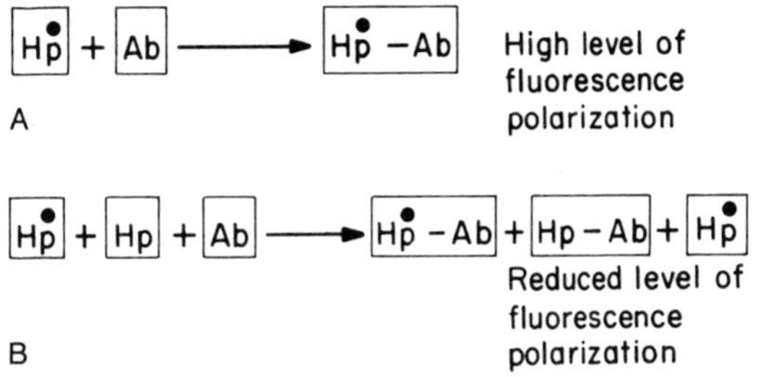

A

B

FIGURE 15-6. Fluorescence polarization immunoassay. (*A*) When the fluorescent labeled hapten (Hṗ) combines with the antibody (Ab), a complex is formed. When this complex is excited with polarized light, a high level of fluorescence polarization is detected. (*B*) In the test system, patient hapten (Hp) competes with Hṗ for the Ab; thus, a lower level of fluorescence polarization is detected.

(1) $$\text{NADH} + \text{FMN} + H^+ \xrightarrow[\text{dehydrogenase}]{\text{NADH}} \text{NAD} + \text{FMNH}_2$$

$$\text{FMNH}_2 + \text{RCHO} + O_2 \xrightarrow[\text{luciferase}]{\text{bacterial}} \text{FMN} + \text{RCO}_2\text{H}$$
$$+ H_2O$$
$$+ \text{photon of light}$$

(2) $$\text{Luciferin} + \text{ATP} \xrightarrow[\text{Mg}^{+2}]{\text{firefly}\atop\text{luciferase}} \text{oxyluciferin}$$
$$+ \text{PP}_i + CO_2$$
$$+ \text{AMP}$$
$$+ \text{photon of light}$$

Dose Response Curves (Standard Curves)

Competitive Assays

As the concentration or dose of unlabeled ligand increases in a competitive assay, the amount of labeled ligand (tracer) complexing with the binding reagent decreases. Most separation techniques allow the bound tracer to be measured. When no unlabeled ligand is present, maximum binding by the tracer is possible; this is referred to as B_0, B_{max}, or maximum binding. The data are plotted in one of three ways, as shown in Figure 15-1: bound/free versus the arithmetic dose of unlabeled ligand; % bound versus the log dose of unlabeled ligand; and logit bound versus the log dose of the unlabeled ligand.

The bound fraction can be expressed in several different formats. Bound/free (B/F) is the counts per minute (CPM) of the bound fraction compared with the CPM of the unbound fraction. Bound/total (B/T) is the CPM of the bound fraction compared with the CPM of maximum binding by the tracer (B_0) added to each tube. Percent bound (%B) is the percentage of CPM of the bound fraction compared with the total CPM. Logit transformation is the mathematical relationship where

$$\text{logit } (B/B_0) = \log_e \left(\frac{B/B_0}{1 - (B/B_0)} \right)$$

When using special logit graph paper on which B/B_0 is plotted on the ordinate and the log dose of the unlabeled ligand is plotted on the abscissa, a straight line with a negative slope is produced.[1]

Immunometric Assays

In immunometric assays the amount of unlabeled antigen in the patient sample, control, or standard is directly related to the amount of bound label that is measured. In radiolabeled assays the CPM is measured; in enzyme-labeled assays the absorbance is measured. As shown in the dose-related curve in Figure 15-7, with a limited range, the response (CPM or absorbance) is directly related to the amount of unlabeled antigen present.

Qualitative Tests

Some assays are qualitative and do not require a standard curve. These assays rely on a comparison of the unknown specimen and a calibrator. In these tests it is sufficient to detect the presence or absence of the analyte in the sample. A standard material, the calibrator, generates the minimum response (most often CPM or absorbance) needed to establish the cut off point for the presence of an analyte; the response of the control and patient sample is compared with the response of the calibrator. When the response of the patient sample or control is greater than that of the calibrator, the patient sample or control is considered positive for the analyte. Likewise, when the response of the patient or control is less than that of the calibrator, the specimen is negative. An example of a qualitative assay is a sandwich enzyme immunoassay to detect rubella antibody to assess susceptibility or resistance to rubella infection. If sufficient rubella antibody is present, an individual has already been exposed to the virus, has mounted a specific immune response, and is resistant to rubella virus

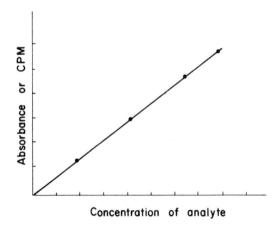

FIGURE 15-7. Immunometric dose response curve. As the concentration of the unlabeled antigen increases, the amount of label that is measured increases.

infection. In this case, it is sufficient to know that antibody is present; it is unnecessary to know the quantity of antibody present. By comparing the absorbance reading of the patient specimen to that of the low positive control (or calibrator), the immune status of the patient is determined. If the patient sample absorbance is greater than that of the low positive control, the patient sample contains sufficient antibody to be considered immune to rubella virus infection; if the patient sample absorbance is less than the low positive control, insufficient antibody is present, so the patient is susceptible to rubella virus infection.

Interferences and Sources of Error

The sensitivity of ligand assays suggests that minor variations in technical manipulation can be a significant source of error. Therefore, most ligand assay procedures require that each patient specimen, control, and standard be tested in duplicate to minimize manipulative variation, especially pipetting.

Heterogeneous assays require a separation step, the most critical step. In solid-phase assays, washing is the separation step; incomplete washing leads to incomplete removal of free labeled reagent, which results in a false positive reaction in a qualitative assay or a falsely elevated quantitative result.

Each laboratory develops confidence in an immunoassay procedure by adequately evaluating each method to assure its accuracy, sensitivity, and precision prior to its adoption. Each assay, whether an in-house assay or a commercially prepared kit, has many variables, such as antibody purity, antibody affinity, antibody specificity, and type of assay. What is the technique of separation? In a solid-phase assay what is the shape and surface area of the solid phase? How are the molecules attached to the solid phase?

How long are the incubation periods? What is the sequence of adding reagents in the assay? Once a particular assay is chosen, the reproducibility of results must continuously be monitored to assure the quality performance of the assay. Consideration must be given to interlaboratory variation, proper functioning of the instrumentation (pipets, spectrophotometers, gamma counter), and environmental conditions. Finally, accurate interpretation of patient results requires that a valid reference interval be established by each laboratory.

Detection of Human Chorionic Gonadotropin

The following discussion about human chorionic gonadotropin (hCG) highlights the development and progression of immunoassays.[17,18] The first molecular marker of pregnancy, hCG is produced by trophoblastic cells of the placenta. The first assay to detect hCG was a bioassay in which the biologic effect of hCG, its ability to induce the formation of corpus luteum in female mice, was observed. In the 1960s, agglutination immunoassays, which are faster and easier to perform, replaced the bioassays. Examples of agglutination assays include hemagglutination inhibition, latex agglutination inhibition, hemagglutination, and latex agglutination. The agglutination inhibition methods require the premixing of patient urine with hCG antiserum, then particles (erythrocytes in the hemagglutination inhibition method or latex particles in the latex agglutination inhibition method) coated with hCG are added. Patient hCG, if present, will neutralize the antiserum, which prevents it from agglutinating hCG-coated particles; therefore, lack of agglutination with the hCG-coated particles indicates the presence of hCG in the patient specimen (a positive test). In the latex agglutination or hemagglutination methods, the particle is coated hCG antibody. When patient specimen containing hCG is added, it binds to the antibody and cross-links the particles, resulting in macroscopic agglutination.

The specificity of all immunoassays is controlled by the specificity of the antibody used in the assay. It must be remembered that the four glycoprotein hormones (thyroid stimulating hormone, luteinizing hormone, follicle stimulating hormone, and human chorionic gonadotropin) have the same dimeric structure: All have identical α subunits and differ only in their β subunit. The β subunit of luteinizing hormone, structurally the most similar to hCG, shows 80% homology with the β subunit of hCG. The similarity of glycoprotein hormones, especially luteinizing hormone, may permit the glycoprotein hormones to cross-react in an assay designed to measure hCG, depending on the antiserum used. To develop an assay specific for hCG, the antibody must recognize the unique section of the β subunit or recognize an epitope present only on an intact hCG molecule.

Monoclonal antibody technology has allowed easier production of well-characterized antibodies; thus, specific assays with little or no cross-reaction with the glycoprotein hormones have been developed. Improved specificity has made available assays with greater sensitivity, mostly RIA and EIA methods. Some assays detect hCG by using two different antibodies, one recognizing an epitope on the α chain and the other on the β chain, whereas other assays are engineered to recognize an epitope present only on the intact molecule. Protein does not interfere in these RIA and EIA methods, so urine or serum may be used. Methods include double antibody precipitation RIA and sandwich ELISA antigen assay. Recently developed antigen capture assays using membranes are popular because they are easier to perform, have better sensitivity, and require less time to perform. Urine or serum containing hCG is passed through a filter membrane on which specific antibody is immobilized; hCG is captured. After applying the enzyme-labeled second antibody and the appropriate substrate, the color developed in the patient test is compared with the intensity of color generated by the standard. Some assays are read by viewing colored circles or a symbol such as a plus "+" (indicating the presence of hCG) or minus "−" (indicating the absence of hCG).

hCG concentration is expressed in mIU/mL, IU/mL, or ng/mL, where 1 mIU/mL = 0.08

Table 15-5: Selected Kits to Detect Human Choriogonadotropin

Kit	Manufacturer	Method	Sensitivity
Sensitex	Roche	Tube LAI	250 mIU/mL
Neo-Pregnosticon	Organon Teknika	Tube HA	75 mIU/mL
Pregnosis	Roche	Slide LAI	1500 mIU/mL
TANDEM® ICON™ II HCG (urine)	Hybritech, Inc.	Membrane EIA	20 mIU/mL
Test Pack™ HCG-Urine	Abbott Laboratories	Membrane EIA	25 mIU/mL
HCG-B Combi RIA	NMS Pharmaceuticals, Inc.	RIA	3 mIU/mL

LAI = latex agglutination inhibition
HA = hemagglutination
EIA = enzyme immunoassay
RIA = radioimmunoassay

ng/mL.[18] The First International Reference Preparation of Human Chorionic Gonadotropin for Immunoassay made available in 1975 from the World Health Organization serves as the reference for all hCG immunoassays; the concentration of the reference preparation is 650 IU/ampoule. The sensitivity of several commercially available methods appears in Table 15-5; this sensitivity is stated by the manufacturer and may differ from other reported values.[19]

The level of hCG in normal pregnancy changes during gestation. The detectable level of hCG increases sharply during the first trimester, peaks about 70 days after the last menstrual period, declines slightly to a plateau, and remains constant for the second and third trimesters. Generally, urine levels of hCG are sufficient to diagnose normal pregnancy; however, in the event that a urine pregnancy test is negative and pregnancy is still suspected, a second specimen should be collected and retested. In early pregnancy, hCG levels double rapidly and should soon reach a detectable level.

hCG is also measured to diagnose ectopic pregnancy and to evaluate a threatened spontaneous abortion. In ectopic pregnancy the hCG level is less than that in uterine pregnancy, in the range of 150 to 800 mIU/mL; those tests with lower sensitivity are particularly useful to diagnose this potentially life-threatening condition. Lower than expected levels or decreasing levels of hCG in the first trimester are associated with spontaneous abortion.

hCG is measured to evaluate trophoblastic tumors, testicular tumors, and some nontrophoblastic tumors. Trophoblastic tumors, such as hydatidiform mole and choriocarcinoma, secrete high levels of hCG in the range of 5000 to 6,000,000 mIU/mL. To quantitate these levels, it may be necessary to dilute the specimen sequentially for agglutination assays or to use a quantitative EIA or RIA method. High levels of hCG may also be associated with multiple pregnancies, eclampsia, polyhydramnios, and erythroblastosis fetalis. Testicular choriocarcinomas, seminomas, teratomas, and embryonal carcinomas

are associated with elevated levels of hCG. When monitoring tumor activity, quantitating the β subunit is preferred because tumors may produce free β chains as well as intact hCG molecules.

Other Applications

Ligand assay is well suited to measure substances found in small quantities in serum or fluids or to measure small molecules. Hormones are potent biologic mediators found in very low concentration in the blood. Most commonly, thyroid hormones are measured. Ligand assays are useful to monitor therapeutic drugs that are small molecules in low serum concentration. Drug dosage, such as that of digoxin, must be closely monitored and adjusted to therapeutic, but not toxic, levels. Infectious agents that are difficult or impossible to culture (such as *Chlamydia trachomatis*) or for which evidence of current infection is needed quickly (*Hemophilus influenza*) are likely organisms to be monitored by immunoassay. The versatility, ease and speed of performance, sensitivity, and specificity of immunoassays account for the variety of tests currently performed in the clinical laboratory and for the projection that immunoassays will expand in the future.

References

1. Travis JC: Fundamental of RIA and Other Ligand Assays: A Programmed Text, p 48. Anaheim, Radioassay Publishers, Division of Scientific Newsletters, Inc., 1979

2. Howanitz JH, Howanitz PJ: Immunoassay and related techniques; Tumor markers. In Henry JB (ed): Clinical Diagnosis and Management by Laboratory Methods, 17th ed, p 283. Philadelphia, WB Saunders, 1984

3. Rubenstein KE, Schneider RB, Ullman EF: "Homogeneous" enzyme immunoassay, a new immunochemical technique. Biochem Biophys Res Comm, 47:846, 1972

4. Zuk RF, Ginsberg VK, Houts T, et al: Enzyme immunochromatography: A quantitative immunoassay requiring no instrumentation. Clin Chem 31:7,1144, 1985

5. Weiss AJ, Blankenstein LA: Membranes as a solid phase for clinical diagnostic assays. Am Clin Prod Rev, p 8, June, 1987

6. Valkirs RF, Barton R: Immunoconcentration™: A new format for solid phase immunoassays. Clin Chem 31:1427, 1985

7. Rubenstein AS, Hostler RD, White CC, et al: Particle entrapment: Application to ICON™ immunoassay. Clin Chem, 32:6,1072, 1986

8. Powsner ER: Basic principles of radioactivity and its measurement. In Tietz NW (ed): Fundamentals of Clinical Chemistry, 3rd ed, p 124. Philadelphia, WB Saunders, 1987

9. Engvall E, Perlmann P: Immunochemistry, 8:871, 1971

10. Van Weemen BK, Schuurs AHWM: Immunoassay using antigen-enzyme conjugates. FEBS Letters, 15, 232, 1971

11. Nakamura RM, Robbins BA: Analytical fluid-phase fluorescence immunoassays. In Rose NR, Friedman H, Fahey JL (eds): Manual of Clinical Laboratory Immunology, 3rd ed, p 116. Washington, DC, American Society for Microbiology, 1986

12. Alpert NL: Time-Resolved Fluorescence Immunoassay. Clinical Instrument Systems, 9:2,1, 1988

13. Déchaud H, Bador R, Claustrat F, et al: New approach to competitive lanthanide immunoassay: Time-resolved fluoroimmunoassay of progesterone with labeled analyte. Clin Chem 34:3,501, 1988

14. Tiffany TO, Burtis CA: Fluorometry, nephelometry, and turbidimetry. In Tietz NW (ed): Fundamentals of Clinical Chemistry, 3rd ed, p 66. Philadelphia, WB Saunders, 1987

15. Buhles WC: Fluorescence immunoassays. In Rippey JH, Nakamura RM (eds): Diagnostic Immunology: Technology Assessment and Quality Assurance, p 59. Skokie, College of American Pathologists, 1983

16. Boguslaski RC: Luminescent Immunoassays. In Rippey JH, Nakamura RM (eds): Diagnostic Immunology: Technology Assessment and Quality Assurance, p 47. Skokie, College of American Pathologists, 1983

17. Sheehan C. Current status of pregnancy testing. Am J Med Technol, 49:7,485, 1983

18. Krieg AF, Wenk RE: Pregnancy tests and evaluation of placental function. In Henry JB (ed): Clinical Diagnosis and Management by Laboratory Methods, 17th ed, p 493. Philadelphia, WB Saunders, 1984

19. Buck RH, Norman RJ, Reddi K, et al: Various Methods for Determining Urinary Choriogonadotropin Evaluated for the Early Diagnosis of Ectopic Pregnancy. Clin Chem, 32:5,879, 1986

CHAPTER 16

Nephelometry

Alice K. Chen

Nephelometry is a direct method of measuring light scattered by particles suspended in solution. Nephelometry, based on the classic antigen–antibody precipitin reaction first described by Heidelberger and Kendall,[1] is now routinely used to quantitate specific proteins. With stable, reliable commercial instruments and reagents readily available, nephelometry provides great advantages over the standard techniques of radial immunodiffusion (RID) and immunoelectrophoresis (IEP). Quantitation of specific protein by nephelometry is now accurate, precise, fast, easy to perform, and fully automated. With good sensitivity and specificity, it has become a standard method not only in the research laboratory but in the clinical laboratory as well. It is most commonly used for measuring plasma proteins such as immunoglobulins, complement components, and other specific proteins. This chapter will discuss the basic principles of nephelometry and its application to immunology. For more detail, manuals and review articles are readily available in the literature.[2–4]

Principle of Nephelometry

The Nature of Light Scattering

The interaction of light with particles in solution can be measured by nephelometry or turbidimetry. When light strikes particles, it can be transmitted through the solution and be absorbed, reflected, or scattered by the particles. Turbidimetry is the measurement of light transmitted through a suspension of particles. A spectrophotometer can often be used for turbidity measurement. Nephelometry is a direct measurement of light scattered by the particles; the instrument detects the scattered light at angles away from the incoming light source (incident light). The low intensity of scattered light, sometimes not visible to the naked eye, can be measured by a sensitive detector. If a solution to be measured for light scattering absorbs or reflects negligible amount of the incoming light, nephelometry can be used to determine specific proteins with a greater detection range and better sensitivity than turbidimetry.

In immunonephelometry the nature of light scattering can be classified into two types, depending on the diameter (d) of the particles relative to the wavelength (λ) of light passing through the solution. As shown in Figure 16-1, small particles, such as albumin, IgG, and IgM ($d \leq 0.05\ \lambda$), produce Rayleigh light scattering that is symmetric in the forward and backward directions. A minimum scatter is observed at 90° from the incident light. Larger molecules or antigen–antibody complexes, with diameters comparable to the wavelength, produce Rayleigh–Debye light scattering. In this case, the light scattered has greater intensity in the forward direction when the detection angle, θ, approaches zero. For both types of light scattering, the intensity of scattered light is always proportional to the intensity of incident light and inversely related to the fourth power of the light wavelength. Using light in the blue-green region ($\lambda = 400$ to 500 nm) and, depending on particle sizes, immune complexes such as IgG, IgA, and IgM precipitins and serum lipoprotein produces Rayleigh–Debye and Rayleigh scattering. Using a laser light source and a forward angle detection of scattered light, therefore, produces greater signals and, hence, greater sensitivity in nephelometry.

Kinetics of Fluid Phase Precipitation

The interaction of antigen and antibody in solution depends on many factors, most important of which is their relative concentrations. The initial interaction is the primary binding of antigen to the antibody molecules. Since most reactions in solution are reversible, when the antibody is in excess and the antigens are polyvalent, secondary rearrangement of bindings between the two species occurs and cross-linking of the antigen–antibody complexes leads to slow formation of a lattice. At this stage, the complex is large and

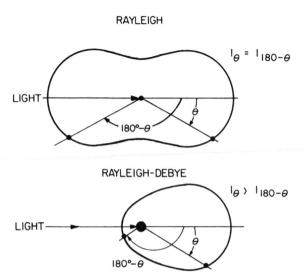

FIGURE 16-1. Angular distribution patterns for Rayleigh light scattered from small particles, and Rayleigh-Debye scattering from somewhat larger particles. (From Sternberg JC. Rate nephelometry. In Rose NR, Friedman H, Fahey JL (eds): Manual of Clinical Laboratory Immunology, 3rd ed. Washington, DC: American Society for Microbiology, 1986, p. 34. Used by permission.)

can produce Rayleigh–Debye scattering of visible light. If the antibody concentration remains in excess, the secondary rearrangement continues, which eventually forms aggregates, forms a visible precipitation, and settles out of the solution. As shown in Figure 16-2, maximal lattice is formed at the antigen–antibody equivalence zone. If more antigen or antibody is added to the lattice, the additional antigen or antibody will break up the lattice aggregates to produce a large amount of smaller antigen–antibody complexes. For any antibody dilution, two different antigen concentrations, one in the antibody excess zone and one in the antigen excess zone, can produce the same amount of lattice and light scattering signal. Nephelometry is often used to quantitate antigen concentrations in the presence of excess antibody so that the amounts of lattice aggregate and light scattering are proportional to the antigen

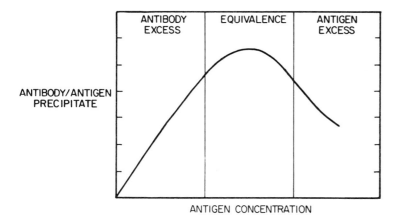

FIGURE 16-2. The quantitative precipitin curve generated by adding increasing amounts of antigen to a solution of antibody and measuring antibody–antigen complexes by nephelometry. (Reprinted from Ref. 3, p. 123, by courtesy of Marcel Dekker, Inc.)

concentration in test specimens. To prevent a reaction in antigen excess, a check of free antibody is built into the assay procedures.

Figure 16-3 shows a typical immunoprecipitin reaction as monitored by nephelometry under the antibody excess condition. When the specimen is diluted with buffer and added to the cuvet, a small background light scattering due to sample blank is pro-

duced. The sources of this background scattering are proteins and lipoproteins in the specimen, particles or dust present in the reagents, or stray light. The small background signal is usually independent of the detection angle and can be minimized by using nephelometric grade antisera and a high dilution of the specimens. The addition of antiserum into the cuvet initiates the antigen–antibody binding reaction, and

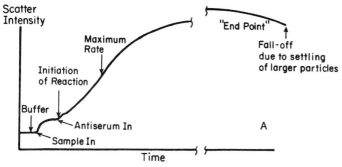

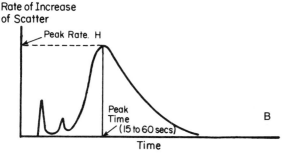

FIGURE 16-3. Time course of the immunoprecipitation reaction. (A) Variation of intensity of scattered light versus time. (B) Rate of increase of scatter versus time. (From Sternberg JC. Rate nephelometry. In Rose NR, Friedman H, Fahey JL (eds): Manual of Clinical Laboratory Immunology, 3rd ed. Washington, DC: American Society for Microbiology, 1986, p. 34. Used by permission.)

a short period of slow complex formation is reflected in the slow increase of light scattering. This is followed by a rapid increase in scatter intensity, because of acceleration in the immunoprecipitin formation. The amount of scattered light reaches a plateau and falls off when the precipitin starts to aggregate and settle out of the solution. The rate of increase of scattering and the height of the plateau reached are directly related to the antigen concentration and the dilution of the antiserum. Nephelometry, based on the antigen–antibody reaction rate and the plateau stage, is used for kinetic and end point assays, respectively, to measure the antigen concentrations in clinical specimens.

The antigen–antibody interaction not only is controlled by the antiserum affinity and avidity, the buffer, pH, and ionic strength of the assay solution,[5] but also can be greatly enhanced by the presence of nonionic, hydrophilic polymers. These polymer molecules, more hydrophilic than the antigen or antibody molecules, attract water molecules from the antigen and antibody and subsequently increase the chance of antigen–antibody reaction. Polyethylene glycol (PEG) is now routinely used in nephelometry assays. It speeds up the reaction rate, increases the slope of the precipitin curve in the antibody excess zone, and pushes the equivalence zone to a higher antigen con-

centration. This results in nephelometry of considerably greater sensitivity, wider detection range, and faster assay. The PEG is especially effective with low-avidity antisera.

Instrumentation

The basic components of a nephelometer are shown in Figure 16-4. Typically, the instrument includes a light source, a collimating system to focus the light, a monochromator, a cuvet, and a photomultiplier tube. The light source varies from simple, inexpensive tungsten lamps to mercury lamps, xenon arc lamps, and high-intensity lasers. The nephelometer basically requires the same components as a fluorometer, except in nephelometry, the wavelength of the incident light does not need a very narrow bandwidth. In fact, a fluorometer can be used for nephelometric measurement simply by using the same filter or wavelength for the incident light and the scattered light. A high-quality spectrophotometer using photomultiplier tubes sometimes is modified in its detection angle for nephelometric assays.

Nephelometers with the highly intense, single wavelength, narrowly focused laser light source allow a greater signal to be measured and do not

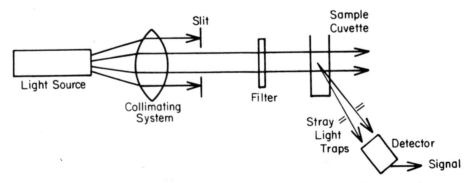

FIGURE 16-4. Schematic of basic components of a nephelometer (Reproduced by permission from Frings CS, Gauldie J. Spectral techniques. In Kaplan LA, Pesce AJ (eds): Clinical Chemistry: Theory, Analysis and Correlation. St. Louis: CV Mosby, 1984, p. 69.)

require the collimating system, but the scattered light is more susceptible to fluctuations of particle size, since the antigen–antibody complex size changes with reaction time. An instrument with a conventional lamp, such as a tungsten light source, has light of wider bandwidth, produces signals proportional to the average size of the precipitin, and is therefore less susceptible to particle size change and produces a more reproducible kinetic or rate measurement. As shown in Figure 16-1 for Rayleigh and Rayleigh–Debye scattering, small front angle detection can more than double the amount of light scattering measured by an instrument with a 90° angle of detection.

Some commercial clinical instruments designed for nephelometric assays and automated analyzers suitable for nephelometric analysis are listed in Table 16-1. All the instruments are highly automated, and the initial cost of purchasing could be an important factor to consider. The Beckman ICS, a microprocessor-controlled nephelometer, either can be used in the kinetic or rate mode, which bypasses the problems of background interference, or can be used in the manual mode for end point analysis. It has a tungsten light source and measures scattering at a front angle of 70°. Using the reagents made specifically for the instrument, the instrument operates with single-point calibration. This is achieved by using an optically read card that comes with each reagent kit to control the instrument's operation. A series of sixfold dilutions of calibrator and test sample is carried out automatically. Using a predetermined curve-fitting program, light-scattering signals are converted to concentrations. The instrument automatically checks antigen excess, checks out-of-range specimens, and provides instructions for reassays. When used in the kinetic mode, the instrument does not wait for the plateau response, and therefore it has a short turnaround time. The nature of continuous monitoring of the reaction rate, on the other hand, allows fewer specimens to be processed per hour. The Beckman ICS can be used for discrete or batch analysis with up to six tests per specimen and produces consistently low coefficient of variance (CV) at all levels of immunoglobulin.[6]

Instruments utilizing end point analysis are more susceptible to specimen matrix interference, require a long incubation time (10 minutes to an hour), but handle a greater number of samples per hour. Because of the incubation time required for the plateau response, they have a longer turnaround time and therefore are not practical for stat analysis. For laboratories where automated analyzers—such as centrifugal, continuous-flow, or fluorescence immunoassay analyzers—are available, nephelometric immunoassay can be performed on these analyzers with little difficulty. For example, the Abbott TDx fluorescence polarization analyzer has been used for nephelometric analysis of IgG, IgA, IgM, and transferrin with automatic antigen excess check. The calibration curve can be stored for up to 2 weeks.[7]

Limitations of Light-Scattering Methods

As shown in Figure 16-2, for each antibody dilution, two different antigen concentrations, one in the antibody excess zone and one in the antigen excess zone, will produce the same amount of antigen–antibody lattice and, thus, intensity of light scattered. Antigen excess is more frequently encountered in monoclonal immunoglobulins, C-reactive protein, and β_2 microglobulin.[3] To validate assay results, antigen excess must be checked in all nephelometric assays. One way to check antigen excess is to assay the specimens at two different dilutions. Or assays can be checked for antigen excess by adding more antibody to the assay mixture. The increase in reaction rate or plateau response can be used to check if assays were performed in the desired antibody excess region. Samples with antigen excess are then reassayed at a greater dilution.

Like all other immunoassays, nephelometry is

Table 16-1: Automated Clinical Instruments Available for Light-Scattering Analysis

	Technicon AIP	Behring Autolaser LN	Beckman Automated ICS	Reaction Rate Analyzer	Centrifugal Fast Analyzer
Nephelometer (N) (angle) or turbidometer (T)	N (90°)	N (5°–12°)	N (70°)	T	T
Endpoint (E) or kinetic (K) analysis of reaction	E + blank	E + blank	K	K or E	K or E
Light source (wavelength, nm)	Mercury arc (357 nm)	Laser (632.8 nm)	Tungsten lamp (400–550 nm)	Variable: ultraviolet to 700 nm	Variable: ultraviolet to 700 nm
Calibration	Standard curve	Standard curve	Single point, reagent lot	Standard curve, reagent lot	Standard curve, reagent lot
Samples/hour	120	120–240	30–50	20–40	300
Reaction time	10 min	1 hour (no PEG)	30 sec	1–2 min (kinetic)	1–2 min (kinetic)
Sensitivity	5 mg/L	—	1 mg/L	—	—
Precision (CV)					
Within-run	2%–5%	—	2%–5%	—	—
Between-run	5%–10%	—	5%–10%	—	—
Capital outlay	++	+++	+++	+++	++++
Original monitoring capability	0	±	+++	±	±
Other type of analysis	++	+	+	+++	++++

From: Frings CS, Gauldie J: Spectral techniques. In Kaplan LA, Pesce AJ (eds): Clinical Chemistry: Theory, Analysis and Correlation, St. Louis, CV Mosby Co, 1984. Adapted from Deverill I, Reeve WG: J Immunol Methods 38: 191–204, 1980.

subject to interferences and limitations. Spurious light scattering due to dust particles or endogenous particles such as lipoprotein may limit the assay sensitivity of the end point method, but often this can be eliminated by kinetic measurement. The endogenous light-scattering materials are less soluble in PEG solution; therefore, samples can be treated with PEG and centrifuged before the assay with antisera. Some turbid specimens may have to be filtered before their assay by nephelometry. The use of PEG as an enhancer can also cause nonspecific precipitation of macromolecules in samples. Proteins, lipoproteins, heparin, immunoglobulins, and endogenous immune complexes will affect the true reaction rate or the end point plateau light scattering.

Nonspecific side-reactions can be initiated by rheumatoid factor or the C1q component of the complement system. Rheumatoid factor is an IgM antibody directed against the Fc portion of an IgG molecule and will react with IgG, thus decreasing the IgG concentration in the patient sample and antibody reagent. The C1q molecule has six sites that recognize the Fc portions of IgG and IgM. When IgG or IgM are the serum protein to be quantitated, C1q can bind to the immunoglobulin, so that it is unavailable in the nephelometric reaction. In addition, C1q can bind to the nephelometric antiserum reagent, thereby neutralizing it. Both side-reactions will decrease the specific reaction measured. Rheumatoid factor can be denatured by pretreating samples with dithiothreitol or mercaptoethanol, which break the interchain disulfide bonds of the IgM molecule. C1q can be denatured by heating the sample for 30 minutes at 56°C.

Freezing and thawing of samples may cause protein denaturation or aggregation of immunoglobulins, which will cause high sample blank values or background light scattering. Sample matrix interference can be reduced by diluting the sample with reagent buffer containing PEG before antibody is added to the assay mixture.

The detection limit of nephelometric immunoassay is typically in the mg/L range. This is comparable to the sensitivities of radial immunodiffusion, immunoelectrophoresis, enzyme immunoassay, or fluorescence immunoassay. With automation, the precision or CV of nephelometry has been improved to the order of 2% to 5%.[8] Accuracy is more difficult to achieve. For each analyte to be measured, accuracy is determined by the quality of antisera as well as specimens used. Common to all immunoassays, calibrator or standards may be difficult to obtain or not available at all. Whenever available, calibrators or standards certified by international or professional organizations such as the World Health Organization (WHO) and College of American Pathologist (CAP) is strongly recommended.

Methods

Endpoint Nephelometry

In the immunoprecipitation reaction, the time to reach plateau light scattering may vary from a few minutes to 1 hour, depending on reaction conditions. After correction for background light scattering, this plateau for each sample is often directly proportional to its antigen concentration. The steps in an actual assay include the following: (1) Reagents, specimens, and antisera are first mixed together; (2) the background signal is measured; (3) incubation of the mixture continues until the plateau is reached; (4) the plateau or endpoint signal is measured; (5) a final signal is generated after correcting for background interference; and finally (6) the antigen concentration is determined using a calibration curve. Because of considerable variation between samples, there must be a background correction in end point nephelometry. The background interference due to sample blank will limit the sensitivity of end point nephelometry. The antisera avidity and affinity determine the incubation time and the height of the plateau reached for each assay.

Kinetic Nephelometry

For most nephelometric immunoassays, the peak rate of light scattering usually occurs in less than 1 or 2 minutes. The kinetics of the antigen–antibody complex formation are shown in Figure 16-3. The speed of reaction depends on the concentration of antigen and the affinity and titer of the antisera. In antibody excess the peak rate increases as the antigen concentration increases. The calibration curve of peak rate, or two-point reaction rate, versus antigen concentration may not necessarily be linear. This nonlinear relationship can be determined and stored in the instrument for data analysis. The time required to reach the peak reaction rate is inversely proportioned to the sample antigen concentration. Nephelometric assays operated in the kinetic mode need continuous monitoring of the reaction, starting when antibody is added and continuing to antigen excess check. The kinetic assay does not require the long incubation time for the immune complex reaction to reach the plateau. It generally requires antiserum of higher affinity and avidity than the endpoint method. The kinetic method is more sensitive to such factors as pH, buffer, and polymer enhancers. In the kinetic method, a conventional lamp with a wider bandwidth produces reaction rates that are more reproducible than rates measured with a laser. This is due to the fact that scattering signals from a single-wavelength laser source is more susceptible to the changing size of the immune complex during its initial formation stages.

Nephelometric Inhibition Immunoassay

Although the basic principles of nephelometric inhibition immunoassay (NIIA) were first reported by Pauling in 1942,[9] application of this immunoassay for haptens and drugs was only developed when automated nephelometers became available in the 1970s.[10,11] Haptens of molecular weight less than 4000 d cannot be measured directly by nephelometry because the monovalent nature of haptens prevents the lattice formation. Haptens covalently conjugated to carrier proteins can react with antisera directed against the hapten to form a lattice of sufficient size to be easily detected by nephelometers. Haptens will form soluble complexes with the antihapten antiserum. In NIIA, hapten is added to a mixture of a fixed amount of hapten conjugate and a limited amount of specific hapten antibody; the hapten will bind to the antibody and inhibit the lattice formation of hapten conjugate with antibody. Using reactants at concentrations close to equivalence and with the addition of enhancers, NIIA has been used in end point and rate assay of therapeutic drugs. This competition of hapten and its conjugates for antibody binding in NIIA allows homogeneous (nonseparation) immunoassay for haptens. The amount of light scattered is inversely related to the concentration of hapten in the specimen.

The precision of NIIA compares well with other drug assays. Like all immunonephelometry, the test is subject to sample matrix effect and nonspecific side-reactions.[10]

Particle-Enhanced Immunoassay

The latex agglutination test was first developed in 1956 by Singer and Plotz.[12] It is still widely used in semiquantitative serologic tests to detect rheumatoid factor, C-reactive protein, and antibodies to infectious agents. In immunonephelometry the sensitivity of protein assays depends on the number of immune complexes needed to produce precipitin for light scattering. When the reagents are immobilized onto an inert particle and retain their immunoreactivities, greater sensitivity can be achieved by monitoring the agglutination of the reagent particles. In essence, inert particles are used as building blocks to create light-scattering immunoprecipitin.

Polymer latexes, such as polystyrene latex, with diameters of 0.1 to 0.2 μm are coated with antigen or antibody. Antibody fragments and haptens can be covalently attached to particle surface for direct nephelometric immunoassay or indirect competitive NIIA. The performance characteristics of particle-enhanced immunoassays are reported to be comparable to the performance of enzyme immunoassay and radioimmunoassay.[13] Glycine buffers and surfactants are frequently used in particle reagents to improve shelf life by reducing self-aggregation of latex particles.

Applications

Measurement of immunoglobulins, complement components, C-reactive protein, and many other serum proteins is now routinely performed by automated nephelometry in many clinical laboratories. Commercial kits are readily available for IgG, IgA, IgM, C3, C4, and other specific proteins. Kinetic laser nephelometry has been used to evaluate other specific serum proteins, including clotting factors, prothrombin, antiprothrombin, and many abnormal proteins.[14] The antisera used should be nephelometric grade with affinity higher than that required for radial immunodiffusion. The titer and avidity of the antisera determine the dilution of antisera for sensitive standard curves and the useful range of the assay. Many monoclonal antibodies will not precipitate antigens. This can be overcome by using a mixture of antibodies against different antigenic determinants.[15]

Accuracy in immunoassays depends on the heterogeneity of the calibrator and the antigen tested. Immunoglobulins can be extremely heterogeneous, with large variations in size and subclass. This makes accuracy difficult to achieve. The WHO International Reference Preparation of human immunoglobulins, IgG, IgA, and IgM, is accepted as a primary standard against which many commercial calibrators or secondary standards are calibrated.[15]

Serum Immunoglobulin

Numerous techniques and commercial reagents are available for nephelometric determination of serum IgA, IgG, and IgM. With a maximum sensitivity of 1 mg/L, normal serum concentrations of IgD and IgE are too low to be detected by nephelometry. The advantages of nephelometry are good precision, accuracy, ease of assay, low cost, and fast turnaround time. Nephelometric assay has gradually replaced RID as the preferred method.[15,16] The correlation coefficient between nephelometry and RID methods is reported to be greater than 0.9. The range of CV for nephelometry is 0.6% to 10%. Among more than 1000 laboratories that participated in the CAP survey during 1982 and 1984, the Beckman ICS nephelometer produced the best precision, with CV between 3.7% and 5.6% for mid-level to high-level specimens and an overall CV for 5121 results of 4.8%. End point nephelometry, with a CV of 10.3%, is less satisfactory.[6,15]

Rate nephelometric determination of κ/λ ratio can distinguish monoclonal and polyclonal hypergammaglobulinemia; this distinction may be difficult using serum protein electrophoresis.[17]

Although nephelometry has been accepted as a standard laboratory procedure, when used to compare and evaluate new tests, problems may occur in nephelometric detection and characterization of immunoglobulin abnormalities in light-chain disease and polymeric IgG, IgD, and IgE. Nephelometric quantitation is limited by the subtypes of immunoglobulins in the calibrator and the specificity of the antisera used. Myeloma proteins and polymeric IgA of very large molecular mass could be underestimated by a factor of 10.[18] Some commercial kits may lead to incorrect or inconclusive results. Confirmation of results by immunoelectrophoresis is a good practice.

Cerebrospinal Fluid Immunoglobulin Synthesis

Although serum specimens are used more frequently, cerebrospinal fluid (CSF) and other body fluids can also be used in nephelometry. Daily determination of IgG synthesis in CSF of multiple sclerosis and neurologic patients was found to have diagnostic sensitivity, specificity, and a predictive value of 96% to 98%.[19] Nephelometric determination of CSF IgG/albumin ratio has both accuracy and precision comparable to RID.

Rheumatoid Factor

Measurement of rheumatoid factors (RF) has been greatly improved with the introduction of automated nephelometers. Rheumatoid factors are determined in immunonephelometry in a reverse technique whereby serum RF is measured using antigen (IgG) as the reagent. The results compared favorably with latex slide agglutination tests and latex tube dilution methods using Cohn fraction II as the source of IgG antigen. Nephelometric tests of RF by laser nephelometry and rate nephelometry were reported to have 86% to 105% recovery and CV is less than 5%.[20,21]

Specimens can be stored at 2° to 8°C for up to 5 days. Sera stored longer than 5 days should be frozen at or below −20°C. Repeated thawings denature proteins and should be avoided.

Circulating Immune Complexes

Nephelometry has been used successfully to quantitate circulating immune complexes by measuring the IgG in the complexes. When compared with the C1q-binding test, the correlation coefficient is 0.83.[22] To increase the assay sensitivity, immune complexes can be concentrated from serum by precipitation with PEG prior to assay using C1q.

Complement Components

Complement components are measured in immune complex diseases and in other conditions, such as inflammatory reactions and congenital deficiency. Nephelometric assays are used for complement components C3, C4, C3d, and Factor B.[23] The antisera should be nephelometric grade or filtered to remove large scattering particles. Complement components are detected as antigens and not by their function. In inflammatory conditions, because of the increased rate of synthesis and the short half-life of complement components, serial determinations in an individual to monitor changes in concentration are more informative than single measurements. Nephelometric determination of C3d is a better method to detect complement consumption; it provides more rapid and accurate quantitative results than does immunofixation.

In addition to clinical applications, nephelometry has become an important research and manufacturing tool to monitor quality of immunoreagents, to determine antisera titer and avidity, and to characterize modified antisera.[24,25]

Conclusion

Nephelometry has been accepted as a routine clinical laboratory method for immunoassay of immunoglobulins, immune complexes, complement components, abnormal serum proteins, and small compounds, such as hormones and drugs. Compared with RID and IEP, nephelometric immunoassay is convenient, nonisotopic, fast, and easily automated. Nephelometry instruments in general are expensive, but many automated chemical analyzers, such as centrifugal analyzers and enzyme analyzers, are readily available for nephelometric and turbidimetric immunoassay. With a good-quality control program and use of high-quality calibrators and reagents, nephelometric immunoassay can produce reliable results.

References

1. Heidelberger M, Kendall FE: A quantitative study and a theory of the reaction mechanism. J Exp Med 61:563, 1935

2. Sternberg JC: Rate nephelometry. In Rose NR, Friedman H, Fahey JL (eds): Manual of Clinical Laboratory Immunology, 3rd ed, p 33. Washington, DC, American Society for Microbiology, 1986

3. Whicher JT, Perry DE: Nephelometric methods. In Butt WR (ed): Practical Immunoassay: The State of the Art. Clin Biochem Anal 14:117, 1984

4. Normansell DE: Quantitation of serum immunoglobulins. CRC Crit Rev Clin Lab Sci 17:103, 1982

5. Merrack JR, Richards CB: Light-scattering studies of the formation of aggregates in mixture of antigen and antibody. Immunology 20:1019, 1971

6. Ritchie RF, Rippey JH: Performance on immunoglobulins IgG, IgA and IgM tests in CAP survey specimens. Am J Clin Pathol 78:644, 1982

7. DeGrella RF, Combs GL, Coffee EE, et al: A nephelometry system for the Abbott TDx analyzer. Clin Chem 31:1474, 1985

8. Frings CS, Gauldie J: Spectral techniques. In Kaplan LA, Pesce AJ (eds): Clinical Chemistry: Theory, Analysis and Correlation, p 67. St. Louis, CV Mosby, 1984

9. Pauling L, Pressman D, Campbell DH, et al: The serological properties of simple substances II: The effects of changed conditions and of added haptens on precipitation reactions of polyhaptenic simple substances. J Am Chem Soc 64:3003, 1942

10. Gauldie J, Bienenstock J: Automated nephelometric analysis of haptens. In Ritchie RF (ed): Automated Immunoanalysis, 1, p 321. New York, Marcel Dekker, 1978

11. Cambiaso CL, Riccomi H, Masson PL, et al: A new technique for the immunoassay of haptens: nephelometric inhibition immunoassay (NINIA). Protides Biol Fluids Proc Colloq 21:585, 1973

12. Singer JM, Plotz RM: The latex fixation test-applications to rheumatoid arthritis. Am J Med 21:888, 1956

13. Galvin JP: Particle-enhanced immunoassays. In Rose NR, Friedman H, Fahey JL (eds): Manual of Clinical Laboratory Immunology, 3rd ed, p 38. Washington, DC, American Society for Microbiology, 1986

14. Girolami A, Ruzza G, Saggin L, et al: The role of laser nephelometry in the study of abnormal clotting factors: Characterization of two abnormal antithrombins (ATIII Padua and ATIII Padua 2). Am J Clin Pathol 81:323, 1984

15. Check I, Piper M: Quantitation of immunoglobulins. In Rose NR, Friedman H, Fahey JL (eds): Manual of Clinical Laboratory Immunology, 3rd ed, p 138. Washington, DC, American Society for Microbiology, 1986

16. Jackson G: Immunoglobulin quantitation. In Pesce AJ, Kaplan LA (eds): Methods in Clinical Chemistry, p 735. St. Louis, CV Mosby, 1987

17. Renckens AL, Jansen MJ, van Munster PJ, et al: Nephelometry of the kappa/lambda light-chain ratio in serum of normal and diseased children. Clin Chem 32:2147, 1986

18. Levinson SS, Goldman JO, Markyvech L, et al: Inaccurate measurement of a polymeric IgA myeloma protein by nephelometric and fluorometric instrumentation. Clin Chem 32:2112, 1986

19. Valenzuela R, Mandler R, Goren H: Immunonephelometric quantitation of central nervous system IgG daily synthesis in multiple sclerosis. Am J Clin Pathol 78:22, 1982

20. Finley PR, Hicks MJ, Williams RJ, et al: Rate nephelometric measurement of rheumatoid factor in serum. Clin Chem 25:1909, 1979

21. Weinblatt MD, Schur PC: Rheumatoid factor detection by nephelometry. Arthritis Rheum 23:777, 1980

22. Feldkamp CS, Levinson SS, Perry M, et al: Anti-IgG combined with rate nephelometry for measuring polyethylene glycol-precipitated circulating immunocomplexes. Clin Chem 31:2024, 1985

23. Sun T, Stagias J: Detection of complement activation in immunocomplex diseases: six methods compared. Clin Chem 32:2170, 1986

24. Sittampalam G, Wilson GS, Byers JM: Characterization of antigen-enzyme conjugates: Theoretical considerations for rate nephelometric assays of immunoreactions. Anal Biochem 122:372, 1982

25. Hudson GA, Ritchie RF, Haddow JE: Method for testing antiserum titer and avidity in nephelometric systems. Clin Chem 27:1838, 1981

CHAPTER 17

Cellular Assays

Dorothy J. Fike

Mononuclear cells of the immune system may be divided into subsets by identifying specific cell surface markers. Many different procedures are used to identify the markers, some of which are flow cytometry for the enumeration of B cells and T-cell subsets using specific monoclonal antibodies for each; cytotoxicity testing, for the detection of HLA-A, -B, and -C antigens; and the mixed-lymphocyte culture for the detection of the HLA-D antigens. It is important to enumerate T and B cells, because an increase or decrease may indicate specific diseases. HLA antigen detection is very important for the survival of an organ in transplantation.

Other procedures are used to assess the cell function. It is not sufficient to enumerate the cells, since in some individuals the number of cells may be normal or increased but the cells may not function properly producing disease instead. Some procedures used to assess function are lymphocyte transformation, mixed-lymphocyte culture, the formation of lymphocyte activation products, cell-mediated cytotoxicity, and neutrophil functional assays. In some

procedures, a purified sample of cells must be prepared, whereas a purified sample is not required in other procedures. It is important that specific sample requirements be followed for accurate results.

Cell Separation Techniques

The most common procedure used for the separation of mononuclear cells is density gradient centrifugation. Ficoll-Hypaque, a commonly used density gradient preparation that is available commercially, requires that the blood sample be defibrinated or collected with preservative-free heparin. A total white blood cell count and differential performed on the blood sample prior to the separation allows the calculation of the white cell count.[1] Generally, diluted blood is carefully added to a tube containing the density gradient preparation to ensure that no blood mixes with the density gradient preparation. If blood mixes with the preparation, separation will be poor. After centrifugation, four layers can be identified:

The plasma will be on top, followed by mononuclear cells, the density gradient preparation, and finally the red cells and granulocytes (Fig. 17-1). If the tube is disturbed by braking the centrifuge or mixing the tube as it is removed from the centrifuge, the cell layers will be destroyed.[2] Granulocytes can be harvested from the density gradient separation by removing the supernate and lysing the red cells using an ammonium chloride solution; the neutrophils remain intact.[1] The separated cells may be used to detect specific cell markers.

Some methods to identify cell markers use whole blood. Whole blood is incubated with a fluorescent labeled monoclonal antibody to identify a specific type of cell. The red blood cells are lysed. The remaining cells are washed and the specific cells are counted by fluorescence microscopy or flow cytometry. Functional studies do not use whole blood because red cell or plasma proteins may interfere with the assay.[3]

Lymphocyte Subset Enumeration

Lymphocytes are divided into two major types, T cells and B cells. T cells are further divided into subsets, each with unique surface markers and functions. Monoclonal antibodies were used to discover distinct surface markers of the subsets. In 1983 a meeting was held by the First International Workshop on Human Leukocyte Differentiation Antigens to standardize the nomenclature of surface markers defined by different monoclonal antibodies. This group established the "cluster of differentiation" (CD) nomenclature that defined the different cellular antigens; periodically, meetings are held to refine and expand the CD designations.[3] Table 3-1 gives a partial listing of CD designations.

Cells in various stages of differentiation also have unique antigenic markers on their surface. During T-cell maturation, CD2 appears on early thymocytes and mature circulating lymphocytes. In the thymus, thymocytes mature into functional, circulating T lymphocytes. CD2 appears on the early thymocyte and persists on other cells in the maturation series, including peripheral blood T cells. The second stage of T-cell development, the common thymocyte, is marked by the simultaneous expression of CD2, CD3, CD4, and CD8. Mature thymocytes are identified by the presence of CD3 (T-cell antigen receptor) on their surface and the restricted expression of the functional markers CD4 and CD8.[4]

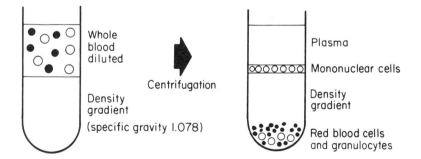

FIGURE 17-1. The separation of lymphocytes using a density gradient is performed by adding the diluted whole blood to a tube containing a density gradient with a specific gravity of 1.078. The tube is centrifuged and four layers are obtained. The lightest layer is plasma, which is on top. The mononuclear layer is located between the plasma layer and the density gradient layer. Red cells and granulocytes are the most dense and are located on the bottom of the tube.

Some T-cell subset types may not have a specific CD number. The CD designation is assigned after a specific monoclonal antibody to the marker has been produced. CD4, the T-cell helper/inducer subset, has two distinct cell types: the helper cell, which influences the B cell to produce antibody, and the inducer cell, which influences the induction of mature helper cells and suppressor cells. No monoclonal antibody has been produced that uniquely defines each cell type, so both cell types are given the designation CD4.[3] When a unique monoclonal antibody can define a specific marker on the surface of each type, a new CD will be assigned to each type.

Types of lymphocytes and subsets of lymphocytes may be quantitated manually or by flow cytometry. Differentiating between T and B cells can be done manually using rosetting techniques. T cells have a receptor for sheep red cells (SRBC), E-rosette receptor (CD2). When SRBC are incubated with purified lymphocytes, the SRBC will bind to the E-rosette receptor, thus identifying a T cell. At least three SRBC must adhere to the lymphocyte surface to be considered a rosette. When visualized by light microscopy, lymphocytes with rosettes and nonrosetted cells are counted. The percentage of T cells can be calculated. B cells can also be enumerated manually using a rosetting procedure in which antibody-coated sheep cells (EA-rosette) or antibody and complement-coated sheep cells (EAC-rosette) are used.[3] The production of monoclonal antibodies, discovery of subsets of T cells, and the labor-intensive nature of rosetting techniques have discouraged their use on a routine basis.

Flow cytometry is the method of choice for T- and B-cell analysis. This technique utilizes monoclonal antibody conjugated with a fluorescent dye and a photometer to measure the light energy emitted from cells. Simultaneous analysis of surface markers, cell volume, and cell size is now possible. The three most commonly used fluorescent labels are fluorescein and phycoerythrin (both of which are excited by light energy at 490 nm) and rhodamine (excited by light energy at 545 nm). A sample may be incubated with one or two different monoclonal antibodies to detect one or two different cell surface markers. This single- or two-color staining technique is a direct staining method.

In the indirect staining method, the monoclonal antibody is either unconjugated or conjugated with biotin. After incubation with the lymphocytes, a fluorochrome-labeled avidin or fluorochrome-labeled anti–mouse immunoglobulin is added to stain the cells. The indirect staining method is more sensitive than the direct staining method, and the procedure requires more time to perform.[5]

Once the sample is labeled, it is placed in the flow chamber for analysis (Fig. 17-2).[6] When the cell interrupts the beam of light from a neon or argon laser or mercury arc lamp, forward light scatter and side scatter at approximately a 90° angle are measured using a detector. Forward light scatter is a measure of the cell size or cell volume, whereas side scatter is a measure of cellular granularity.[5] Figure 17-3 is a histogram of a single analysis. The number of cells is obtained. Each cell type will be in a separate area of the histogram, depending on the cell size. In measuring forward light scatter, cell debris, lymphocytes, and large granular lymphocytes with monocytes will be measured (Fig. 17-3A). If wide-angle light scatter is measured, only lymphocytes and large granular lymphocytes with monocytes will be measured, since cell debris does not have any granularity (Fig. 17-3B). Measuring the two parameters of forward light scatter and side scatter will yield a dot display as seen in Figure 17-4.[5]

The number of cells that have a particular marker is also determined. The fluorescent dye causes stained cells to emit a fluorescent pulse, which is detected by the second detector. A histogram of the fluorescent readings may be seen in Figure 17-5.[6] A percentage of the cells fluorescing is obtained and the actual number of cells of a particular type must

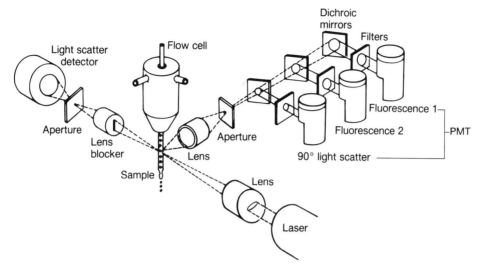

FIGURE 17-2. In the flow cytometer the cells flow through a laser light source one by one. The light is scattered by the presence of the cell. The amount of light scattered may be detected using a photomultiplier tube (PMT). Other photomultiplier tubes are used to detect the presence of fluorescence if a particular fluorescent-labeled antiserum is used to detect a specific cell marker.

be calculated from the cell count done initially. A two-parameter analysis of the wide-angle light scatter and the log of the intensity of either the red or green light emitted may also be obtained. Similar to the previous two-parameter analysis, a dot display is obtained. This two-parameter analysis is to check the accuracy of the gate setting. (A gate is the setting on the instrument that allows a particular set of cells to be analyzed.[5]

Two-color staining, the use of two different antibodies, each conjugated with a fluorescent dye that emits light of a different color, requires more con-

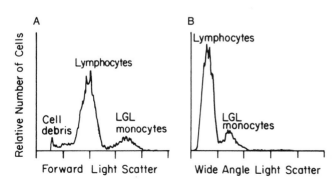

FIGURE 17-3. When only one parameter is measured, a histogram of the cell number is obtained. (A) When forward light scatter is measured using Ficoll-Hypaque separated cells, cell debris is detected in the first peak, the number of lymphocytes is determined in the second peak, and the number of large granular lymphocytes (LGL) and monocytes is found in the third peak. (B) When wide-angle scatter is used, there is no longer a peak for cell debris. The first peak determines the number of lymphocytes, whereas the second peak is the number of large granular lymphocytes and monocytes.

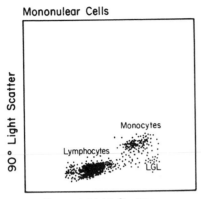

Mononuclear Cells

FIGURE 17-4. When the two parameters of 90° light scatter and forward light scatter are used together, a dot display is obtained rather than a histogram. Lymphocytes, large granular lymphocytes (LGL), and monocytes are found in a particular area of the dot display based on their size and granularity.

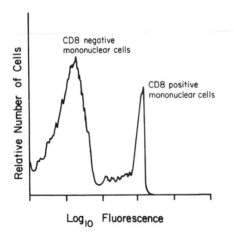

FIGURE 17-5. If mononuclear cells are stained with CD8 antiserum conjugated with fluorescein-isothiocyanate (FITC) and assayed using a flow cytometer, a histogram is obtained. The CD8-negative mononuclear cells are unstained and are the first peak seen on the histogram. The CD8-positive cells are enumerated in the second peak observed on the histogram.

trols than single-color staining. The gates for each marker must be accurately placed for correct analysis. Although two-color staining can yield greater information about the cells being studied, it should be done with extreme care.[5]

T-Cell Subset Analysis

Most CDs are related to T-cell subsets, which are differentiated to assess the immune competence of an individual. Once the percentage of cells is obtained from the flow cytometric analysis, the absolute number of cells in each subset may be calculated if the total number of lymphocytes is known; therefore, it is important that the total and differential white blood count be accurate. Since the reference range of each cell subset has not been established, each laboratory must establish its own range. Control populations should include a large sample of healthy men and women. The reference range should be those values that fall within the 5th and 95th percentile of all values obtained.[7]

The most frequently measured T-cell subsets in clinical settings are the helper T cells that express CD4 and suppressor T cells that express CD8. The ratio of CD4-positive cells and CD8-positive cells can be calculated; however, this ratio may not be accurate, because other cells may express CD4 or CD8. A decrease in CD4-positive cells and CD8-positive cells may be seen in primary and secondary immunodeficiencies. In primary immunodeficiency, cellular defects may be due to the condition itself, whereas in secondary immunodeficiency, an infection causes a decrease in some cell types. Table 17-1 lists some conditions in which CD4- and/or CD8-positive cell concentrations are altered. If a drug alters the CD4- or CD8-positive cell concentrations, the effect may vary with dosage and route of administration. T-cell subset quantitation is important in solid organ transplantation to monitor the effect of immunosup-

Table 17-1: Alterations in CD4- and CD8-Positive Lymphocytes

Condition	CD4	CD8
Multiple sclerosis	↓ or N	N
Systemic lupus erythematosus	↓	↓
Corticosteroids	↓	N
Cyclophosphamide	↓	↓
AIDS	↓	N (may be ↑ early)
CMV mononucleosis	↓ (transient)	↑ (lasts months to years)
EBV mononucleosis	N	↑ (transient)
P. falciparum malaria	↓ (transient)	N
Severe bacterial infections	↑ (relative)	—

There are several conditions in which the number of CD4- or CD8-positive lymphocytes is altered. (↑ indicates an increased number, ↓ indicates a decreased number, and N indicates no change.)

pressive therapy. In bone marrow transplantation the donor marrow is tested before transplantation to determine the number of cells that may cause a graft versus host reaction (mature T cells). Generally, mature T cells are removed prior to transplantation to minimize graft versus host disease. If these cells remain after immunosuppression of the marrow, suppression is insufficient. After transplantation, quantitation of T-cell subtypes is used to indicate the success of the transplantation. The total number of T cells, as well as that of CD4- and CD8-positive cell populations, is important.[7]

Other CD markers are used to study leukemia and lymphoma by identifying the cell line and stage of maturation of the aberrant cell. Some CD markers found on malignant cells are CD5, CD6, CD7, CD10, and CD15. The common acute lymphocytic leukemia antigen (CALLA) is recognized by CD10 antiserum. CD markers are found on other tumors that aid in the identification of the type of malignancy and, in some cases, the prognosis of the disease.[3,7,8]

B-Cell Analysis

The most useful surface marker on mature B cells is the surface immunoglobulin (sIg), which is synthesized by the B cell and serves as the antigen receptor. Flow cytometry can be used to quantitate mature B cells by identifying sIg. Because precursor B cells do not express sIg on their surface, flow cytometry cannot be used to quantitate precursor B cells. Most frequently, sIg is of the IgM and IgD classes with varying amounts on each cell. Some B cells also express surface IgG or IgA. Therefore, the antibody used in flow cytometric analysis should be a mixture of anti-immunoglobulin heavy chain types and light chain types to detect all B cells. The distribution of fluorescence intensity is the same for κ and λ light chains.[3,9] Polyspecific fluoresceinated antisera may also be used to manually quantitate B cells with a fluorescent microscope. This manual procedure is not as accurate as those assays done on the flow cytometer.[9]

In some diseases it may be beneficial to use a specific monoclonal antibody to determine the number of a specific cell type. Normally, CD5 is found on T cells; however, in cases of chronic lymphocytic leukemia, CD5 is found on the surface of neoplastic B cells. CD5 is also present on the surface of B cells following bone marrow transplantation.[9]

There are several technical problems when using sIg to quantitate B cells, because other cell types may also have immunoglobulin on their surface. Normal B cells, natural killer (NK) cells, activated T cells, and all phagocytic cells have Fc receptors that can bind circulating immunoglobulin. An incubation period of 1 hour at 37°C without serum prior to labeling the cells with fluoresceinated antiserum will remove immunoglobulin from the surface of cells that have not synthesized the immunoglobulin.[9]

Another problem associated with the B-cell enumeration is capping and shedding of sIg. When anti-immunoglobulin is added to the cell suspension, the initial uniform distribution of sIg rapidly disappears and is replaced by clumping of sIg on the cell surface. This process is slowed when cells are labeled and washed at cold temperatures. The labeled antibody should be the F(ab')$_2$ fragment, so that labeled antibody cannot nonspecifically bind to cells via the Fc receptor.[9]

It is important to enumerate B cells in normal individuals and patients with primary immunodeficiencies, some lymphomas, and neoplasms, such as multiple myeloma. In some cases of hypogammaglobulinemia, the number of B cells is within the reference range, even though the serum immunoglobulin concentration is decreased. Monoclonal antibodies may be used to detect the presence of a clonal prolif-

eration of B cells. Sometimes antiserum specific for κ or λ light chains is used to detect a clonal proliferation; if clonal proliferation is present, the usual two-to-one κ to λ ratio will not be present. A clone will express κ or λ chains as part of the sIg but not both.[9]

Enumeration of Other Cells in the Immune System

Natural killer (NK) cells can be enumerated by flow cytometry. NK cells express CD2, CD7, CD8, and CD16 on their surface. CD2, CD7, and CD8 antigens are shared by other T lymphocytes. Since NK cells are larger than other lymphocytes, it is possible to detect NK cells in the large granular lymphocytes (LGL) region of a double scatter plot (see Fig. 17-4). CD16 detects the Fc receptor on the surface of cells, and although it identifies NK cells, it also identifies other cells with Fc receptors, so that interpretation of results may be difficult. It may be important to assess the number of NK cells during immunosuppressive treatment or post–bone marrow transplantation. NK cells are the first lymphocytes to return, and the presence of NK cells in the blood indicates that the bone marrow is being reconstituted.[7]

Monocytes are approximately one third of the cells found in Ficoll–Hypaque mononuclear preparations. One method used to enumerate monocytes uses latex bead ingestion. Monocytes phagocytize the latex beads, and cells that have ingested these particles are counted. Surface markers, such as complement receptors may also be used to enumerate monocytes and macrophages.

Antibodies to the CR3 (the receptor for the C3b component of complement) may also be used to quantitate cells of the immune system. Most normal monocytes and granulocytes express this receptor on their surface. Because cell preparation for each cell type is different (see Fig. 17-1), the flow cytometer histogram would detect one cell type at a time. Some individuals may lack the CR3 receptor on monocytes and granulocytes, though these cells are present in normal quantities.[1]

Assays to Assess Cell Function

In addition to quantitating cell types, it is important to determine the ability of the cell to function. Some individuals have a normal cell number, but the cells fail to provide immunity, and repeated infections are present. Some techniques used to assess cell function are lymphocyte transformation, presence of lymphokines, cytotoxicity studies, chemotactic assays, and phagocytic assays.

Lymphocyte Transformation

Lymphocyte transformation is the ability of lymphocytes to proliferate in response to a stimulus. Measuring lymphocyte transformation is useful to assess and monitor function in congenital defects or immunosuppressive therapy, to identify transplantation antigens, to detect lymphokines, and to diagnose prior exposure to antigens. In all cases, the lymphocytes are incubated with a stimulus, and the ability of the cell to respond is measured by the percentage of lymphoblasts present or by the increase in DNA synthesis. In the former method the percentage of lymphoblasts is detected by light microscopy. The latter method measures tritiated thymidine, a radiolabeled DNA precursor, that is incorporated into actively replicating cells. This method is preferred, since radioactive decay is recorded by a scintillation counter rather than by subjective microscopic analysis by an individual.[2]

Mitogens, substances that induce mitosis in T or B cells, are used as the stimulus in lymphocyte transformation. Human studies using mitogens do not have the same specific T- and/or B-cell response that is found in mice. Phytohemagglutinin (PHA) and concanavalin A (Con A) stimulate predominantly T cells, whereas pokeweed mitogen (PWM) stimulates predominantly B cells. Lipopolysaccharide (LPS) does not appear to be a potent B-cell stimulator in humans. Staphylococcal protein A (SpA) stimulates B cells but triggers the response by interacting with the Fc receptor on the cells rather than the antigen receptor (Table 17-2).[3]

Lymphocytes are purified by Ficoll–Hypaque separation. Fresh or previously frozen cells are incubated with the mitogen in the assay. Culture conditions should support optimal growth of the lymphocytes; to enrich the culture medium human AB serum is added. Other heterologous serum may nonspecifically stimulate the cell. Optimal DNA synthesis usually occurs within 2 to 4 days, although 5 to 7 days may be required for an optimal response. DNA synthesis indicates that the lymphocytes responded to the mitogen, underwent blast transformation, and incorporated the tritiated thymidine into the newly synthesized DNA. Incorrect results may be obtained if optimal conditions are not met. Some conditions that cause suboptimal proliferation are inadequate number of cells, incorrect incubation time period, incorrect concentration of mitogen, and pres-

Table 17-2: Mitogens for Lymphocyte Transformation

Mitogen	Relative Specificity
PHA	T cells
Con A	T cells (different subset from PHA)
PWM	B cells, T-cell-dependent
SpA	B cells, T-cell-independent

ence of an inhibitory factor in the media or serum. Controls are run to assess each variable separately.[2,3]

In addition, specific soluble antigens may also be used for lymphocyte transformation. Fewer cells are transformed than those responding to mitogens because only those cells that have been sensitized to the specific antigen can respond. The assay procedure is the same as that for mitogens; thus, the same problems may occur. In normal individuals, the response to an antigen with skin testing or *in vitro* antigen assays is comparable; however, in some cases, the *in vitro* test is more sensitive.[3] Figure 17-6 illustrates the results of lymphocyte transformation.

Mixed-Lymphocyte Culture

The mixed-lymphocyte culture (MLC), a variation of lymphocyte transformation, is primarily used to detect major histocompatibility antigens (see Chapter 2). In the MLC, lymphocytes are used to stimulate a second source of lymphocytes. The MLC procedure may be used as a "one-way" or "two-way" responder cell assay, though the most practical technique is the "one-way" MLC. In the one-way MLC the stimulator cell is irradiated so that it serves as the antigen stimulus and the responder cell can react

to the stimulator cell, whereas in the two-way MLC, either cell type can respond to the other. The two-way MLC yields little information and is rarely used. In any MLC, the culture conditions, incubation time, and assessment of cell division are the same.[3,10]

To define the HLA-D antigen type of a patient by one-way MLC, homozygous typing cells (HTC) that serve as the stimulator cell are inactivated by irradiation or treatment with mitomycin C, so they are unable to respond or divide. HTC are lymphocytes that express only one HLA-D antigen on their surface. When incubated with patient lymphocytes, the patient lymphocytes will respond to those HTC that express HLA-D antigens that are not present on the patient's lymphocytes. A second application of the MLC is in transplantation compatibility. Compatibility between the recipient and donor allows better survival of the grafted tissue. In solid organ transplantations, the donor cells are inactivated and then exposed to patient lymphocytes, so that any response is by the patient lymphocytes. The inactivated cell is the stimulator cell, and the untreated cell is the responder cell.

After inactivation of the stimulator cell, the two cell types are incubated in the culture medium for a minimum of 4 days. Radiolabeled DNA precursor is added to the cells, and the cells are incubated for at

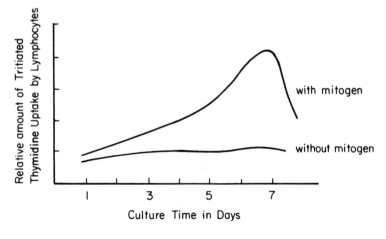

FIGURE 17-6. In the lymphocyte transformation procedure, the cells that are transformed with mitogen incorporate the radioactive DNA precursors into the cell. The amount of radiation observed in these cells reaches a peak in days 5 to 6 of the assay.

least 6 to 12 hours. The cells are harvested, and the amount of radiolabel in the cells is measured (Fig. 17-7).[3,10] Interpreting the assay may be difficult because of the variation in antigen concentration on the stimulator lymphocyte. In some situations the responder cell may not have sufficient tritiated thymidine counts to indicate whether the antigen is present or not. The significance of a moderate response is not understood.[3,10]

Lymphocyte Activation Products

The presence of lymphokines released by activated lymphocytes is evidence of lymphocyte function. Some lymphokines that are assayed are macrophage migration inhibitory factor (MIF), leukocyte inhibi-

tory factor (LIF), and leukocyte adherence inhibition (LAI).

There are two methods to assay migration inhibition: the direct, or one-step, procedure and the indirect, or two-step. In the one-step procedure the lymphocytes are in the presence of mononuclear cells. When a specific antigen is added, the lymphocytes produce the MIF or LIF lymphokines, thus inhibiting the migration of monocytes or granulocytes, respectively (Fig. 17-8). In the two-step procedure, the lymphocytes are cultured with antigen and the supernate-containing lymphokines is collected; this supernate is then used to assay the migration inhibition of a cell. The test procedure may be carried out in a capillary tube or agarose gel.[11]

The LAI technique may be one- or two-step procedures using a hemocytometer, test tube, or micro-

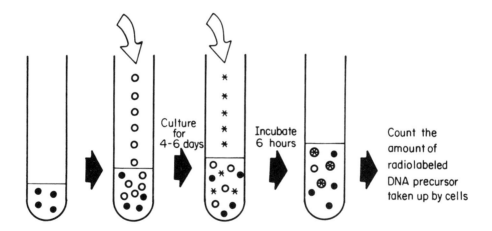

● = Irradiated Stimulator Lymphocytes
O = Responder Lymphocytes
* = Radiolabeled DNA Precursor (Titiated Thymine)

FIGURE 17-7. Irradiated stimulator lymphocytes are incubated with responder lymphocytes in cell culture for 4 to 6 days. After this incubation, radiolabeled DNA precursor, generally tritiated thymidine, is added to the culture and reincubated for an additional 6 hours. After the second incubation, the amount of radiation present in the cells is measured. If the stimulator lymphocytes and responder lymphocytes have different HLA antigens present on the cell surface, the amount of radiation present in the cells will be increased.

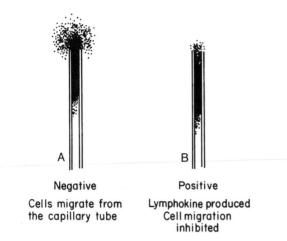

Negative

Cells migrate from
the capillary tube

Positive

Lymphokine produced
Cell migration
inhibited

FIGURE 17-8. Migration inhibition tests are functional assays that detect the presence of lymphokine production. (A) In a negative test, lymphokine is not produced. The mononuclear cells are not inhibited from migrating from the capillary tube and cells will be observed in the area around the capillary tube. (B) In a positive test, lymphokine is produced. The mononuclear cells are inhibited from migration and no cells will be observed in the surrounding area.

titer plate. When the lymphocytes produce LAI, the migration of leukocytes is inhibited. The cells that adhere to the surface of a hemocytometer chamber after it is washed are counted. In the test tube method, cells that do not adhere are counted. In the microtiter method, cells adhering to the side of the well are stained and counted.[11]

Cytotoxicity

Evidence of cellular function may also be observed by cytolysis or cytotoxicity. Some techniques that incorporate cellular destruction of cells are the cytotoxicity test to detect class I human leukocyte antigens (HLA), natural killer activity, cell-mediated lympholysis, and macrophage tumoricidal activity. Cell lysis may be due to the interaction of antibody and complement or to the specific action of some cells.

HLA Detection

As with lymphocyte transformation techniques, one major use of the cytotoxicity technique is in transplantation. The HLA antigens detected by this procedure are HLA-A, -B, -C, -DR, and -DQ. After lymphocytes are separated by the density gradient procedure, the cells are added to a microtiter tray in which each well contains one specific antibody. After a short incubation, rabbit complement is added and the tray is incubated again. If an antigen is located on the lymphocyte surface, the specific antibody in the well will attach to the cell, complement will be activated, and the cell will lyse. The cells are stained with a supravital stain, such as trypan blue or eosin; the latter is generally preferred because it stains the cells more consistently. Stained cells are counted using a light or inverted microscope (Fig. 17-9).[2,13] Cells that stain are those with the specific HLA antigen on their surface to which the antibody has bound. When complement lyses the cell, holes in the membrane allow the stain to enter the cell. Thus, dead cells allow the stain to enter the cell, whereas live cells exclude the stain.

To distinguish between cytolysis due to complement activity and that resulting from spontaneous cell death, a cell control that contains lymphocytes and non–immune blood group AB serum is used to establish a cut-off percentage for a positive test. Since antibody affinity and avidity may vary, several different antibodies against the same antigen are used in the microtiter tray.[12,13] The upper limit of acceptable spontaneous cell death in the cell control is 5%; values higher than this may indicate old cells, improperly handled cells (improper centrifugation or improper pH and tonicity of reagents), or rabbit antibodies in the complement that react with human cells. Sources of error are related to evaluation of the percentage of stained cells, uneven distribution of cells (the number of cells was not the same in each of the wells or the cells were not evenly distributed in the well), debris that stains, bubbles that stain, and

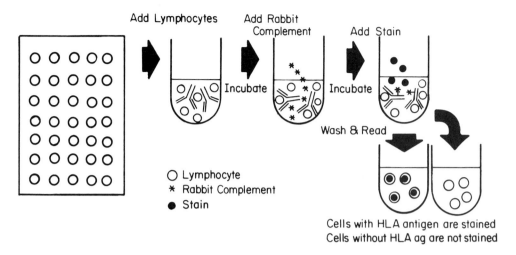

Add Lymphocytes   Add Rabbit Complement   Add Stain

Incubate   Incubate

Wash & Read

○ Lymphocyte
* Rabbit Complement
● Stain

Cells with HLA antigen are stained
Cells without HLA ag are not stained

FIGURE 17-9. The microcytotoxicity test to detect MHC class I molecules is done using a microtiter tray. Each well contains a specific antibody and the purified lymphocytes are added to each well. Rabbit complement is added and the tray is incubated to allow antigen, antibody, and complement to react. If the class I antigen is present on the lymphocyte, antibody will react with the antigen and the complement cascade will cause the lysis of the lymphocyte. Eosin is added and will enter cells that have been lysed. The tray is washed free of all stain that is not cell bound. Each well is read microscopically for the presence of eosin-stained cells.

old serum in the wells; the latter is only a problem in laboratories reusing old plates.[13]

The cytotoxicity procedure can also be used to detect HLA-A, -B, and -C antibodies in the patient serum. Patient serum is incubated with a panel of lymphocytes with known antigens on their surface. The remainder of the procedure is the same. Antibodies to HLA antigens may be produced during pregnancy and following blood transfusions and organ transplantation. If an organ recipient has an HLA antibody and the organ to be transplanted expresses the same antigen, the survival time of the transplanted organ will be short. Therefore, it is preferable to transplant an organ without the antigen to extend the survival time.[14]

Cell-Mediated Cytotoxicity

Natural killer cells (NK), T cells, and monocytes may be cytotoxic to other cells, but the mode of action is independent of complement. Monocytes may be cytotoxic to tumor cells. This tumor cell–dependent cellular cytotoxicity may be detected using purified monocytes in a microtiter tray. The monocytes are incubated with and without target tumor cells, which are radiolabeled with ^{125}I iododeoxyuridine. If the monocytes are functional, they will kill the target cells. After washing the dead cells from the microtiter wells, the remaining cells are lysed to release the radioactive label, which is then measured.[15]

NK cells kill other cells by an antibody-dependent mechanism. Though the cytolytic mechanism is not clear, antibody is present yet complement is not involved. Antibody-dependent cell-mediated cytotoxicity (ADCC) will destroy tumor cells or cells that contain microorganisms. Other cells (macrophages, granulocytes, and a lymphocyte subpopulation) will participate in ADCC; but the major cell involved is the NK cell. In the assay to demonstrate ADCC, the target cell (a radiolabeled bacterially infected cell or tumor cell) is coated with antibody; then purified NK cells are added that attach to the target cells. After incubation and washing to remove lysed cellular material, the remaining intact cells are lysed and the radiolabel is measured. The percent of specific cytotoxicity is calculated.[16]

Cytotoxic T cells may lyse cells, independent of antibody, through cell-mediated lympholysis (CML). The procedure for assessing CML is similar to that of the MLC. A one-way MLC culture is prepared and a ^{51}Cr radiolabeled target cell that is HLA identical to the stimulator cell in the MLC is added. The cytotoxic effect is reflected by measuring the radiolabel in the supernate from the specific target cell. A control using nonspecific target cells is also performed. The CML activity is the percentage of the radioactivity in the control cells versus the radioactivity in the specific target cells.[3]

Neutrophil Function Assays

Neutrophil activity requires cellular and humoral immunity. Since it is complex, several different assays should be performed to assess the parameters of neutrophil function: motility, chemotaxis, ingestion, and intracellular killing.

An unstimulated neutrophil exhibits random motility, which may be assessed using the capillary tube method. Purified neutrophils are placed in a capillary tube, and the motility is observed microscopically by checking the leading edge of the leukocytes at hourly intervals. The distance that the cells move from the starting point is measured. Cells with normal motility move from the capillary tube.[3]

The movement of neutrophils in a specific direction is the result of chemotactic stimuli and may be measured using a Boyden Chamber. Neutrophils are placed in the upper chamber, which is separated from the lower chamber by 5-μm-porosity filter paper. The cells are placed in the upper chamber; the lower chamber contains a chemotactic agent. After incu-

bation the filter paper is stained and stained cells on the lower side of the filter paper are counted.[3,17] Those neutrophils that respond to the chemotactic agent will be counted. The incubation period is very important, since a short incubation period may not detect all cells with chemotactic ability, and an incubation period that is too long may allow cells to detach from the lower surface, resulting in a lower level of measured chemotactic ability.[17]

The main function of neutrophils is to phagocytize cells containing microorganisms. The neutrophils' phagocytic ability may be evaluated by counting ingested particles when a saturating dose of particle is used.[18]

Neutrophils are incubated with *Escherichia coli* lipopolysaccharide-coated oil droplets containing oil red O stain. The particles must first be treated with fresh human serum, which enables C3 to bind to the surface of the particle, facilitating particle ingestion by neutrophils. Following incubation of the cells and particles, the mixture is centrifuged to remove the floating, uningested particles that contain oil red O stain. The intracellular oil red O is extracted from the cells, and the concentration is read spectrophotometrically.[18]

Intracellular killing of microorganisms depends on many enzymes and agents. A procedure that is useful for determining if the neutrophils can kill microorganisms is the nitroblue tetrazolium (NBT) dye reduction test. NBT is a clear yellow, water soluble compound that forms formazan, a deep blue dye, when it is reduced. NBT may be attached to latex particles or other particles. When the neutrophil ingests latex-NBT, a change in color suggests that the cell has the ability to kill microorganisms. The blue dye present in the cell may be extracted and read spectrophotometrically.[3,18]

Summary

To assess immunocompetent cells, both cell numbers and their ability to function must be determined; in

Table 17-3: Cellular Assay Procedures

Procedure	Reagents Used	Assessment
Flow cytometry	Specific antibody to detect cell markers	Number of T$_H$, T$_S$, and B lymphocytes; NK cells; granulocytes; and other cells
Latex bead ingestion	Latex beads	Number of monocytes
Lymphocyte transformation	Mitogen or specific antigen	Ability of lymphocyte to respond to a stimulus
Mixed-lymphocyte culture	Recipient and donor lymphocytes	Detects compatibility of HLA-D antigens
	Patient lymphocytes and homozygous typing cells	Detects HLA-D antigens
Migration inhibition	Monocytes, granulocytes	Ability of lymphocyte to produce chemotactic factors
Cytotoxicity		
Microcytotoxicity	Antibodies	Detects HLA-A, -B, -C, -DR antigens
	Antigens	Detects HLA antibodies
Cell-mediated		
Monocytolysis	Tumor cells	Ability of monocytes to kill cells
ADCC	Tumor cells or cells containing bacteria	Ability of NK cells to lyse cells
Lympholysis	Labeled target cell	Ability of cytotoxic T cells to lyse cells
Boyden chamber	Chemotactic agent	Ability of neutrophils to respond to a chemotactic agent
Phagocytosis	*E. coli* polysaccharide with oil red O stain	Ability of neutrophils to phagocytize
Nitroblue tetrazolium test	Nitroblue tetrazolium	Ability of neutrophils to effect intracellular kill

some cases, cell numbers may be adequate, yet repeated infections may be present.

T- and B-lymphocyte numbers may be determined using specific monoclonal antibodies against cell surface markers, such as CD4 (helper T cells), CD8 (suppressor T cells) and sIg (B cells). When specific antibody is conjugated to a fluorescent dye, the cells may be enumerated using the flow cytometer.

Detection of HLA antigens on cells is important in transplantation. Class I antigens are detected using the cytotoxicity test procedure. The presence of class II antigens is determined using the mixed-lymphocyte culture (MLC). The survival of the transplanted organ is better when class I and class II antigens of the recipient match those of the donor.

Cell function may be assessed using a variety of test procedures. Lymphocyte transformation is used to determine the ability of the lymphocyte to respond to various mitogens or antigens. Other lymphocyte functions that may be assessed are lymphokine production such as migration inhibition tests and the ability to kill other cells using cell-mediated lympholysis (CML). The NK cell function of cytolysis is assessed using antibody-dependent cell-mediated cytotoxicity (ADCC).

The functional ability of neutrophils is important to assess. Test procedures to detect mobility, chemotaxis, ingestion of particles, and killing are used.

Table 17-3 is a summary of all procedures discussed in this chapter.

References

1. Winchester RJ, Ross GD: Methods for enumerating cell populations by surface markers with conventional microscopy. In Rose NR, Friedman H, Fahey JL (eds): Manual of Clinical Laboratory Immunology, 3rd ed, p 212. Washington, DC, American Society for Microbiology, 1986

2. Maluish AE, Strong DM: Lymphocyte proliferation. In Rose NR, Friedman H, Fahey JL (eds): Manual of Clinical Laboratory Immunology, 3rd ed, p 260. Washington, DC, American Society for Microbiology, 1986

3. Stites DP: Clinical laboratory methods for detection of cellular immune function. In Stites DP, Stobo JD, Wells JV (eds): Basic and Clinical Immunology, 6th ed, p 285. Norwalk, Appleton and Lange, 1987

4. Reinherz EL, Schlossman S: The differentiation and function of human T lymphocytes. Cell 19:821, 1981

5. Jackson AL, Warner NL: Preparation, staining and analysis by flow cytometry of peripheral blood leukocytes. In Rose NR, Friedman H, Fahey JL (eds): Manual of Clinical Laboratory Immunology, 3rd ed, p 226. Washington, DC, American Society for Microbiology, 1986

6. Downing JR, Benson NA, Braylan RC: Flow cytometry: Applications in the clinical laboratory. Lab Management, 22:29, 1984

7. Giorgi JV: Lymphocyte subset analysis measurements: Significance in clinical medicine. In Rose NR, Friedman H, Fahey JL (eds): Manual of Clinical Laboratory Immunology, 3rd ed, p 236. Washington, DC, American Society for Microbiology, 1986

8. Parker JW: Flow cytometric analysis of lymphoproliferative disorders using monoclonal antibodies. Lab Med 16:21, 1985

9. Ault KA: Flow cytometric evaluation of normal and neoplastic B cells. In Rose NR, Friedman H, Fahey JL (eds): Manual of Clinical Laboratory Immunology, 3rd ed, p 247. Washington, DC, American Society for Microbiology, 1986

10. Dubey DP, Yunis I, Yunis EJ: Cellular typing: Mixed lymphocyte response and cell mediated lympholysis. In Rose NR, Friedman H, Fahey JL (eds): Manual of Clinical Laboratory Immunology, 3rd ed, p 847. Washington, DC, American Society for Microbiology, 1986

11. Borish L, Liu DY, Remold H, et al: Production and assay of macrophage migration inhibition factor, leukocyte migration inhibitory factor and leukocyte adherence activation factor. In Rose NR, Friedman H, Fahey JL (eds): Manual of Clinical Laboratory Immunology, 3rd ed, p 282. Washington, DC, American Society for Microbiology, 1986

12. Schwartz BD: The major histocompatibility HLA complex. In Stites DP, Stobo JD, Wells JV (eds): Basic and Clinical Immunology, 6th ed, p 50. Norwalk, Appleton and Lange, 1987

13. Sullivan KA, Amos DB: The HLA system and its detection. In Rose NR, Friedman H, Fahey JL (eds): Manual of Clinical Laboratory Immunology, 3rd ed, p 835. Washington, DC, American Society for Microbiology, 1986

14. Zacharey AA, Murphy NB, Smerglia AR, et al: Screening sera for HLA antibodies. In Rose NR, Friedman H, Fahey JL (eds): Manual of Clinical Laboratory Immunology, 3rd ed, p 824. Washington, DC, American Society for Microbiology, 1986

15. Rosenwasser LJ: Monocyte and macrophage function. In Rose NR, Friedman H, Fahey JL (eds): Manual of Clinical Laboratory Immunology, 3rd ed, p 321. Washington, DC, American Society for Microbiology, 1986

16. Herberman RB: Natural killer cell activity and antibody dependent cell-mediated cytotoxicity. In Rose NR, Friedman H, Fahey JL (eds): Manual of Clinical Laboratory Immunology, 3rd ed, p 308. Washington, DC, American Society for Microbiology, 1986

17. Maderazo EG, Ward PA: Leukocyte chemotaxis. In Rose NR, Friedman H, Fahey JL (eds): Manual of Clinical Laboratory Immunology, 3rd ed, p 290. Washington, DC, American Society for Microbiology, 1986

18. Southwick FS, Stossel TP: Phagocytosis. In Rose NR, Friedman H, Fahey JL (eds): Manual of Clinical Laboratory Immunology, 3rd ed, p 326. Washington, DC, American Society for Microbiology, 1986

CHAPTER 18

Syphilis

Ann Marie McNamara

Syphilis

Treponema Pallidum

The etiologic agent of syphilis is the bacterium *Treponema pallidum*, subspecies *pallidum*. This aerobic bacterium is a member of the order Spirochaetales, the family Treponemataceae, and the genus *Treponema*. These spirochetes are long, thin, spiral-shaped, unicellular organisms that are 5 to 15 μm long and 0.09 to 0.18 μm wide[1] (Fig. 18-1). These bacteria are loosely coiled, with 6 to 24 coils (average 14). Spirochetes are unique among bacteria in that their characteristic corkscrew motility is produced by internal periplasmic flagella located between the outer membrane and the periplasmic cylinder (body) of the spirochete.[2]

Two species of the genus *Treponema* infect humans: *T. pallidum* and *T. carateum*, the causative agent of pinta. *T. pallidum* is further divided into three subspecies: *T. pallidum*, subspecies *pallidum*, the causative agent of syphilis; *T. pallidum*, subspecies *pertenue*, the causative agent of yaws; and *T. pallidum*, subspecies *endemium*, the causative agent of nonvenereal endemic syphilis.[3] Unless noted otherwise, *T. pallidum* refers to subspecies *pallidum* throughout the remainder of this chapter. A third species of the genus is *T. paraluis-cuniculi*, the causative agent of rabbit syphilis. All the treponemes infecting humans are identical serologically, sharing similar surface macromolecules and antigens. The three other treponemal diseases (yaws, pinta, and endemic syphilis) are distinguished from syphilis based on their geographic localization and clinical disease syndromes, since the treponemes causing them are morphologically and serologically indistinguishable with current diagnostic methods. Evidence suggests that these three pathogenic treponemes are variants of a single prototype organism whose different clinical syndromes developed in response to host or environmental influences.[3]

In addition to the pathogenic treponemes, a number of nonpathogenic treponemes have been isolated

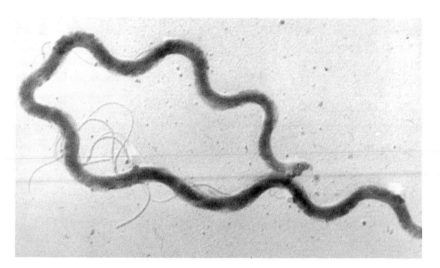

FIGURE 18-1. Electron micrograph of *Treponema pallidum*. (Courtesy of CDC Slide Archives.)

from the human body, particularly from the oral cavity. *Treponema retgerri* is an example of a nonpathogenic treponeme. Nonpathogenic and pathogenic treponemes can be distinguished by the failure of pathogenic treponemes to reproduce in standard laboratory conditions. However, pathogenic treponemes are capable of surviving and retain their mobility in enriched and chemically defined media for up to 7 days at 25°C and up to 48 hours at 37°C.[1] Intratesticular passage of treponemes in rabbits is necessary to maintain a source of treponemes for laboratory studies. This makes research into the biology and pathogenesis of treponemes difficult.

Little is known about the interaction between *T. pallidum* and the human host. There is evidence that the complex symptomatology of syphilis is influenced by both humoral and cell-mediated immune responses. The body produces antitreponemal and anticardiolipin antibodies, initiates an inflammatory response (involving lymphocytes, plasma cells, and macrophages), forms immune complexes, walls off the organism in lesions, and enters a latency (remission) stage of the disease.[3]

Clinical Features

Epidemiology

In 1986 the incidence of primary and secondary syphilis was approximately 11 cases per 100,000 population.[4] Annually, approximately 1.5 million serologic tests are reactive for syphilis in the primary, secondary, and latent stages.[5] Syphilis is transmitted by four main routes: sexual contact, transfusion of fresh human blood, direct inoculation, and through the placenta (congenital syphilis).

The most common route of acquiring syphilis is through sexual intercourse. Most cases occur in the sexually active age group (15 to 30 years old), nonwhites, and homosexual men. Transmission can occur through the act of sexual intercourse itself, kissing, or touching active lesions.

Transmission of syphilis through blood transfusions or blood products is rare in the United States. This is due to the low incidence of syphilis in the United States, combined with the fact that under current blood bank storage conditions, *T. pallidum* cannot survive longer than 24 to 48 hours (at 4°C).[6]

Disease Stages

Incubation Period. *T. pallidum* enters the human body through abrasions in the skin or by penetrating intact mucous membranes. Once inside the human host, the bacterium begins to multiply. Within hours it enters the lymphatics and/or the bloodstream and is disseminated to the various organs of the body.[1] This stage occurs from 0 to 33 hours postinfection and lasts from 9 to 90 days (average of 3 weeks).[5] During the incubation period there are no clinical symptoms of the disease and all serologic tests are negative. Negative skin tests and depressed mitogenic responses indicate that T-cell immunity is impaired.

Primary Syphilis. The primary stage of syphilis begins with the appearance of the initial lesion called a chancre. The chancre is usually a firm, eroded, painless papule with raised, indurated margins that progresses to a clean-based, nonbleeding, painless ulcer.[1] Generally, chancres appear at the site of inoculation after a 2- to 3-week incubation period. They are commonly found in the genital and perianal regions or extragenitally on the lips, tongue, nipples, tonsils, and fingers. Often they are single lesions, although multiple lesions can occur. Within a week of the appearance of the chancre, regional lymph nodes become enlarged (although painless). These enlarged lymph nodes are termed satellite bulboes. The chancre heals spontaneously within 3 to 6 weeks; however, the lymphadenopathy persists.[1] The patient usually enters an asymptomatic period following the healing of the chancre, although some patients begin to develop symptoms of secondary syphilis during the primary stage.

In the early primary stage patients are seronegative, as humoral antibodies generally begin to develop from 1 to 4 weeks after the appearance of the chancre. Darkfield microscopy examination of the lesion fluids for the presence of spirochetes can confirm the diagnosis prior to the development of antibodies. If nontreponemal screening tests are negative but the patient presents with a lesion characteristic of syphilis, the nontreponemal screening test should be repeated after 1 week, 1 month, and 3 months before ruling out a diagnosis of syphilis.[7] Cellular immunity remains depressed at this stage.

Secondary Syphilis. Secondary syphilis marks the disseminated stage of the disease. This stage is characterized by skin rashes and the demonstration of large numbers of treponemes throughout the body. Almost any type of skin rash (except vascular rashes) can be seen in secondary syphilis, with the rash being quite marked on the palms and soles, rarely on the face. The patient also presents with low-grade fever, malaise, pharyngitis, laryngitis, weight loss, arthralgia, and generalized painless lymphadenopathy.[1] Highly infectious lesions called mucous patches develop on the mucous membranes. These erosions are silver-gray in color with a red periphery and contain numerous spirochetes. Because of the large numbers of spirochetes in the bloodstream, these bacteria are disseminated to the organs of the body, including the central nervous system. At this stage of syphilis all serologic tests are positive and T-cell responses become normal. The diagnosis of secondary syphilis should also be considered when a prozone phenomenon (a false negative test in persons with high titers) results in a negative nontreponemal test result.

Latency. Latent syphilis is a stage of acquired or congenital syphilis without signs and symptoms of the disease, but with positive nontreponemal and treponemal antibody tests. Latency is divided into two stages: early latency (less than 1 year after initial infection) and late latency (more than 1 year after infection). In at least 25% of untreated syphilis cases, signs and symptoms of relapses into secondary syphilis occur during early latency.[5] A patient is considered to have early latent syphilis if there is a history of lesions consistent with untreated primary or secondary syphilis, or if the patient has had a nonreactive, nontreponemal reagin test within the last year.[5] During late latent syphilis the patient becomes more resistant to reinfection and to relapses.[1]

Spirochetemia is reduced during latency, although the patient remains infectious. When lesions are present, syphilis may still be transmitted by sexual contact; otherwise blood transfusions and congenital transfer are the main routes of transmission during latency. Serologic tests are reactive during the latency stage and are the only means of diagnosing latent syphilis when clinical symptoms are absent.

Tertiary Syphilis. Tertiary syphilis is a slowly progressive inflammatory disease that can produce clinical illness 2 to 40 years after initial infection. This stage has been called gummatous syphilis, neurosyphilis, or cardiovascular syphilis.[1] Gummas are lesions of syphilis that resemble tuberculosis and may occur in the skin, bones, mucosa, muscles, and organs of the body.[8] These lesions are believed to be the result of delayed hypersensitivity reactions and contain few treponemes. Penicillin rapidly resolves gummatous lesions.[1] Cardiac anomalies contribute to the morbidity and mortality in tertiary syphilitic patients. Most commonly, syphilitic aortitis, aortic valve insufficiency, and thoracic aneurysm and rupture occur.[8] Central nervous system (CNS) involvement results from the multiplication of treponemes in CNS lesions. Neurosyphilis may present in asymptomatic or symptomatic stages and often causes blindness and/or insanity. The symptomatic phase may present with symptoms of endarteritis obliterans, general paresis, or tabes dorsalis.[1] Nontreponemal reagin tests are less sensitive than treponemal tests for detecting tertiary syphilis. Neurosyphilis can be confirmed by a positive Venereal Disease Research Laboratory-cerebrospinal fluid (VDRL–CSF) test (described later).

Congenital Syphilis. Transfer of *T. pallidum* across the placenta can occur in any untreated mother in any stage of syphilis. Generally, the severity of congenital infection correlates to the clinical stage of the mother, the most severe cases occurring when the mother has early primary or secondary syphilis. Clinical outcome may be late abortion, stillbirth, neonatal death, neonatal disease, or latent infection.[1] Treatment of the mother during the first 4 months of pregnancy almost always prevents congenital syphilis.[1] Signs of early congenital syphilis include rhinitis (snuffles) and a diffuse maculopapular desquamatous rash, particularly about the mouth and on the palms and soles. The child may also have hemolytic anemia, jaundice, hepatosplenomegaly, and bone involvement.[1] Signs of late syphilis, after 1 year of age, include corneal involvement, deafness, and abnormal bone and tooth development.[1] Treponemes are present in almost every tissue of the infant. A definitive diagnosis may be made by darkfield examination of skin lesions or nasal discharge for the presence of *T. pallidum* and by increasing antibody titers in quantitative nontreponemal tests.[8]

Diagnosis

The diagnosis of syphilis is based on recognition of the clinical signs and symptoms in the various disease stages of syphilis, darkfield examination of fluid from syphilitic lesions for spirochetes, and syphilis serologic testing. The most important of these three is syphilis serology, because of the transient and sometimes nonspecific symptoms of the disease, and the lack of well-trained darkfield microscopists who must be able to distinguish between pathogenic and nonpathogenic spirochetes in patient samples.

Treatment

The treatment of choice for all stages of syphilis (early syphilis, secondary syphilis, tertiary syphilis, neurosyphilis, congenital syphilis, syphilis during pregnancy) is penicillin. For penicillin-allergic patients, the alternative drug of choice is tetracycline. Since tetracycline has been shown to have adverse effects on the human fetus, pregnant women who are allergic to penicillin should be treated with erythromycin.[9] Recent studies have shown that the Nichols strain of *Treponema pallidum* can accept penicillinase-producing plasmids, so antibiotic therapy may change in the future.[6]

Serologic Diagnosis

General Principles

Infection of humans by *T. pallidum* leads to the production of two major types of antibodies: nonspecific (reagin) antibodies and specific treponemal antibodies. Nonspecific antibodies are measured in "nontreponemal" screening tests for syphilis, whereas specific treponemal antibodies are measured in "treponemal" confirmatory tests for syphilis.

The nontreponemal tests for syphilis detect the presence of nonspecific antibodies directed against lipid antigens of the treponemes' outer membrane, or against lipid antigens produced by interaction of the treponeme and the human host. Since these lipid antigens are present in other diseases (SLE, autoimmune diseases, pregnancy, some chronic infections of the elderly, and drug addicts) and in normal tissue,

the antibodies they elicit are not specific for syphilis, and the tests that detect them are useful only as screening tests for the disease. The antigen for the nontreponemal tests is a cardiolipin–lecithin–cholesterol antigen. The antibody that reacts with this antigen has been termed *reagin*. Reagins are immunoglobulins of the IgG and IgM classes.

Although nontreponemal tests are inexpensive, rapid, and easy to perform, they may be insensitive in detecting primary, latent and tertiary infections (Table 18-1). They may be particularly insensitive in early primary syphilis before reagin antibodies have had a chance to form. Since reagins are nonspecific, false positive tests may occur. The proportion of falsely reactive nontreponemal tests has been estimated at 3% to 40%,[9] depending on the type of test used and the incidence of syphilis in the test population studied. For this reason all positive nontreponemal tests for syphilis are confirmed by a treponemal test in which patient sera are tested for antibodies developed specifically against *T. pallidum*. Nontreponemal tests are also useful in monitoring effectiveness of therapy, in determining reinfection in patients with a history of syphilis, and in the diagnosis of congenital syphilis.

Table 18-1: Percentage of Patients Reactive in Serologic Tests for Syphilis*

Test	Stages of Syphilis				
	Primary	Secondary	Latent	Tertiary	Congenital
VDRL	70–80	100	75–90	62–75	88
RPR	~80	100	75–90	~75	100
FTA-ABS	85–92	100	97	97–100	100
MHA-TP	65–78	100	98–99	94–98	100
TPI	57	99	97	92	NA
ELISA†	82–100	100	72–100	83–100	NA

* Percent rounded to nearest whole number. Compiled from bibliography sources.
† Bio-Enzabead ELISA, Organon Teknika Corp. Lower percentages reflect test results read visually vs. use of a spectrophotometer.

Treponemal confirmatory tests determine the presence of specific antitreponemal antibodies in the patient's serum. The antigens used in these tests are the nonpathogenic *T. phagedenis* biotype Reiter treponeme or *T. pallidum* antigens. Treponemal tests are most useful in confirming latent and tertiary disease states (see Table 18-1), and once positive, remain reactive for the life of the patient. Since all pathogenic treponemes show cross-reactions in these tests, the different treponemal diseases (syphilis, bejel, yaws, and pinta) cannot be distinguished by serologic means alone, but must rely on geographic location, clinical signs and symptoms, and positive serologic tests. The treponemal tests may be divided into four categories: the *Treponema pallidum* immobilization test, fluorescent antibody tests, hemagglutination tests, and enzyme-linked immunoassays.

Nontreponemal Screening Tests

VDRL Slide Test

The standard nontreponemal test is the Venereal Disease Research Laboratory (VDRL) slide test. The principle of this test is to examine microscopically patients' heat-treated sera (source of reagin antibodies) for ability to flocculate (form antigen–antibody complexes in suspension) with an antigen containing 0.03% cardiolipin, 0.9% cholesterol, and 0.21% lecithin (VDRL antigen).[10] This test may be either qualitative or quantitative, and each step in the testing has been meticulously described and must be strictly adhered to.[10] Results are reported as nonreactive (no clumping), weakly reactive (small clumps), or reactive (medium or large clumps). Since prozone reactions occur in which undiluted serum gives partial or complete inhibition of reactivity and corresponding diluted serum is reactive, weakly reactive results in the qualitative VDRL test should be followed by a quantitative VDRL test to rule out this phenomenon. The VDRL test generally becomes positive in 1 to 3 weeks after the appearance of the chancre. The antibody titer then increases during the secondary stage and begins to fall during latency. Although largely replaced by newer nontreponemal tests for syphilis, the VDRL–cerebrospinal fluid (VDRL–CSF) test is the only test used to diagnose neurosyphilis.

The nontreponemal tests that follow are all modifications of the VDRL test. The main modification has been the addition of choline chloride and ethylenediamine tetracetic acid (EDTA) to the VDRL antigen. These two chemicals allow non-heat-inactivated serum to be used in place of the heat-inactivated serum and stabilize the antigen, respectively. Another modification of these tests is the use of compounds to increase the visibility of the flocculation reaction. The ability to perform these tests on disposable microscope slides or paper cards makes them simpler and less expensive to perform than the standard VDRL test. All reactive qualitative nontreponemal tests should be followed by a quantitative nontreponemal test of the same type as differences in the titers may be obtained using each of these various tests. A rise in titer in a quantitative nontreponemal test may indicate recent infection or reinfection. Quantitative nontreponemal tests are also useful in monitoring the antibody titer in congenital syphilis. Newborns are monitored with quantitative nontreponemal tests for the first 6 months of life. A rise in antibody titer is diagnostic; however, an infant who was not infected *in utero* should show a decrease in antibody titer after 3 months as maternal antibody levels decrease. An important use of quantitative nontreponemal tests is in monitoring the effectiveness of therapy. Brown *et al*[11] showed that there is at least a fourfold decrease in titer by 3 months after appropriate treatment for primary and secondary syphilis. Antibody titers may decline until no serologic reaction is detectable; however, low titers may persist when the patient is in the latent stage.[12]

Unheated Serum Reagin Test

The unheated serum reagin test (USR) is a microscopic flocculation test that uses the choline chloride–EDTA-modified VDRL antigen.[13] This test is primarily used as a screening test or for monitoring efficacy of treatment. The principle is that unheated serum (qualitative test) or unheated serum dilutions (quantitative test) are mixed with the modified VDRL antigen suspension on glass slides. The slides are then rotated mechanically and read microscopically for flocculation. Results are read as nonreactive, weakly reactive, or reactive as in the VDRL test. All reactive qualitative USR tests should be followed by a quantitative USR test.

Rapid Plasma Reagin Card Test

The rapid plasma reagin card test (RPR) is a macroscopic flocculation test that uses the modified VDRL antigen and charcoal particles to aid in visualizing the flocculation reaction with the naked eye. These modifications allow the use of non-heat-treated serum and eliminate the use of a microscope, resulting in a fast, easy-to-read nontreponemal test. Performing the test on cardboard with designated test circles makes the test disposable for screening large numbers of samples. There are two different formats for RPR card testing: the RPR teardrop card test and the RPR circle card test. The RPR teardrop card test was designed as a screening test for field use. Fingerstick blood plasma is mixed with a modified VDRL antigen suspension containing charcoal particles on a disposable card within a teardrop-shaped circle. The card is rocked by hand and the results are read as reactive (flocculation) or nonreactive (no flocculation). This test is only qualitative.[14] The RPR circle test, however, can be read as a qualitative or a quantitative test for both screening and diagnostic purposes, respectively.[15] In contrast to the RPR teardrop card test, the RPR card test uses patient serum and is rotated on a mechanical rotator. Results are read as reactive or nonreactive.

Reagin Screen Test

The reagin screen test (RST) is another macroscopic flocculation test that can be read qualitatively and quantitatively for the screening and diagnosis of syphilis.[16] This test uses the modified VDRL antigen with added Sudan Black B, a lipid-soluble diazo dye,

for visualization of the flocculation reaction. Results are read as reactive (flocculation) or nonreactive (no flocculation).

Confirmatory Treponemal Tests

Treponema Pallidum Immobilization Test

The *Treponema pallidum* immobilization (TPI) test was once the standard test against which all treponemal tests were compared. This test has since been replaced by newer confirmatory tests that are more sensitive, less difficult to perform, and less expensive. The TPI test was the first serologic treponemal test developed in 1949 by Nelson and Mayer.[17] The purpose of this test was to measure the ability of antibody and complement to immobilize a suspension of live treponemes as visualized under darkfield microscopy. Live, motile *Treponema pallidum* from a testicular lesion in a rabbit is mixed with patient sera and guinea pig complement. The mixture is incubated in an atmosphere of 5% carbon dioxide and 95% nitrogen. An aliquot is then examined under a darkfield microscope for immobilization of the *T. pallidum* present. If 50% or more treponemes are immobilized the test is positive. Less than 20% immobilization constitutes a negative test, and the range between 20% and 50% immobilization represents a "doubtful" result. Antibiotics in the patient sera will also immobilize the treponemes present, resulting in a false positive test. Interpretation of TPI test must also take into account the patient's stage of syphilis, since reactivity to the TPI test develops slowly and the sensitivity of the TPI test in the primary stage is approximately 50% (see Table 18-1).

Fluorescent Treponemal Antibody Absorption Test

Syphilis has traditionally been diagnosed by examining serous exudates from primary and secondary syphilitic lesions by darkfield microscopy for the presence of *T. pallidum*. Distinguishing *T. pallidum* by its characteristic morphology and motility from other nonpathogenic human commensal treponemes is exceedingly difficult, requiring a trained microscopist and resulting in a sensitivity of approximately 75%.[18] As an alternative to darkfield microscopy, *T. pallidum* may be detected in a fluorescent treponemal antibody absorption test (FTA-ABS). In this indirect fluorescent antibody test, dried Nichols strain *T. pallidum* grown in rabbit testes is used as the antigen. This material is smeared onto glass slides, air dried, and acetone fixed. Heat-inactivated patient serum (antibody) is then mixed with "sorbent," a culture of Reiter treponemes that removes antibodies to group antigens common to *T. pallidum* and the nonpathogenic treponemes. This step makes the test more specific in detecting *T. pallidum* antibodies. Absorbed patient serum is then added to the antigen smears, and fluorescein–isothiocyanate-labeled antihuman gamma globulin is added. If antitreponemal antibody is present in the patient's serum, green fluorescent treponemes are visible under the fluorescence microscope. Positive reactions are graded from 1+ to 4+ by comparing with appropriate 1+ to 4+ control sera. Nonreactive tests lack fluorescent treponemes. A modification of the FTA-ABS test for use with epifluorescence microscopes is the fluorescent treponemal antibody absorption doublestaining test (FTA-ABS-DS). This procedure utilizes a rhodamine-labeled, class-specific, anti–human IgG primary stain and the fluorescein-labeled antitreponemal globulin as a counterstain. In this test treponemes exhibit specific red fluorescence. Farshy *et al* have shown that the FTA-ABS-DS test gives comparable results to the FTA-ABS test with the added advantage of being easier to read, especially with borderline reactive sera.[19]

Newer direct fluorescent antibody tests (DFA-TP) have been developed and have been determined to be as sensitive and specific as darkfield microscopy. In these tests serous lesion exudate (antigen) is collected on a microscope slide, fixed in acetone, and overlayed with either absorbed fluorescein-labeled

polyvalent rabbit antitreponemal antiserum (antibody)[20] or *T. pallidum* specific monoclonal antibodies (antibody).[21] When Evans blue stain is used as a counterstain, treponemes fluoresce green in a red background in a reactive test.

For the diagnosis of congenital syphilis, an FTA-ABS test that detects IgM antibodies (FTA-ABS-IgM) has been developed. This test may be used as a confirmatory test for congenital syphilis but should not be used as a screening test, as the false positive rate of the test is 10% and the false negative rate is greater than or equal to 35%.[22] Congenital syphilis should be diagnosed with a quantitative VDRL test at this time.

Fluorescent antibody tests are the most widely used confirmatory treponemal tests for syphilis. This is due to their advantages over darkfield microscopy and their sensitivity in detecting syphilis, particularly in the early stage of the disease (see Table 18-1).

Hemagglutination Assays: MHA–TP, HATTS, and TPHA

Three hemagglutination assays for the detection of antibodies to syphilis are currently available: the microhemagglutination assay for antibodies to *Treponema pallidum* (MHA-TP), the hemagglutination treponemal test for syphilis (HATTS), and the *T. pallidum* hemagglutination assay (TPHA). Each is produced by a different manufacturer and differs in the types of erythrocytes employed in these indirect hemagglutination assays. The MHA-TP uses tanned formalin-fixed sheep erythrocytes, whereas the HATTS and TPA use gluteraldehyde-stabilized turkey erythrocytes. The sensitivity and specificity of these tests are virtually identical, and the choice of one as a confirmatory test depends on the preference of the user. All these tests, however, give comparable test results to the FTA–ABS test in all stages of syphilis except the primary stage. In the primary stage, the FTA-ABS or nontreponemal tests are better choices (see Table 18-1). Each of these hemagglutination assays is performed by mixing erythrocytes sensitized with an ultrasonicate of *T. pallidum* with absorbed patient serum in either microtiter plate wells or in test tubes. Unsensitized cells in a second well or tube acts as a control. The tests are incubated at room temperature and agglutination of the sensitive cells constitutes a positive test. The unsensitized control cells and negative test results fail to agglutinate, forming a button of erythrocytes in the well or test tube bottom.

Enzyme-Linked Immunosorbent Assay

Enzyme-linked immunosorbent assay (ELISA) tests have recently been developed for the diagnosis of syphilis. The commercially available Bio-Enza Bead (Organon Teknika Corp.) test kit uses Nichols strain *T. pallidum* antigen fixed to metal beads. Patient serum provides the antibody source, and the detection system is horseradish peroxidase–conjugated anti–human IgG (second antibody) and 2,2′-azinodi (3-ethyl-2,3 dihydro-6-benzthiazoline-sulfonate, the enzyme substrate). Results are read visually[22] or on a spectrophotometer at a wavelength of 690 nm for green color development.[23] Results obtained in this ELISA test were found to be comparable with results obtained in the FTA-ABS test (see Table 18-1).[23–25] The major advantage of ELISA tests over immunofluorescent and hemagglutination tests for syphilis is their ability to be read spectrophotometrically, which eliminates the subjective judgments of visual methods. In addition, ELISA methodology makes screening large numbers of sera possible in sexually transmitted disease clinics and public health departments.

Summary

Syphilis is caused by the bacterium *Treponema pallidum* subspecies *pallidum*. Following an incubation period, the disease presents as three clinical stages in the adult (primary, secondary, or tertiary syphilis) or via transplacental transmission as congenital syphilis in the neonate. Each stage can be diagnosed by appropriate use of darkfield microscopy or serologic testing. Two major antigens elicit the production of antibodies in syphilis: lipid antigens and specific treponemal antigens. Lipid antigens elicit the production of nonspecific, reagin antibodies detected by nonspecific nontreponemal tests for syphilis. Because these lipid antigens are present in some normal tissue and in disease states other than syphilis, nontreponemal tests may give false positive results and therefore act only as screening tests for syphilis. Patient sera giving positive reagin tests or patients whose sera give negative reagin test results but who have signs and symptoms of syphilis are further evaluated using treponemal tests for syphilis. Treponemal tests are confirmatory and highly specific tests for syphilis, because they detect antigens produced by *T. pallidum*.

Bibliography

1. Tramont EC: *Treponema pallidum* (Syphilis). In Mandell GE, Douglas RG Jr, Bennett JE (eds): Principles and Practices of Infectious Diseases, 2nd ed, p 1323. 1985

2. Johnson, RC: Spirochetes. In Howard B, Klaas J, Rubin S, et al (eds): Pathogenic Microbiology, p 503. 1986

3. Baseman JB: The biology of *Treponema pallidum* and syphilis. Clin Microbiol Newsletter 5:157, 1983

4. US Dept Health and Human Services: Progress Toward Achieving the National 1990 Objectives for Sexually Transmitted Diseases. Surveill Summ 36:173, 1987

5. Fiumara NJ, Finegold S: The surgical diagnosis: Ruling out VD, Part 2. Syphilis. Infections in Surgery 3:359, 1984

6. Wilcox RR, Guthe T: *Treponema pallidum*. A bibliographic review of the morphology, culture, and survival of *T. pallidum* and associated organisms. Bull WHO 35:1, 1966

7. US Dept Health Education and Welfare: Criteria and techniques for the diagnosis of early syphilis. Centers for Disease Control, 1980

8. Larsen SA, Beck-Sague CM: Syphilis. In Balows A, Hausler WJ Jr, Lennette EH (eds): The Laboratory

Diagnosis of Infectious Diseases: Principles and Practice. New York, Springer-Verlag (in press)

9. US Dept Health and Human Services: 1985 STD treatment guidelines. Centers for Disease Control, 1985

10. US Dept Health Education and Welfare, National Communicable Disease Center, Venereal Disease Program: Manual of tests for syphilis. Centers for Disease Control, 1969

11. Brown ST, Zaidi A, Larsen SA, Reynolds GH: Serological response to syphilis treatment: A new analysis of old data. JAMA 2593:1296, 1985

12. Fiumara NJ: Serological response to treatment of 128 patients with late latent syphilis. Sex Transm Dis 6:243, 1979

13. Portnoy J, Bossak HN, Falcone VH, et al: Rapid reagin test with unheated serum and new improved antigen suspension. Public Health Rep 76:933, 1961

14. Portnoy J, Brewer JH, Harris A: Rapid plasma reagin test for syphilis. Public Health Rep 72:761, 1957

15. Falcone VH, Stout GW, Moore MBM: Evaluation of rapid plasma reagin (circle) card test. Public Health Rep 79:491, 1964

16. March RW, Stiles GE: The reagin screen test: A new reagin card test for syphilis. Sex Transm Dis 7:66, 1980

17. Nelson RA Jr, Mayer MM: Immobilization of *Treponema pallidum in vitro* by antibody produced by syphilitic infection. J Exp Med 89:369, 1949

18. Daniels KD, Ferneyhough HS: Specific direct fluorescent antibody detection of *Treponema pallidum.* Health Lab Sci 14:164, 1977

19. Farshy CE, Kennedy EJ, Hunter EF, et al: Fluorescent treponemal antibody absorption double staining test evaluation. J Clin Microbiol 17:245, 1983

20. Jue R, et al: Comparison of fluorescent and conventional darkfield methods for the detection of *Treponema pallidum* in syphilitic lesions. Am J Clin Pathol 47:809, 1967

21. Hook EW III, Roddy RE, Lukehart SA, et al: Detection of *Treponema pallidum* in lesion exudate with a pathogen specific monoclonal antibody. J Clin Microbiol 22:241, 1985

22. Kaufman RE, Olansky DC, Weisner PJ: The FTA-ABS (IgM) test for neonatal congenital syphilis: A critical review. J Am Venereal Dis Assoc 1:79, 1974

23. Stevens RW, Schmitt ME: Evaluation of an enzyme-linked immunosorbent assay for treponemal antibody. J Clin Microbiol 21:399, 1985

24. Moyer NP, Hudson JD, Hausler WJ: Evaluation of the Bio-EnzaBead Test for Syphilis. J Clin Microbiol 25:619, 1987

25. Larsen SA, Hamble EA, Cruce DD: Review of the standard tests for syphilis and evaluation of a new commercial ELISA, the Syphilis Bio-Enzabead test. J Clin Lab Anal 1:300, 1987

19

Rubella Virus Infection and Serology

Rosemarie Matuscak

Virus

Size and Composition

The rubella virus, composed of single-stranded RNA, is a member of the family Togaviridae.[1] It is a roughly spherical particle with a diameter between 60 and 70 nm. The virion contains a dense core surrounded by a lipid bilayer covered with short, fine projections.[1,2] Only one serotype of rubella virus is known,[1,3] and it remains immunologically distinct from any other described group.[1]

Rubella virus contains two major structural subunits, one associated with the viral envelope and one associated with the nucleoprotein core. Several major and minor polypeptides have been identified in purified rubella virus.[4] Each of these polypeptides is immunologically active, but infectivity has not been associated with a distinct antigenic site.[1]

Isolation and Identification

Although the rubella virus may be propagated in a variety of primary cell cultures and cell lines,[5,6] rubella infections are routinely diagnosed through serologic methods that are less time-consuming and cumbersome. Primary cell lines, especially monkey kidney, are superior for viral isolation, whereas continuous cell lines produce higher levels of virus and are generally better for antigen production.[6] Growth of the virus has not been reproduced in embryonated eggs, suckling mice, or adult rabbits.[4,5,7]

Antigenicity

The virus contains a hemagglutinin, associated with the viral envelope,[6,8] that reacts with newborn chick, goose, and pigeon red blood cells at 4°C and 25°C, but not at 37°C.[9] Both the red blood cells and serum of individuals infected with rubella virus contain a nonspecific β-lipoprotein inhibitor to hemagglutination.[6]

The major complement-fixing activities are associated primarily with the envelope, although some activity is also associated with the nucleoprotein core.[6] Both the hemagglutinin and the complement-fixing antigens can be detected through serologic testing.

Viral Replication

Viruses replicate inside host cells. A typical replication cycle occurs in a stepwise process that includes the following phases: (1) attachment, (2) penetration, (3) uncoating, (4) biosynthesis, and (5) maturation and release. Although this is a typical cycle, variations occur, depending on the type of viral nucleic acid and the viral group.[10]

Attachment, the first step in infection, occurs when a surface site on the virion, or virus particle, binds to a receptor site on the host cell. Attachment of the virion is reversible in some circumstances. For infection to occur, the second step, penetration of the virus into the host cell, must follow. This process may involve several mechanisms: (1) fusion of the viral envelope with the host cell membrane, (2) direct penetration of the membrane, (3) interaction with receptor sites on the cell membrane, or (4) viropexis, or phagocytosis.[10,11]

After entering the host cell the viral nucleic acid must be uncoated or released from its surrounding envelope or capsid. Uncoating of the envelope occurs at the cell surface in certain viruses. Generally, this is an enzymatic process that either uses preexisting lysosomal enzymes or involves the synthesis of new enzymes. Following uncoating, biosynthesis of nucleic acid and various viral proteins is necessary. Viral synthesis occurs in either the nucleus or the cytoplasm of the host cell, depending upon the type

of viral nucleic acid and the viral group. In RNA viruses, such as the Rubella virus, synthesis occurs in the cytoplasm. In most DNA viruses, however, the viral nucleic acid is replicated in the host cell nucleus, whereas the viral protein is replicated in the cytoplasm. In the final step of viral replication, maturation or assembly of the viral particles occurs. The mature particles are then released by budding through the cell membrane or by cell lysis.[10,11]

Disease

German Measles

Rubella, a mild, contagious illness characterized by an erythematous maculopapular rash, is observed primarily in children 5 to 14 years old and in young adults.[1,12] The disease, commonly called German or 3-day measles, may be asymptomatic or involve a 1- to 5-day prodromal period of malaise, headache, cold symptoms, low-grade fever, and suboccipital lymphadenopathy.[12]

In children the first sign of illness is the appearance of a rash.[12] However, in adolescents and adults the rash is preceded by the prodromal period, which occurs approximately 14 to 21 days after exposure to the virus. The rash appears first on the face, spreads downward,[6,12] and clears in a similar fashion within 1 to 5 days.[12] The rash is characterized by discrete pink–red lesions that may or may not coalesce. Lesions that coalesce form a uniform red blush that generally appears on the trunk and resembles the rash of mild scarlet fever.[12] The rash may also be confused with that induced by certain drugs. Therefore, rendering a diagnosis of rubella solely on clinical grounds is unreliable, especially during periods between epidemics.[1]

The portal of entry for rubella virus is the upper respiratory tract, perhaps through the lymphoid tissue, where it establishes intracellular reproduction in a susceptible host.[8] Within 9 to 11 days following onset of infection, detectable levels of virus may be demonstrated in nasopharyngeal secretions, urine, cervix, and feces.[8] Shedding of the virus is most prolonged and reaches highest levels through pharyngeal secretions.[8]

Arthritis may be a complication of rubella infection in adolescents and young adults involving the knees, ankles, or elbows. The arthritis may resemble the type observed in cases of rheumatic fever or rheumatoid arthritis.[8] Other complications may include transient arthralgias (15% to 52% of cases), encephalitis (1 in 6000 cases), and thrombocytopenic purpura.[1,12] The prognosis of rubella without complications is excellent, since the disease is benign and self-limited.

Congenital Rubella

Although recognized by German authors in the mid-eighteenth century as a clinical entity,[8] it was not until 1941 that Sir Norman Gregg discovered a causal relationship between maternal infection during pregnancy and congenital defects.[13] Maternal infection may result in spontaneous abortion, stillbirth, or infection of the fetus.[13] Infection of the placenta may occur without fetal involvement.[8] Fetal infection during the first trimester of pregnancy and, to a lesser extent, the second trimester, may result in congenital defects. As many as 85% of infants infected during the first 8 weeks of gestation have detectable defects by 4 years of age.[8] The classical abnormalities associated with the rubella syndrome include congenital heart disease, cataracts, and neurosensory deafness.[14,15] After 20 to 24 weeks of gestation, congenital abnormalities are rare. Defects may not be apparent until late childhood, with the most common manifestations being ocular defects and deafness.[16,17]

Infants born with the rubella syndrome usually have a low birth weight. Other symptoms, such as thrombocytopenia, hepatitis, long bone lesions, retinitis, encephalitis, interstitial pneumonitis, psychiat-ric disorders, thyroid disorders, and diabetes mellitus, may also be present in a variety of combinations.[1,12] The virus can be isolated readily from the throat and less frequently from the feces and urine[18] and may persist up to a year in infected infants.[12]

Immunologic Response

Antibodies to rubella virus appear as the rash fades, with both IgG and IgM reaching detectable levels at this time.[1,6] Antibodies to IgG persist throughout life, whereas antibodies to IgM usually decline after 4 to 5 weeks.[1,6] Fetal infection is usually accompanied by early placental transfer of maternal IgG. In addition, substantial levels of fetal IgM are produced by midgestation (Fig. 19-1).[8] Since levels of IgM are generally increased at birth in infected infants, screening for congenital infection may be accomplished by quantitating IgM.

Although reinfection with the virus can occur it is almost always asymptomatic and can be detected by a rise in IgG antibodies.[1,6,19] Viremia has been detected in volunteers with low rubella titers after experimental challenge with rubella vaccine.[20] This demonstrates that viremia can indeed occur after reinfection. Although studies have shown that rubella vaccine virus can cross the placenta and infect the fetus during early stages of development, the risk of congenital malformations appears to be low to nonexistent.[21]

Laboratory Testing

Tests Available

Reliable serologic techniques for the detection of rubella antibodies provide the methods of choice for the (1) determination of immunity to rubella, (2) diagnosis of congenital rubella, and (3) diagnosis of acute

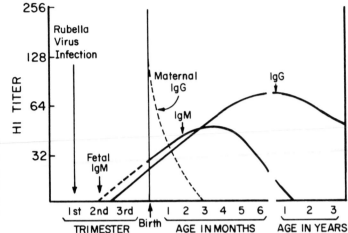

FIGURE 19-1. Antibody responses in an infant congenitally infected with rubella virus. (From Chernesky MA, Mahony JB: Rubella virus. In Rose NR, Friedman H, Fahey JL (eds): Manual of Clinical Laboratory Immunology, 3rd ed, p 537. Washington, DC, American Society for Microbiology, 1986.)

rubella infection.[1,3] Methods currently available include passive hemagglutination (PHA), hemagglutination inhibition (HI), radial hemolysis, latex agglutination, solid-phase immunoassay (SPIA), neutralization, mixed hemadsorption, complement fixation (CF), and time-resolved fluoroimmunoassay. Of these methods, PHA and CF do not show peak titers until later in the disease (Fig. 19-2). More than 95% of rubella antibody testing in the United States is being performed with commercially prepared test kits that are evaluated and monitored by the Centers for Disease Control.[1]

Clinical Indications

Determining Recent Infection

Sera Available at Onset of Symptoms. A rapid and accurate serologic diagnosis is needed to investigate a pregnant patient who was exposed to the rubella virus. If signs and symptoms develop, two serum specimens should be collected. An acute-phase serum is obtained at the onset of symptoms and a convalescent serum obtained within 5 to 7 days. Both specimens should be tested in parallel on the same day using the same test and appropriate controls.[1,3] Otherwise, changes in titer may merely reflect variation in testing rather than true antibody levels.[6] A

fourfold or greater rise in antibody titer together with clinical symptoms is diagnostic of a recent rubella infection.[1,3]

The HI antibodies reach peak titers in 10 to 20 days, whereas CF antibodies appear approximately a week later, do not reach as high a level, and decline more rapidly.[1] The CF test may be useful in cases where the acute-phase serum was collected too late to show a rise in HI titer.[3]

Sera Not Available at Onset of Symptoms. Testing for specific IgM antibody in serum that has been collected several days after onset of symptoms may aid in retrospectively establishing a diagnosis of rubella.[1,3] In this case, all serologic tests will show a titer. However, titers of IgM antibody wane rapidly and may disappear within 4 weeks. Therefore, a negative result does not exclude the possibility of a recent rubella infection.

Diagnosing Congenital Infection

Although congenital infection may be confirmed by isolating the virus from throat washings, urine, and other body fluids, isolation may require repeated attempts.[1] Therefore, serologic testing is the recommended method. Testing for the presence of specific IgM antibody is indicated for any neonate of low birth weight who also presents with any of the symptoms associated with congenital rubella.[3,20] The

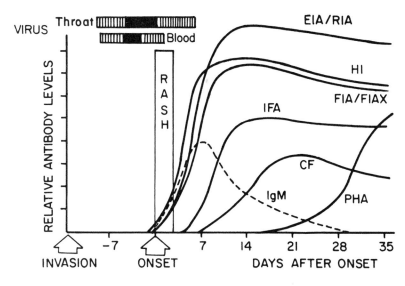

FIGURE 19-2. Schema of immune response in acute rubella infection. RIA, radioimmunoassay; FIA/FIAX, fluorescence immunoassay. (From Herrmann K: Rubella virus. In Lennette EH, Balows A, Hausler WJ JR, Shadomy HJ (eds): Manual of Clinical Microbiology, 4th ed, p 783, Washington, DC, American Society of Microbiology, 1985.)

demonstration of IgM antibody in the infant is diagnostic of congenital infection, because these antibodies do not cross the placenta.[1,3]

Specific rubella IgG antibodies may be produced by the infant *in utero*. However, since maternal IgG crosses the placenta, it is difficult to differentiate between passively transferred antibody and specific antibody produced by the infant.[6] Persistence of specific rubella IgG antibody beyond 6 to 12 months of age indicates that the antibody is being produced by the infant and is, therefore, retrospective evidence of congenital infection.

Determining Immune Status

The most widely used tests for determining rubella immunity status are the HI, PHA, enzyme immunoassay and indirect immunofluorescence methods.[22] Detectable levels of antibody are indicative of past infection with the rubella virus. Individuals with detectable antibody levels are considered immune.

Hemagglutination-Inhibition Test

A hemagglutination inhibition (HI) test for the detection of rubella antibody was first described in

1967.[9] A standardized reference HI procedure was developed in 1970 and has been adopted by the National Committee for Clinical Laboratory Standards and the World Health Organization as the reference method.[1] Serologic tests for rubella should be compared with the HI test for accuracy before being employed for diagnostic purposes. Both IgM and IgG antibodies can be detected using the HI test.[22]

Principle

Rubella virus has the ability to agglutinate chick erythrocytes. When patient serum containing rubella antibody is incubated with rubella antigen, binding occurs. To determine whether binding has occurred, chick erythrocytes are added. Any unbound rubella antigen present is free to agglutinate the chick RBCs.

Procedure

Antigen Preparation. Rubella antigen is prepared in BHK-21 or Vero cell cultures and may be purchased commercially.[6]

Erythrocytes. Erythrocytes (indicator cells) used in the test proper and antigen titration procedure are obtained from 1- to 3-day-old unfed baby chicks.[1,6,9] These cells may be stored for up to 2 weeks in Alsever solution without loss of sensitivity.[1,6] Indicator cells are 0.25% suspensions. The cells used to adsorb patient sera for natural agglutinins are 50% suspensions.

Antigen Titration. To determine the proper dosage of antigen, titration is necessary. Satisfactory rubella antigens range in titer from 4 to 1024. An excess amount of antigen will result in low antibody titers, whereas an insufficient amount gives rise to falsely elevated titers.[6]

Titration is performed by preparing serial twofold dilutions of test antigen in V-type microtiter plates and incubating at 4°C with indicator cells. Plates are read for agglutination. The highest dilution producing complete agglutination is called 1 HA unit. The reciprocal of the highest dilution producing complete agglutination is the titer of the antigen. The dilution of antigen to be used for the HI test must contain 4 HA units and is, therefore, fourfold dilution lower.

Removal of Nonspecific Inhibitors. Before the HI test is performed, nonspecific β-lipoprotein inhibitors and nonspecific agglutinins must be removed.[3,4,20] This is accomplished by incubating all sera and controls with heparin–$MnCl_2$ or dextran sulfate–$CaCl_2$[9] to remove the nonspecific inhibitors and by adsorbing with 50% chick erythrocytes to remove natural agglutinins.[1,3,6]

HI Test. The HI test involves preparing serial twofold dilutions of treated serum and incubating at 4°C with antigen (4 HA). Plates are then incubated with indicator cells and read after 15 to 20 minutes at room temperature.

Antigen Back-titration. To ensure that the antigen dilution used in the HI test is correct, an antigen back-titration is performed simultaneously with the HI test by preparing serial twofold dilutions of the antigen preparation (4 HA units).

Interpretation

The test is valid, providing the antigen back-titration confirms that between 2 and 8 HA units were used and controls show that nonspecific inhibitors and ag-

glutinins were removed. The endpoint is read as the highest dilution of serum that completely inhibits hemagglutination.

Recent rubella infections are demonstrated by a fourfold or greater rise in titer between acute and convalescent (paired) sera. Interpretations of the HI antibody titer on single specimens do not present diagnostic information. High titers (≥512) may be observed in immune individuals with no recent rubella infection.[4] HI titers ≥ 8 indicate immunity to rubella disease.

Passive Hemagglutination (PHA)

Principle

In the passive hemagglutination (PHA) test, stabilized human red blood cells are coated with soluble rubella virus antigen. These sensitized erythrocytes agglutinate in the presence of specific rubella antibody.[1,3,6,23]

Procedure

Patient and control sera are diluted in phosphate buffered saline (PBS), mixed with antigen-coated red blood cells, and incubated at room temperature for 2 hours to allow the cells to settle.[1]

Results and Interpretation

The plates are read for the presence or absence of agglutination. A button of erythrocytes forming at the bottom of the V-shaped well in the microtiter plate indicates a negative reaction (absence of antibody or susceptibility to rubella infection). Agglutination or a dispersal of erythrocytes indicates a positive reaction (presence of antibody or immunity to rubella).[1,3,6]

Advantages

An advantage of the PHA test is that sera do not require treatment for removal of nonspecific reactants prior to testing. The test can be performed rapidly and correlates well with HI test results in over 98% of cases.[1] The PHA test is most useful in detecting rubella immunity status and is sensitive to IgG antibodies.[22]

Solid-Phase Immunoassays

Solid-phase immunoassay (SPIA) methods are useful in the detection and quantitation of both IgG and IgM rubella antibodies, depending on the antiglobulin conjugate used.[22,24,25] Most commercially available SPIA kits are enzyme immunoassays. However, solid-phase radioimmunoassays have been developed.[26]

Indirect Immunoassays

Immunoassays that employ rubella virus antigen adsorbed to a solid phase (plate or beads) are known as indirect or antigen-capture assays. After incubation with patient serum, rubella-specific antibody binds to the antigen on the solid phase. Rubella-specific antibody is subsequently detected by incubation with anti–human antibodies that are enzyme-labeled[24,27] or radiolabeled.[26]

The indirect method is effective for detection of IgG antibody, but false positive and false negative reactions may be encountered when assaying for IgM. False positive reactions may appear with IgM rheumatoid factor (IgM-RF) and specific IgG.[28] Immune IgG binds to the antigen and IgM-RF binds to the IgG. The IgM-RF will then bind to the labeled anti–human antibodies, causing a false positive result.[29] High titered IgG may cause false negative results by competing with the IgM antibody for the antigen coated on the solid phase.[29,30] These can be minimized by pretreatment of the serum to remove the IgG or the IgM-RF or by employing a direct immunoassay described below.[29]

Direct Immunoassays

Direct immunoassays or antibody capture assays employ a solid phase coated with anti–human IgM antibodies.[30–32] After incubation with patient serum, patient IgM antibodies bind to the anti–human IgM antibodies on the solid phase. Specific rubella antibodies are then detected by incubation with rubella antigen, followed by another incubation with enzyme-labeled or radiolabeled rubella antibody (anti–rubella conjugate).

Interpretation

No standard method of reporting results of enzyme immunoassay tests exists. Therefore, results must be interpreted according to the instructions in the specific test employed.[22]

Sucrose Density Gradient Ultracentrifugation

Specific IgM antibodies to rubella can be detected by several techniques other than solid-phase immunoassay.[26] These include indirect fluorescent antibody, adsorption of IgG with staphylococcal protein A,[33] or physical separation of IgG and IgM by sucrose density gradient ultracentrifugation.[34] The method of choice for detection of IgM antibodies is sucrose density gradient ultracentrifugation of serum followed by HI assay of the IgG or IgM fractions.

Principle

Patient serum is sedimented through a sucrose density gradient to fractionate serum, thus separating IgM and IgG antibodies. The antibody-rich fractions are then tested for specific rubella antibodies.

Procedure

Serum to be tested is layered on top of a linear sucrose gradient and centrifuged. The gradient is prepared by layering 37% to 12.0% (wt/vol) solutions of sucrose in PBS, pH 7.4, in a cellulose nitrate tube and allowing overnight diffusion at 4°C.[3,26] After centrifugation, fractions of serum are collected from the bottom of the tube using a needle-type fraction collector.[3,6,26]

Results

Nonspecific inhibitors remain in the top fractions,[34] whereas IgM antibodies concentrate in the bottom fractions and IgG antibodies separate primarily in the middle portions.[3,6] Fractions are then tested for specific antibody using the HI procedure.

Interpretation

Because IgM antibodies do not cross the placenta, detection of these antibodies in infant sera is evidence of congenital infection.

Rubella Vaccination

Vaccines

Three strains of a live, attenuated rubella vaccine were developed and licensed in 1969. Each of these vaccines has been proved safe with low rates of fever, rash, arthritis, and lymphadenopathy as side-effects in recipients. However, arthralgia has been reported in as high as 40% of female vaccinees.[19] In January 1979, the RA 27/3 vaccine strain (rubella abortus, 27th specimen, third explant, grown in human diploid fibroblast culture) became the product generally available in the United States.[19]

Vaccine Distribution

The rubella immunization program was instituted after a worldwide rubella epidemic that occurred from 1962 to 1965. Beginning in 1969, federal support was given to the immunization program and within 3 years, more than 45 million doses were administered to nonpubescent children.[19] Within this time the incidence of rubella in the general popula-

tion greatly declined (Fig. 19-3).[35] However, since 10% to 15% of adults in the continental United States have no detectable levels of rubella antibody, the potential for outbreaks of the disease still exists.[22]

Reinfection

Subclinical reinfection has been detected in persons with natural or vaccine-induced immunity after challenge with wild-type rubella virus. Reinfection is demonstrated by at least a fourfold rise in pre-existing antibody titer and is more likely to occur in previously immunized persons with low levels of antibody.[12] Although rubella vaccine viruses can cross the placenta and infect the fetus, no congenital rubella syndrome defects have been observed.[36] None of the three rubella vaccine strains have proved to be teratogenic.

Vaccination Practices

Immunization should be administered after 12 months of age, or if given in combination with the measles and mumps vaccines (MMR), not until 15 months of age. If the rubella vaccine is given before age 12 months, maternal antibodies present in the infant may interfere with immunization.[37]

Vaccine should be administered to children and adults who are negative for rubella antibody or who have no history of immunization. No adverse reactions have occurred in individuals receiving the vaccine following previous immunization.

Contraindications

A potential risk to the fetus of acquiring congenital rubella syndrome following vaccination cannot be totally eliminated. Therefore, pregnancy remains a contraindication to rubella vaccination.[36] In addition,

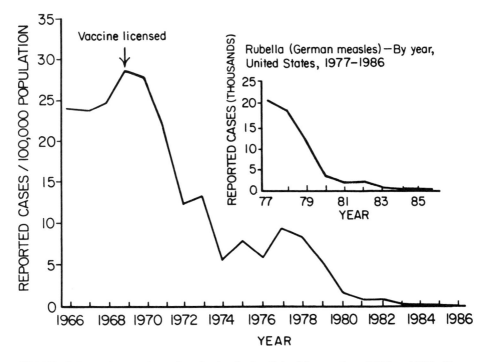

FIGURE 19-3. Incidence of rubella infection in the United States from 1966 to 1986. (From Centers for Disease Control, Summary of Notifiable Diseases, United States, 1986. Surveill Summ 35:35, 1986.)

women of child-bearing age should prevent pregnancy for 3 months after vaccination.[19] However, rubella vaccination of a pregnant woman should not ordinarily be a reason to consider abortion, because the risk of congenital rubella syndrome is extremely low.[36]

Additionally, rubella vaccination is not recommended for persons with impaired immunity, persons receiving radiation treatments, or persons being treated with corticosteroids, alkylating drugs, or antimetabolites.[37]

References

1. Herrmann KL: Rubella virus. In Lennette EH, Balows A, Hausler WJ Jr, et al (eds): Manual of Clinical Microbiology, 4th ed, p 779. Washington, DC, American Society for Microbiology, 1985

2. Alford CA Jr, Neva FA, Weller TH: Virologic and serological studies on human products of conception after maternal rubella. N Engl J Med 271:1275, 1964

3. Chernesky MA, Mahony JB: Rubella Virus. In Rose NR, Friedman H, Fahey JL (eds): Manual of Clinical Laboratory Immunology, 3rd ed, p 536. Washington, DC, American Society for Microbiology, 1986

4. Oker-Blom C, Kalkkinen N, Kaariainen L, et al: Rubella virus contains one capsid protein and three envelope glycoproteins, E12, E2a, and E2b. J Virol 46:964, 1983

5. Parkman PD, Buescher EL, Artenstein MS: Recovery of rubella virus from army recruits (27750). Proc Soc Exp Biol Med 111:225, 1962

6. Herrmann KL: Rubella virus. In Lennette EH, Schmidt NJ (eds): Diagnostic Proceedings for Viral, Rick-

ettsial, and Chlamydial Infections, 5th ed, p 725. American Public Health Association, Washington, DC, 1979

7. Weller TH, Neva FA: Propagation in tissue culture of cytopathic agents from patients with rubella-like illness (27749). Proc Soc Exp Biol Med III:215, 1962

8. Alford CA Jr, Griffiths PD: Rubella. In Remington JS, Klein JO (eds): Infectious Diseases of the Fetus and Newborn Infant, 2nd ed, p 69. Philadelphia, WB Saunders, 1983

9. Stewart GL, Parkman PD, Hopps HE, et al: Rubella-virus hemagglutination-inhibition test. N Engl J Med 276:554, 1967

10. Kucera LS, Myrvik QN: Pathways and classes of virus replication. In: Fundamentals of Medical Virology, 2nd ed, p 27. Philadelphia, Lea & Febiger, 1985

11. Tortora GJ, Funke BR, Case CL: Viruses. In: Microbiology: An Introduction, 2nd ed, p 339. Menlo Park, CA, Benjamin/Cummings, 1986

12. Rubella (German measles). In Krugman S, Katz SL (eds): Infectious diseases of children, 7th ed, p 315. St. Louis, CV Mosby, 1981

13. Wesselhoeft C: Rubella (German measles). N Engl J Med 236:978, 1947

14. Cooper LZ, Ziring PA, Ockerse AB, et al: Rubella: Clinical manifestations and management. Am J Dis Child 118:18, 1969

15. Dudgeon JA: Congenital rubella: Pathogenesis and immunology. Am J Dis Child 118:35, 1969

16. Forrest JM, Menser MA: Congenital rubella in schoolchildren and adolescents. Arch Dis Child 45:63, 1970

17. Peckham CS: Clinical and laboratory study of children exposed in utero to maternal rubella. Arch Dis Child 47:571, 1972

18. Phillips AC, Melnick JL, Yow MD, et al: Persistence of virus in infants with congenital rubella and in normal infants with a history of maternal rubella. JAMA 193:1027, 1965

19. Preblud SR, Serdula MK, Frank JA, et al: Rubella vaccination in the United States: A ten-year review. Epidemiol Rev 2:171, 1980

20. O'Shea S, Best JM, Banatvala JE: Viremia, virus excretion, and antibody responses after challenge in volunteers with low levels of antibody to rubella virus. J Infect Dis 148:639, 1983

21. Modlin JF, Herrmann KL, Brandling-Bennett AD, et al: Risk of congenital abnormality after inadvertent rubella vaccination of pregnant women. N Engl J Med 294:972, 1976

22. Herrmann KL: Rubella. In Lennette EH (ed): Laboratory Diagnosis of Viral Infections, p 481. New York, Marcel Dekker, 1985

23. Safford JW Jr, Whittington R: A passive hemagglutination assay for detecting rubella antibody [Abstr]. Fed Proc 35:813, 1976

24. Gravell M, Dorsett PH, Gutenson O, et al: Detection of antibody to rubella virus by enzyme-linked immunosorbent assay. J Infect Dis 136:S300, 1977

25. Voller A, Bidwell DE: A simple method for detecting antibodies to rubella. Br J Exp Pathol 56:338, 1975

26. Meurman OH, Viljanen MK, Granfors K: Solid-phase radioimmunoassay of rubella virus immunoglobulin M antibodies: Comparison with density gradient centrifugation test. J Clin Microbiol 5:257, 1977

27. Chernesky MA, Wymann L, Mahony JB, et al: Clinical evaluation of the sensitivity and specificity of a commercially available enzyme immunoassay for detection of rubella virus-specific immunoglobulin M. J Clin Microbiol 20:400, 1984

28. Champsaur H, Dussaix E, Taurmier P: Hemagglutination inhibition, single radial hemolysis, and ELISA tests for the detection of IgG and IgM to rubella virus. J Med Virol 5:273, 1980

29. Voller A, Bidwell D: Enzyme-linked immunosorbent assay. In Rose NR, Freedman H, Fahey JL (eds): Manual of Clinical Immunology, 3rd ed, p 99. Washington, DC, American Society for Microbiology, 1986

30. Bonfanti C, Meurman O, Halonen P: Detection of specific immunoglobulin M antibody to rubella virus by use of an enzyme-labelled antigen. J Clin Microbiol 21:963, 1985

31. Vejtorp M: Solid phase anti-IgM ELISA for detection of rubella specific IgM antibodies. Acta Pathol Microbiol Scand Sect B 89:123, 1981

32. Enders G, Knotek F: Detection of IgM antibodies against rubella virus: Comparison of two indirect ELISAs and an anti–IgM capture immunoassay. J Med Virol 19:377, 1986

33. Ankerst J, Christensen P, Kjellen L, et al: A routine diagnostic test for IgA and IgM antibodies to rubella virus: Adsorption of IgG with *Staphylococcus aureus*. J Infect Dis 130:268, 1974

34. Vesikari T, Vaheri A: Rubella: A method for rapid diagnosis of a recent infection by demonstration of the IgM antibodies. Br Med J 1:221, 1968

35. Centers for Disease Control: Summary of Notifiable Diseases, United States, 1986. Surveill Summ 35:35, 1986

36. Centers for Disease Control: Rubella vaccination during pregnancy—United States, 1971–1986. Surveill Summ 36:457, 1987

37. Alexander ER: Rubella. In Fulginiti VA (ed): Immunization in Clinical Practice, p 103. Philadelphia, JB Lippincott, 1982

CHAPTER 20

Epstein-Barr Virus Infection and Serology

Ann C. Albers

Epstein-Barr Virus

The Epstein-Barr virus (EBV), a double-stranded DNA-enveloped virus, belongs to the Herpetoviridae family. Like all herpesviruses, it possesses the characteristic icosahedral nucleocapsid with 162 capsomeres, surrounded by a 120-nm envelope. The virus can be isolated from both lymphoid tissues and epithelial tissues of the nasopharynx. It has only been propagated *in vitro* in B lymphocytes from humans and primates.[1]

EBV produces disease by transforming B lymphocytes, which then become self-perpetuating. Their multiplication is arrested by two mechanisms. One of these is a cellular immune response capable of eliminating most of the infected cells; the other is neutralizing antibodies that prevent the spread of the infection to other B lymphocytes. The atypical (reactive) lymphocytes that are characteristic of infectious mononucleosis (IM) are mostly suppressor–cytotoxic lymphocytes that recognize and kill EBV-infected B lymphocytes.[2]

The worldwide distribution of EBV is so widespread that 80% to 90% of all adults have been infected.[3,4] Transmission is almost exclusively through salivary contact. The virus is excreted orally by both symptomatic and asymptomatic individuals and can be isolated from the saliva of 10% to 20% of healthy adults. Primary infection, with or without disease, will induce production of neutralizing antibodies, usually resulting in lifelong immunity; however, the individual remains infected with the virus and is thus a carrier for life. Epstein-Barr virus can survive for years in peripheral lymphocytes without any disease, but, like other herpesviruses, EBV may become reactivated in the immunocompromised host.

The presentation and course of disease vary with the age at which the primary infection occurs. In childhood it is usually asymptomatic and is rarely associated with classical infectious mononucleosis. In areas of the world where there is poor hygiene and crowded conditions, infection usually occurs early in childhood. When primary infection does not occur until early adolescence or adulthood, 50% to 75% will be symptomatic, usually presenting as IM.[5] The infection is persistent, and disease can be reactivated by immunosuppression.

Isolation of the EBV is time-consuming and not practical for diagnostic purposes; therefore, serology is the basis for laboratory diagnosis of infection and disease. Two kinds of antibodies are used to diagnose infection and disease from EBV. The heterophile antibodies rise and fall rapidly and the virus-specific antibodies persist for the duration of the infection (*i.e.*, the rest of the patient's life).

Diseases

There are many subclinical cases of EBV infection and three diseases known to be associated with the virus. The most important, in terms of number of people affected, is infectious mononucleosis. The other two affect fewer people, but the diseases are more serious: Burkitt's lymphoma and nasopharyngeal carcinoma.

Burkitt's Lymphoma and Nasopharyngeal Carcinoma

A malignant neoplasm of B lymphocytes, Burkitt's lymphoma (BL) is found primarily among children in a restricted area of Africa and in New Guinea. Although BL has a higher incidence in these areas, it is observed sporadically throughout the world. In the rest of the world, however, EBV-associated lymphomas are found primarily in immunocompromised adults. The clusters of this malignancy in two restricted areas prompted a search for viral etiology.

This search culminated with the discovery, in 1964, of EBV, which bears the name of the researchers who first isolated it from BL tumor cells.[6]

Although the association of EBV with BL is strong, EBV has not been demonstrated in the BL tumor cells *in situ;* however, there is immunologic evidence for the presence of virus-specific antigens on the cell surface. Tumor cells *in vitro* produce the virus.

Epstein-Barr virus has been consistently associated with a rare form of squamous cell carcinoma of the nasopharynx; the highest incidence is observed among southern Chinese.

Neither BL nor nasopharyngeal carcinoma is thought to be a primary infection. Environmental and genetic factors appear to affect the development of these two human malignancies.[4]

Infectious Mononucleosis

A disease of the reticuloendothelial system, IM has a broad spectrum of clinical presentations, ranging from asymptomatic to severe, although it is rarely life threatening. The heterophile-positive IM is caused by EBV; heterophile-negative IM is induced by other agents, including cytomegalovirus, adenovirus, and *Toxoplasma gondii.*

The incubation period has been estimated to be 4 to 7 weeks.[7] The patient is probably infectious before illness, and based on studies of saliva of IM patients, infectivity continues for several weeks or months. The onset of the disease may be acute or insidious and is characterized by fever, sore throat, and lymphadenopathy. Hepatosplenomegaly, lymphocytosis with many atypical (reactive) lymphocytes, and enlarged cervical lymph nodes are common. The patient may develop a skin rash, and there may be conjunctivitis and central nervous system damage. The white blood cell count increases; there is a decrease in polymorphonuclear cells and a marked increase in monocytes and atypical (reactive) lymphocytes. The acute disease usually persists for about 2 weeks and is followed by a lengthy convalescence. The patients usually develop transient IgM heterophile antibodies, have an abnormal white blood cell picture, and have abnormal liver function tests.

Socioeconomic conditions affect the incidence of IM. In underdeveloped countries, as well as in densely populated countries, most children are infected by their third birthday.[8] In developed countries infection is frequently delayed until early adulthood, with approximately 50% of students entering college in the United States not yet infected.[5] By 30 years of age the prevalence of EBV antibodies approaches 100%, regardless of socioeconomic status.

Chronic illness subsequent to IM, although reported as early as 1948, has been reported with increasing frequency during the past few years.[9-12] This long-term illness is characterized by lymphadenopathy, fever, headache, pharyngitis, and persistent fatigue. Although some patients with this chronic form of IM are immunocompromised, not all are. It appears that there is also a chronic mononucleosis illness that is unrelated to EBV infection.

Laboratory Tests

Serologic evidence for infectious mononucleosis is obtained through examination of patient blood for heterophile or EBV-specific antibodies. The Paul-Bunnell and Davidsohn differential tests detect heterophile antibodies and are almost specific for the disease with few false positives. The rapid tests, however, have a higher rate of false positives. Some patients, especially children, fail to develop classical heterophile antibodies; therefore, EBV-specific tests must be performed for laboratory diagnosis. Heterophile antibodies wane after the initial infection, whereas some EBV-specific antibodies persist for the life of the patient.

Heterophile Antibodies

Heterophile antibodies react with antigens found in species unrelated to the antigen that stimulated their formation. There are many heterophile antibodies: sheep erythrocyte antibodies in IM, the nonimmune antibodies to the ABO blood groups, and nontreponemal antibodies (reagin) in syphilis. Heterophile antibodies, produced in response to the EBV-specific cell surface antigens during IM, react with antigens from several species (*e.g.*, erythrocyte surface antigens of sheep, beef, and horses). Antibodies formed in response to serum of a different animal species are found in serum sickness; these antibodies react with sheep, beef, and horse erythrocytes as well. The first heterophile antibodies described, Forssman, are formed in response to certain bacteria. Forssman antibodies react with sheep and horse erythrocyte antigens, but not with beef erythrocyte antigens.

Paul-Bunnell Presumptive Test[13]

Principle

Heterophile antibodies appear in the acute serum of 85% to 90% of young adults and adolescents who have classical IM.[1] Such antibodies usually reach significant levels by the end of the first week of illness and peak at 2 to 3 weeks.[14] These heterophile antibodies react with erythrocytes of several species, including sheep. Young children are usually seronegative unless they develop the classical disease. Infectious mononucleosis heterophile antibodies are of the IgM class and represent an early response.

Procedure

The Paul-Bunnell presumptive test employs dilutions of heat-inactivated patient serum mixed with a standard concentration of sheep erythrocytes. The dilutions of inactivated patient serum are twofold, beginning with 1:5. Subsequent to preparing serum dilutions, a 2% sheep erythrocyte suspension is added, resulting in twofold dilutions beginning with 1:7. After room temperature incubation, the tubes are read for visible agglutination.

Results

The titer is the reciprocal of the highest dilution of serum showing visible agglutination of the erythrocytes. A titer of 56 or less is normal, whereas a titer of 128 or greater is indicative of the presence of heterophile antibodies.

Interpretation

The Paul-Bunnell is a screening test that detects heterophile antibodies, which are not necessarily specific for IM. If it is negative, no further testing is needed. If it is positive, it indicates that the patient has heterophile antibodies, which are found in IM, serum sickness, and several rheumatic diseases. The false positive rate, approximately 3%, is almost totally due to individuals who maintain persistent, albeit low, heterophile antibody levels long after their illness. The false negative rate, 10% to 15%, is more common among children; these patients' sera should be tested with EBV-specific serology.[15]

Davidsohn Differential Test

Principle

The Davidsohn differential test[16,17] assumes the presence of heterophile antibodies at a titer of at least 56, as determined in the Paul-Bunnell test. Heterophile antibodies of IM will be absorbed by beef erythrocytes and will be absorbed weakly, if at all, by guinea pig kidney cells. The converse is true of Forssman heterophile antibodies, whereas the heterophile antibodies of serum sickness are not absorbed by either guinea pig kidney or bovine erythrocyte antigens (Table 20-1). Therefore, by comparing the agglutinins remaining in the serum after absorp-

Table 20-1: Davidsohn Differential Test Absorption Patterns

Heterophile Antibody	Antibody Absorbed by	
	Guinea Pig Kidney Cells	Beef Erythrocytes
Infectious mononucleosis	no	yes
Serum sickness	yes	yes
Forssman	yes	no

tions with guinea pig and bovine antigens, it is possible to differentiate between these three types of heterophile antibodies.

Procedure

Patient serum is added to a suspension of guinea pig kidney antigen and to bovine erythrocyte antigen; both suspensions are well mixed. After a short incubation period at room temperature, the suspensions are centrifuged. The supernatants are saved for the test, and the antigens are discarded. The supernatants are each 1:5 dilutions of patient serum. They are serially diluted twofold up to one dilution greater than the titer of the positive Paul-Bunnell test. When the 2% sheep erythrocyte suspension is added, the resultant dilutions are 1:7, 1:14, 1:28, and so on. After a room temperature incubation, the tubes are read for visible agglutination.

Results

The two titers are the reciprocals of the highest dilution showing visible agglutination.

Interpretation

The titer in the Paul-Bunnell test is known and is ≥56. In infectious mononucleosis the guinea pig kidney antigen absorption will reduce the Paul-Bunnell titer by no more than three tubes (sixfold or less reduction in titer); and the bovine erythrocyte antigen absorption reduces the Paul-Bunnell titer by four tubes or more (eightfold reduction required). In serum sickness, both absorptions will reduce the titer by at least eightfold. Serum from patients with Forssman antibodies will have an eightfold or greater reduction in titer from the guinea pig kidney antigen, and the beef erythrocyte absorption will be the same as the Paul-Bunnell titer (Table 20-2).

Rapid Tests[18,19]

Principle

A number of rapid, qualitative, differential slide tests are commercially available. They employ differential agglutination by patient serum of horse erythrocytes after the serum has been absorbed with fine suspensions of guinea pig kidney antigen and beef erythrocyte antigens.

Procedure

The differential spot test is performed on a slide. Patient serum or plasma specimens (do not have to be inactivated) are initially mixed separately with guinea pig kidney antigen and with beef erythrocyte antigen; subsequently, each mixture is mixed with horse red blood cells.

Results

The differential spot test is read for agglutination.

Interpretation

The spot test is positive if agglutination with the guinea pig kidney antigen–absorbed serum agglutinated more strongly than did the beef erythrocyte antigen–absorbed serum. The test is negative if no agglutination is observed or if agglutination is stronger in the bovine erythrocyte antigen–absorbed serum than in the guinea pig kidney antigen-abosrbed serum. Positive spot tests must be confirmed with the Paul-Bunnell test to determine the antibody titer. The sensitivity and specificity of the spot tests depend on the manufacturer; the horse cell agglutination procedure is the most sensitive (95% positive in serologically proved IM) and the bovine cell hemolysin procedure is the most specific.[4]

Enzyme-Linked Immunosorbent Assay[20]

In the enzyme-linked immunosorbent assay (ELISA) purified antigen from bovine erythrocyte stroma is attached to the solid phase. The test employs heavy-chain-specific anti-IgM labeled with alkaline phosphatase to detect the heterophile antibody. The quantitative results correlate well with horse erythrocyte agglutination titers.

EBV-Specific Tests

Several tests specific for EBV have been developed. The usual method employed to detect EBV-specific antibodies is immunofluorescence.

Table 20-2: Interpretation of Davidsohn Differential Test Results

	Changes in Paul-Bunnell Titer After Absorption With	
Disease	Guinea Pig Kidney Cells	Beef Erythrocytes
Infectious mononucleosis	≤ sixfold	≥ eightfold
Serum sickness	≥ eightfold	≥ eightfold
Forssman	≥ eightfold	no change

Immunofluorescence Tests[3,21]

There are four EBV-specific antibodies that can be detected by immunofluorescence: IgM and IgG anti–viral capsid antigen (VCA), anti–early antigen (EA), and anti–nuclear antigen (EBNA).

Principle

The immunofluorescence tests are sandwich techniques in which the antigen is fixed to the slide, allowed to react with patient serum and subsequently layered with fluorescent conjugated anti–human IgG or IgM.

Results

The slides are read with a fluorescence microscope. The titer is the reciprocal of the highest dilution showing specific fluorescence.

Interpretation

The most widely used procedure is the test for anti-VCA.[4] Titers of anti–VCA peak 3 to 4 weeks following infection; the IgM becomes undetectable in the circulation by 12 weeks after infection, and the IgG levels decrease but persist for life. Because IgG anti-VCA persists indefinitely, it is the most sensitive indicator of EBV infection. Although high levels of IgG anti-VCA are observed in acute infections, they are not specific for recent infections; increased levels are detected in a variety of other conditions, including immunodeficiency, malignancy, arthritis, systemic lupus erythematosus, and acquired immunodeficiency syndrome (AIDS). IgM anti-VCA is detectable in 97% of patients during the acute phase of IM and is therefore a reliable marker of recent infection.[22]

Antibody to EBV early antigen (anti-EA) is produced concomitantly with IgM anti-VCA and persists for 8 to 12 weeks. Anti-EA is usually associated with recent infection; after the acute phase of infection, anti-EA disappears but reappears as the patient ages.[23]

Table 20-3: Appearance and Duration of Epstein-Barr Virus–Specific Antibodies

Antibody	Time of Appearance	Detectable for
IgM Anti-VCA	onset	12 weeks
IgG Anti-VCA	onset	life
Anti-EA	onset	8 to 12 weeks
Anti-EBNA	2 to 3 months	indefinite

Antibody to the nuclear antigen (anti-EBNA) appears as early as 1 month after infection, but more commonly, 2 to 3 months later, and it persists indefinitely. Presence of anti-EBNA indicates that EBV infection has occurred and that it is not recent. Thus, the presence of anti-VCA IgG or IgM in the absence of anti-EBNA supports the diagnosis of IM (Table 20-3).

Other Changes

Lymphocytosis

When acute IM develops, there may be a leukopenia due to decreased granulocytes; however, usually there will be an increase in white blood cell count (WBC) by the second or third week of illness. The WBC rises to 10 to 20×10^9/L, with $\geq$ 50% mononuclear cells with $\geq$ 10% atypical (reactive) lymphocytes. In the majority of cases, there are 60% to 80% mononuclear cells with > 25% atypical (reactive) lymphocytes. The peripheral blood picture remains abnormal for at least 2 weeks and may persist for months.[14]

When a patient becomes infected with EBV, the initial site of infection is the lymphocytes in the lymphoid tissue of the oropharynx; the host immune response may contain the virus at this point or infection may spread to the rest of the body. If spreading does not occur, infection will not lead to clinical IM. Spreading may occur by viremia or circulation of the infected B lymphocytes. The infected B lymphocytes proliferate and invade many organs of the body.[8] The polyclonal activation of EBV-infected B lymphocytes stimulates the proliferation of T lymphocytes, which are essential in the recovery from IM.[2] The lymph nodes and spleen become enlarged as the WBC increases; most frequently, cervical lymph nodes are involved, although generalized lymphadenopathy is often observed. Splenomegaly occurs in 50% to 60% of patients.[2]

During the incubation period, some infected B lymphocytes are transformed, resulting in a proliferation of B lymphocytes; however, some infected cells lyse, releasing viral antigens. These antigens stimulate the production of antibodies to membrane antigens, viral capsid antigens, and early antigens that can be identified by immunofluorescence testing. The EBNA appears to be derived from transformed cells, not lytic cells; thus, these antibodies are not observed until convalescence.[8]

Liver Function

Clinically apparent jaundice is observed in 5% to 10% of patients with IM, and 10% to 25% have mild hepatomegaly.[2] Abnormal liver function tests are observed in a majority of patients; liver enzymes are raised during the second and third week of the disease. Bilirubin is also increased in most patients. The lactic dehydrogenase usually increased in IM is probably from WBC, not from liver.[2,15]

References

1. Lennette ET: Epstein-Barr virus. In Lennette ET, Balows A, Hausler WJ Jr, et al (eds): Manual of Clinical Microbiology, 4th ed, p 728. Washington, DC, American Society for Microbiology, 1985

2. Crawford DH, Edwards JMB: Epstein-Barr virus. In Zuckerman AJ, Banatvala JE, Pattison JR (eds): Principles and Practice of Clinical Virology, p 111. Chichester, John Wiley & Sons, 1987

3. Henle G, Henle W: Immunofluorescence in cells derived from Burkitt's lymphoma. J Bacteriol 91:1248, 1966

4. Andiman WA: Antibody Responses to Epstein-Barr Virus. In Rose NR, Friedman H, Fahey JL (eds): Manual of Clinical Laboratory Immunology, 3rd ed, p 509. Washington, DC, American Society for Microbiology, 1986

5. Niederman JC, Evans AS, Subrahmanyan MS, et al: Prevalence, incidence and persistence of EB virus antibody in young adults. N Engl J Med 282:361, 1970

6. Epstein MA, Barr YM, Achong BG: Virus particles in cultured lymphoblasts from Burkitt's lymphoma. Lancet 1:702, 1964

7. Henle G, Henle W, Diehl V: Relation of Burkitt's tumor-associated herpes-type virus to infectious mononucleosis. Proc Natl Acad Sci 59:94, 1968

8. Fleisher GR: Epidemiology and pathogenesis. In Schlossberg D (ed): Infectious Mononucleosis, Praeger Monographs in Infectious Disease, Vol 1, p 27. New York, Praeger, 1983

9. DuBois RE, Seeley JK, Brus I, et al: Chronic mononucleosis syndrome. South Med J 77:1376, 1984

10. Isaacs R: Chronic infectious mononucleosis. Blood 3:858, 1984

11. Merlin TL: Chronic mononucleosis: Pitfalls in the laboratory diagnosis. Human Pathol 17:2, 1986

12. Purtillo DT: Epstein-Barr virus: The spectrum of its manifestations in humans. South Med J 80:943, 1987

13. Paul JR, Bunnell WW: The presence of heterophile antibodies in infectious mononucleosis. Am J Med Sci 183:90, 1932

14. Niederman JC: Infectious mononucleosis at the Yale–New Haven Medical Center 1946–1955. Yale J Biol Med 28:629, 1956

15. Henle W, Henle G, Horwitz CA: Infectious mononucleosis and Epstein-Barr virus-associated malignancies. In Lennette EH, Schmidt NJ (eds): Diagnostic Procedures for Viral, Rickettsial and Chlamydial Infections, 5th ed, p

441. Washington, DC, American Public Health Association, 1979

16. Davidsohn I: Serologic diagnosis of infectious mononucleosis. JAMA 108:289, 1937.

17. Davidsohn I, Walker PH: The nature of heterophilic antibodies in infectious mononucleosis. Am J Clin Pathol 5:455, 1935

18. Lee CL, Davidsohn I, Panczyszyn O: Horse agglutinins in infectious mononucleosis, II. The spot test. Am J Clin Pathol 49:12, 1968

19. Lee CL, Davidsohn I, Slaby R: Horse agglutinins in infectious mononucleosis. Am J Clin Pathol, 49:3, 1968

20. Halbert SP, Anken M, Henle W, et al: Detection of infectious mononucleosis heterophile antibody by a rapid, standardized enzyme-linked immunosorbent assay procedure. J Clin Microbiol 15:610, 1982

21. Henle W, Henle G, Horowitz CA: Epstein-Barr virus-specific diagnostic tests in infectious mononucleosis. Human Pathol 5:551, 1974

22. Evans AS, Niederman JC, Cenabre LC, et al: A prospective evaluation of heterophile and Epstein-Barr virus-specific IgM antibody tests in clinical and subclinical infectious mononucleosis: Specificity and sensitivity of the tests and persistence of antibody. J Infect Dis 132:546, 1975

23. Merlin TL: Chronic mononucleosis: Pitfalls in the laboratory diagnosis. Hum Pathol 17:2, 1986

CHAPTER 21

Streptococcal Serology

Ann C. Albers

Organism

All members of the genus *Streptococcus* are gram-positive cocci. Division occurs in only one plane, resulting in cocci in pairs or chains. First described by Pasteur, these catalase-negative, facultative anaerobes comprise a heterogeneous group of homofermentative bacteria whose principal fermentation product is lactic acid.[1]

Streptococcus pyogenes, group A β-hemolytic streptococci, is a major pathogen of this genus. The organism is found only in man, and person-to-person spread is usually by upper respiratory secretions or by direct contact. Group A streptococci constitute the principal bacterial cause of oropharyngitis and are involved in many other suppurative infections, including pyoderma, puerperal sepsis, and acute endocarditis. These organisms are also responsible for the toxigenic condition scarlet fever and for two non-suppurative conditions (*i.e.*, rheumatic fever and acute poststreptococcal glomerulonephritis).

The serogroups of streptococci are determined by the C carbohydrate of the cell wall; all group A streptococci are antigenically identical for this carbohydrate. Group carbohydrates are not known to be associated with any particular disorders.

Serotypes of group A are determined by the proteins in the cell wall (M, T, and R; Fig. 21-1). M antigens are significant in disease association; they are important in adherence of the bacterial cell to the host cells, and antibodies to them are protective.[2] There are at least 80 antigenically distinct M serotypes.[3] Usually, different serotypes of group A are involved in skin infections from those involved in upper respiratory tract infections. These two types of infections do not usually occur simultaneously in the same person. Although serogrouping of streptococci is a routine procedure for many clinical microbiology labs, serotyping is generally limited to a few research labs.

Poststreptococcal Sequelae

Infection with group A β-hemolytic streptococci may be followed by two separate sequela, rheumatic fever (RF) and acute poststreptococcal glomerulonephritis. Rheumatic fever follows streptococcal infection of the throat, and glomerulonephritis follows either streptococcal infection of the throat or streptococcal pyoderma.

Diagnosis of either syndrome requires evidence of antecedent group A streptococcal infection. Most patients no longer have streptococcal infection when they present with RF or acute glomerulonephritis, so evidence of such infections is obtained by serologic assays. The three tests most frequently employed—antistreptolysin O (ASO), antihyaluronidase (AHT), and anti–deoxyribonuclease B (anti-DNase B)—all measure the presence of antibodies to enzymes produced by the organisms during acute infection.

Rheumatic Fever

Rheumatic fever, which is characterized by carditis, chorea, and/or erythema marginatum, follows about 2% to 3% of untreated cases of streptococcal pharyngitis.[4,5] Patients who are treated with antibiotics but who still have organisms recovered from the throat ≥ 3 weeks after acute infection have a similar RF attack rate.[6] Rheumatic fever usually occurs 3 to 4 weeks after group A streptococcal infection in the throat but does not follow skin infection. The syndrome is related to production of antibodies to the streptococci; RF apparently does not develop in patients who fail to produce antibodies to the organisms.[6,7] Because the cholesterol in the skin binds streptolysin O, it is not immunogenic in skin infections.

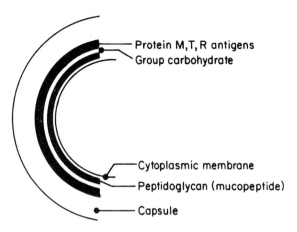

FIGURE 21-1. Layers of the cell wall and capsule of group A streptococcus.

The process that leads from streptococcal infection in the oropharynx to rheumatic fever is not understood. This is a nonsuppurative inflammatory process involving connective tissue and resulting in injury to the heart, joints, and central nervous system. Rheumatic inflammation of the joints (rheumatic polyarthritis) or brain (Sydenham's chorea) rarely results in permanent damage; rheumatic carditis, however, may become chronic and progressively debilitating. It may involve the pericardium, myocardium, and/or endocardium; however, it is the inflammation of the endocardium of the mitral valve that accounts for most of the morbidity and mortality of this disease. The inflammation of the mitral valve continues long after clinical evidence of carditis has disappeared, resulting in progressive scarring and malfunction, with end-stage mitral stenosis.[8]

The pathogenesis of rheumatic fever is not known at this time. There are several theories; the most popular is that the streptococcal infection induces an autoimmune response in the host. The group A streptococci are known to share antigenic determinants with some host cells, tissues, and organs.[9–11] The immune response that is directed against the organisms will cross-react with the host immunodeterminants; thus, these antibodies induced by group A streptococci are also autoantibodies to heart tissue. Patients with acute rheumatic fever have about four times as much of this heart-reactive antibody as patients convalescing from uncomplicated streptococcal infections or acute glomerulonephritis.[12]

Diagnosis of rheumatic fever is by revised Jones criteria which requires supporting evidence of preceding streptococcal infection plus a combination of major and minor manifestations (*i.e.*, carditis, polyarthritis, chorea, erythema marginatum, subcutaneous nodules, previous rheumatic fever or rheumatic heart disease, arthralgia, fever, increased erythrocyte sedimentation rate, C-reactive protein, leukocytosis, and electrocardiographic changes).[13]

Acute Glomerulonephritis

Acute glomerulonephritis, like RF, is a nonsuppurative sequel to group A streptococcal infection. It occurs in quite varied attack rates: 0.03% to 18%.[14] The disease presents with proteinuria, hematuria, hypertension, impaired renal function, and edema, especially about the face and legs. It is thought that this syndrome, like RF, is immunologically mediated. Several theories have been proposed to explain the

disease, but the one most commonly accepted is that the circulating antigen–antibody complexes are deposited in the glomerular basement membrane, where they activate complement, with damage to the glomeruli resulting from complement-mediated lysosomal release from white blood cells. There is an aggregation of platelets and a buildup of fibrin and fibrinogen. These, in turn, cause capillary obstruction, which results in impaired renal function.

Acute glomerulonephritis occurs approximately 10 days after streptococcal infection of the throat or 18 to 21 days after skin infection.[15] It occurs twice as often in males as in females. Many M serotypes can be involved in RF, but only a few specific nephritogenic M serotypes are responsible for acute poststreptococcal glomerulonephritis.

Laboratory Assays

The most reliable laboratory finding to support an antecedent streptococcal infection is isolation of the organism; however, many patients no longer have the organisms when either of the nonsuppurative poststreptococcal sequelae develop. Serologic evidence is then the only means of demonstrating the antecedent infection. The ASO test will be positive in 80% of patients with RF but is rarely positive in patients with acute glomerulonephritis secondary to streptococcal pyoderma. The AHT test is positive in a smaller percentage of RF patients but is also positive in most patients with poststreptococcal glomerulonephritis. The DNase B test is perhaps the most reliable of these three; moreover, it is positive for a longer period of time. It is strongly recommended that a combination of tests be performed for laboratory identification of an antecedent streptococcal infection. The Streptozyme test is a screening test and will give both false negatives and false positives compared with each of the other three assays. The relative reliability of these tests is stated in Table 21-1.

Table 21-1: Relative Reliability of Serologic Tests for Antecedent Group A Streptococcal Infections

Test	RF	AGN*
ASO	+++	0
AHT	++	++
DNase B	++++	++++
Streptozyme	+	+

* Acute glomerulonephritis

ASO Neutralization Test

Streptolysin O is produced by most strains of β-hemolytic group A streptococci. It is responsible, together with streptolysin S, for the hemolysis observed on blood agar. The antibodies to streptolysin O [*i.e.*, anti–streptolysin O (ASO)] neutralize its hemolytic activity. An increase in titer of ASO indicates a recent infection with group A streptococci.

In patients with culture-documented streptococcal infection of the upper respiratory tract, the ASO titer begins to rise after 1 week and peaks at 3 to 6 weeks after infection.[2,16,17] Thus, by the time RF develops, the ASO titer may be declining, particularly in those patients who do not develop any signs of RF for months after the antecedent group A streptococcal infection. In 75% to 80% of patients with RF there will be an increase in ASO titer; consequently, the diagnosis of RF cannot be excluded on the basis of a low ASO titer.[17] Patients with pyoderma and its sequela, acute glomerulonephritis, are less likely to have an increased ASO titer. Streptolysin O is produced by group A streptococci in pyoderma as well as in pharyngitis, but the cholesterol in the skin binds to the enzyme, thus preventing it from becoming an effective immunogen.

Principle

This assay is an enzyme-inhibition (neutralization) reaction. In a patient who has had a recent group A streptococcal infection, the antistreptolysin O antibodies will neutralize the streptolysin O reagent, thus preventing it from hemolyzing human group O red blood cells.

Procedure

Dilutions of patient serum and ASO control are prepared in buffer. To the control and to patient serum dilutions is added streptolysin O reagent. After a short room temperature incubation, 5% group O human red blood cell suspension is added, followed by an incubation at 37°C. Tubes are centrifuged and read for hemolysis.

Results

Tubes are read for hemolysis. Streptolysin O reagent will hemolyze human group O cells; lack of hemolysis is due to the neutralization of the streptolysin O reagent by the antibodies in the patient serum. The titer is the unit of the last tube (*i.e.*, the highest dilution) showing total absence of hemolysis. The reciprocal of the original serum dilution (not the final dilution) in each tube is equal to the Todd unit or the international unit; these two units are the same.

Interpretation

A fourfold increase in titer between acute and convalescent sera is evidence of a recent group A streptococcal infection. It is recommended that this test be performed on paired sera because a wide range of normal values has been reported. Streptococcal infections are fairly common; thus, normal individuals have low titers. The committee for revising the Jones criteria for diagnosis of RF recommended that single titers of at least 250 units in adults and 333 in children over 5 years of age be considered evidence of a recent streptococcal infection.[13] The titer of the ASO is unrelated to the clinical severity of RF.[17]

Antihyaluronidase Test

The enzyme hyaluronidase is produced by group A β-hemolytic streptococci, and antibodies to it, antihyaluronidase, are found in the blood of patients with recent streptococcal infections. The number of patients developing antibodies to this enzyme is somewhat lower than the number developing antibodies to streptolysin O; however, antibodies to hyaluronidase are produced by patients with either throat or skin infections, whereas ASO is produced only following throat infections.

Principle

This test is a neutralization assay in which the antibodies to the enzyme are allowed to neutralize it, thus preventing the subsequent enzymatic breakdown of the substrate, potassium hyaluronate.

Procedure

Serial dilutions of patient serum are prepared and the enzyme, hyaluronidase, is added to each tube. If the patient serum contains antihyaluronidase antibodies, the hyaluronidase will be inactivated. After a short incubation at 37°C, the tubes are cooled and substrate, potassium hyaluronate, is added to each tube. The tubes are reincubated at 37°C and cooled in the refrigerator. To each tube is added 2N acetic acid. If the patient has no antibodies to inactivate the hyaluronidase, it has hydrolyzed the hyaluronate and there will be turbidity after the acid is added. In tubes where the enzyme was inactivated (neutralized) by patient antihyaluronidase antibodies, a mucin clot forms, because the acid reacts with the potassium hyaluronate. The potassium hyaluronate is not destroyed if the hyaluronidase has been inactivated by antibodies, and potassium hyaluronate is therefore available to react with the acid, forming a mucin clot.

Results

The titer is the reciprocal of the highest dilution with definite clot formation. Threads are not considered clot formation.

Interpretation

If both acute and convalescent sera are tested, a fourfold rise in titer is considered evidence of streptococcal infection. If a single convalescent serum is tested, it is considered significant if the titer is >256. Reproducibility of this test is not as good as that of the ASO test and the anti–DNase B test; however, it is superior to ASO in demonstrating an antecedent streptococcal infection in patients presenting with skin-related acute glomerulonephritis.[16]

Anti–Deoxyribonuclease B Test

Streptococcus pyogenes strains are known to produce four DNases—A, B, C, and D.[18] DNase B is produced by nearly all strains of group A streptococci and by some strains of groups C and G. Group B streptococci produce three known DNases that are antigenically distinct from those produced by group A strains. Antibodies to DNase B are produced later than ASO, peaking at 4 to 6 weeks after infection and remaining in the serum for several months.[16] Anti-DNase antibodies are produced by organisms in the throat as well as those of the skin. Thus, anti–DNase B is a more reliable marker of antecedent streptococcal infection than is ASO, particularly in those patients whose symptoms (usually carditis or chorea) of RF are not observed for several months. This test is thought by many to be the single most reliable test to demonstrate antecedent group A streptococcal infection.

Principle

Anti–DNase B test is also a neutralization test. Antibodies in the patients' serum will prevent the enzyme, anti–DNase B (streptodornase) from depolymerizing DNA.

Procedure

Inactivated patient sera and control serum are diluted in buffer and incubated at 37°C, with the enzyme, DNase B, to allow the antibodies, if present, to inactivate (neutralize) the enzyme. Substrate, DNA–methyl green complex, is added to each tube. After overnight incubation at 37°C, the tubes are observed for color. Methyl green is green when combined with DNA. When DNase B hydrolyzes DNA, the methyl green is concomitantly reduced and becomes colorless.[19]

Results

Color in each tube is graded from 0 (no color) to 4+ (green). The titer is the reciprocal of the highest dilution with at least a 3+ reaction.

Interpretation

This test should be performed on paired acute and convalescent sera; a fourfold rise is considered indicative of a recent group A streptococcal infection. Interpretation of results of a single serum specimen depends on the age of the patient. Normal preschoolers have a titer of <120; everyone else has titers of <1360.[20]

Streptozyme

Streptozyme is a screening test marketed by Wampole (Wampole Laboratories, Cranbury, NJ) for detection of antibodies to five streptococcal enzymes: DNase B, hyaluronidase, NADase, streptokinase, and streptolysin O. The slide test is a passive hemagglutination assay that employs sheep erythrocytes coated with the streptococcal enzymes. The reagent is mixed with 1:100 dilution of patient serum. If antibodies to any of these enzymes are present, agglutination is observed. If the test is positive, the patient serum can be further diluted to determine the Streptozyme titer.

Early evaluations of this test kit found good agreement with ASO, antihyaluronidase, and antistreptokinase[21] and with ASO and anti–DNase.[22] However, more extensive evaluation demonstrated that it is not as reliable when compared with ASO and anti–DNase B together to confirm an antecedent streptococcal infection. Gorlubjatnikov *et al* found both false positive and false negative results when compared with ASO and anti-DNase assays.[23] They also reported that agreement rates appear to be age dependent, and as the patient population becomes older, Streptozyme will fail to detect up to 25% of elevated anti–DNase B titers.

References

1. Deibel RH, Seeley HW: *Streptococceae*. In Buchanan RE, Gibbons NE (eds): Bergey's Manual of Determinative Bacteriology, 8th ed, p 490. Baltimore, Williams & Wilkins, 1974

2. Wannamaker LW, Ayoub EM: Antibody titers in acute rheumatic fever. Circulation 21:598, 1960

3. Howard BJ, Ducate MJ: Streptococci. In Howard BJ (ed): Clinical and Pathogenic Microbiology, p 245. St Louis, CV Mosby, 1987

4. Denny FW Jr, Wannamaker LW, Brink WR, et al: Prevention of rheumatic fever: Treatment of the preceding streptococcic infection. JAMA 143:151–153, 1950

5. Wannamaker LW, Rammelkamp CH Jr, Denny FW, et al: Prophylaxis of acute rheumatic fever by treatment of the preceding streptococcal infection with various amounts of depot penicillin. Am J Med 10:673–695, 1951

6. Stollerman GH: Rheumatic fever and streptococcal infection, p 63. Orlando, Grune & Stratton, 1975

7. Markowitz M: Rheumatic Fever, p 1. Philadelphia, WB Saunders, 1972

8. Paterson PY: The enigma of rheumatic fever. In Youmans GY, Paterson PY, Sommers HM (eds): The Biological and Clinical Basis of Infectious Diseases, 3rd ed, p 195. Philadelphia, WB Saunders, 1985

9. Kaplan MH, Svec KH: Immunologic relation of streptococcal and tissue antigens. J Exp Med 119:651, 1964

10. Zabriskie JB, Freimer EH: An immunological relationship between the group A streptococcus and mammalian muscle. J Exp Med 124:661, 1966

11. Husby G, van de Rijn I, Zabriskie JB, et al: Antibodies reacting with cytoplasm of subthalamic and caudate nuclei neurons in chorea and acute rheumatic fever. J Exp Med 144:1094, 1976

12. Zabriskie JB, Hsu KC, Seegal BC: Heart-reactive antibody associated with rheumatic fever: Characterization and diagnostic significance. Clin Exp Immunol 7:147, 1970

13. Committee to Revise Jones Criteria, Stollerman GH (chair): Jones criteria (revised) for guidance in the diagnosis of rheumatic fever. Circulation 32:664, 1965

14. Freeman BA: Burrows Textbook of Microbiology, p 401. Philadelphia, WB Saunders, 1985

15. Facklam RR, Carey RB: Streptococci and aerococci. In Lennette EH, Balows A, Hausler WJ Jr, et al (eds): Manual of Clinical Microbiology, 4th ed, p 154. Washington, DC, American Society for Microbiology, 1985

16. Farmer SG: Immunology of bacterial infections. In Lennette EH, Balows A, Hausler WJ Jr, et al (eds): Manual of Clinical Microbiology, 4th ed, p 898. Washington, DC, American Society for Microbiology, 1985

17. Davis E: Acute rheumatic fever. Practitioner 213:159, 1974

18. Slechta TF, Gray ED: Isolation of streptococcal nuclease by batch adsorption. J Clin Microbiol 2:528, 1975

19. Klein GC, Baker CN, Addison BV, et al: Micro test for streptococcal antideoxyribonuclease B. Appl Microbiol 18:204, 1969

20. Peacock JE, Tomar RH: Manual of Laboratory Immunology, p 50. Philadelphia, Lea & Febiger, 1980

21. Janeff J, Janeff D, Taranta A, et al: A screening test for streptococcal antibodies. Lab Med 2:38, 1971

22. Klein GC, Jones WL: Comparison of the streptozyme test with the anitistreptolysin O, antideoxyribonuclease B, and antihyaluronidase tests. Appl Microbiol 21:257, 1971

23. Golubjatnikov R, Koehler JE, Buccowich J: Comparative study of antistreptolysin O, antideoxyribonuclease B and multi-enzyme tests in streptococcal infections. Health Lab Sci 14:284, 1977

CHAPTER 22

Acquired Immunodeficiency Syndrome

Ann Marie McNamara

The goal of this chapter is to show how immunologic methods can be used in the identification of acquired immunodeficiency syndrome (AIDS), not to provide all the details of how AIDS interferes with the body's immune response. Many articles have reviewed the effects of AIDS on the immune system, and the interested reader is referred to this literature.[1-3]

Human Immunodeficiency Virus

The first case of AIDS was reported to the Centers for Disease Control (CDC) in June 1981.[4] Since then this disease has reached epidemic proportions in the United States, with more than 66,000 cases having been reported in 1988.[5] It has been predicted that the cumulative total number of cases will reach 270,000 in 1991.[6] More than 80% of persons diagnosed as having the disease for 3 or more years have died.[7] To date, there is no cure.

The etiologic agent of AIDS is a human retrovirus known as human immunodeficiency virus (HIV). Retroviruses are RNA viruses that contain reverse transcriptase, an enzyme that makes DNA from the viral RNA. Two types of HIV have been found: HIV-1, the causative agent of AIDS in the United States and Europe, and HIV-2, associated with immunodeficiency and a clinical syndrome similar to AIDS in West Africa.[8]

HIV, formerly known as lymphadenopathy-associated virus (LAV),[9] human T-cell lymphotrophic virus type III (HTLV-III),[10] or AIDS-related virus (ARV),[11] is closely related to a group of nontransforming, cytopathic retroviruses called lentiviruses.

Lentiviruses cause chronic neurodegenerative and wasting diseases in animals, similar to the wasting disease and neurologic disorders produced by HIV in humans. Based on studies of cross-reactions of viral proteins, HIV has been shown to be closely related to simian T-cell lymphotrophic virus type III (STLV-III). STLV-III causes a form of AIDS in African green monkeys, suggesting that HIV originated from a monkey virus prevalent in Africa that adapted to human hosts.

HIV Structure

The HIV virus particle, or virion, is approximately 100 nm in diameter. It consists of three parts: an outer envelope, a core shell of protein, and a cone-shaped inner core that contains the viral RNA (Fig. 22-1).

Small viral surface proteins form a regular geometric structure that resembles a soccer ball in that it consists of pentagons and hexagons combined to form a spherical shape. These proteins are embedded in a lipid bilayer. At regular intervals in this surface structure a large glycoprotein traverses the lipid bilayer membrane and protrudes above the surface in a knoblike structure. This glycoprotein (gp) has two components: gp41 traverses the membrane and gp120 extends beyond the surface as a knob. The names of these proteins are derived from their molecular weight (gp41 = glycoprotein of 41,000 d). The gp120 component is highly immunogenic (it provokes an immune response). The outer envelope also contains human leukocyte antigens. These antigens are derived from human cell membranes when new HIV virions bud from human cells during the process of virus particle formation.

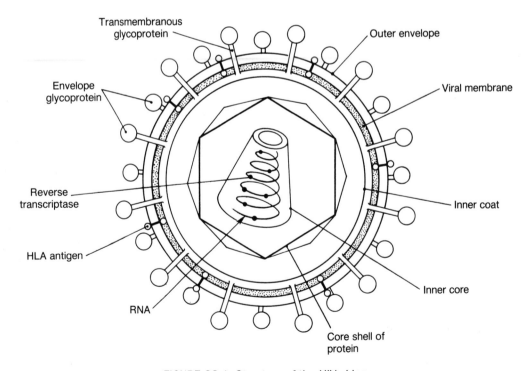

FIGURE 22-1. Structure of the HIV virion.

Beneath the outer envelope lies a protein core composed of viral proteins p24 and p17. Inside the protein core shell lies a cone-shaped central core containing the viral RNA and reverse transcriptase. The reverse transcriptase is unique to retroviruses and allows the viral RNA to be transcribed into DNA for incorporation into the infected human host cells' genome.

HIV Genome

Complete nucleotide sequences of the HIV genome have been determined,[12,13] making it possible to identify viral genes and some of the relationships between viral gene products and the clinical course of AIDS. The HIV genome is unique among retroviruses in its complexity. It has at least five regulatory genes (*tat, art/trs, sor, 3'orf,* and *R*) in addition to the usual structural genes (*gag, pol,* and *env;* see Fig. 22-2).

The *gag* (*g*roup *a*nti*g*en) gene codes for the core proteins. These proteins are cleaved from a large polyprotein of 55 kd (kilodaltons), which is found in high levels in infected cells. The cleavage products form the three core structural proteins, p18, p24, and p15.

The *pol* (*pol*ymerase) gene codes for four enzymes: reverse transcriptase, RNAse, protease, and integrase. Reverse transcriptase transcribes single-stranded RNA into double-stranded DNA. It is an immunogenic protein designated p66/51. RNAse is an enzyme that digests the RNA in RNA–DNA hybrids that form as intermediates in the creation of viral DNA. Protease (p31) cleaves itself from an initial polyprotein and cleaves other enzymes and structural proteins from their polyproteins. Integrase is responsible for inserting the viral DNA into the host DNA.

The *env* (*env*elope) gene codes for the glycoprotein gp160, which is found in infected cells. It is cleaved to form the two envelope glycoproteins gp120, found on the outside of the viral envelope, and gp41, which is embedded in the viral membrane.

The *sor* (*s*hort *o*pen *r*eading frame) gene is related to viral infectivity. It produces a protein, p23, which is present in the filtrate of virus-infected cultures and against which antibodies form in the serum of HIV-infected persons.[14]

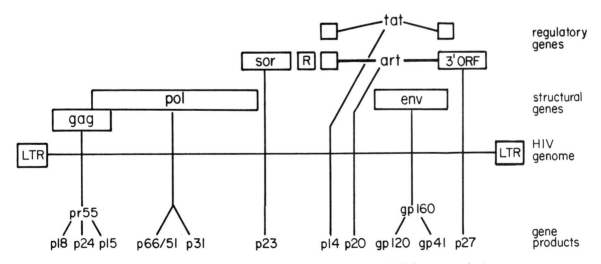

FIGURE 22-2. The HIV genome showing viral genes and viral gene products.

The *tat* (*trans-activation translation*) gene accelerates viral protein production and is required for viral replication. Without *tat* only minimal RNA is produced, and no virus particles are formed.[15] The protein produced by *tat* is p14.

Between *sor* and *tat* on the viral genome lies the *R* (*reading* frame) gene, which codes for an immunogenic product (p15) of unknown function.[16]

The *art/trs* (*anti-repression transactivator*) gene regulates the translation of the viral genome.[17] It produces an anti-repression transactivator protein p20, which regulates the expression of viral gene components.

The *B3'orf* (3' open *reading* frame) gene is responsible for the latency of the virus, slowing down viral reproduction tenfold in CD4 cells. The p27 protein produced by *B3'orf* raises antibodies that have been found in infected persons.[18]

At each end of the viral genome are identical ends (LTR = long terminal repeats) containing a terminator, an enhancer, and a promoter for the process of transcription.

All the protein and glycoprotein gene products (p and gp in Fig. 22-2) appear to be specific for the AIDS virus and may induce an antibody response in an infected person. Studies indicate that the first antibody to be observed in HIV-infected persons is directed against the p24 core protein, followed by a mixture of antibodies, usually including antibodies to the gp41 envelope glycoprotein.[19] In enzyme-linked immunosorbent assays (ELISA) and Western Blot (WB) studies of 280 specimens from AIDS and AIDS-related complex (ARC) patients, 96% of patients had antibodies to p24 and 88% had antibodies to gp41.[20] These antibodies are typically seen in both symptomatic and asymptomatic HIV-seropositive individuals and act as markers of HIV infection. Declining p24 antibody titers occur in the late stages of AIDS, when patients clinically deteriorate (Fig. 22-3). Antibodies to the envelope gene products (gp160, gp120, and gp41) can be detected in nearly all HIV-positive patients, and antibodies to the polymerase gene products (p31, p51, p66) are also commonly detected.[21] Other antibodies are detected less consistently.

HIV Life Cycle

The HIV genome carries within it the genetic information required to reproduce HIV viruses within infected host cells. HIV binds to host cells through a complexing of the gp120 molecule on the viral surface and a receptor molecule: the CD4 molecule on host cells. CD4 molecules are found on the surface of some immune cells (helper T lymphocytes, B cells, monocytes, and macrophages) and on some phagocytic cells found in the nervous system (monocytes and macrophages). Although CD4 receptors have also been identified on some glial cells and neuroleukin receptors have been identified on neurons that are capable of binding gp120, their clinical importance is still uncertain.

After HIV binds to the CD4-containing cell, it penetrates the host cell and loses its outer layers to expose the viral RNA. The viral RNA is transcribed into DNA and inserted into the host genome during cellular division or activation. Host cells can be activated by antigenic challenge or by allogenic stimulation after exposure to blood, semen, or allografts.

Once activated, transcription of viral proteins occurs. Viral RNA and proteins are then assembled at the host cell's cytoplasmic surface to produce a mature virion that escapes the host cell by budding from the host cell membrane (Fig. 22-4). When HIV replication occurs, the CD4 cell is killed, resulting in severe depletion of helper–inducer T lymphocytes. It is the depletion of these cells that correlates to the progressive severity of immune deficiency and to the increased susceptibility to opportunistic disease and malignancies seen in the clinical course of AIDS (Table 22-1).

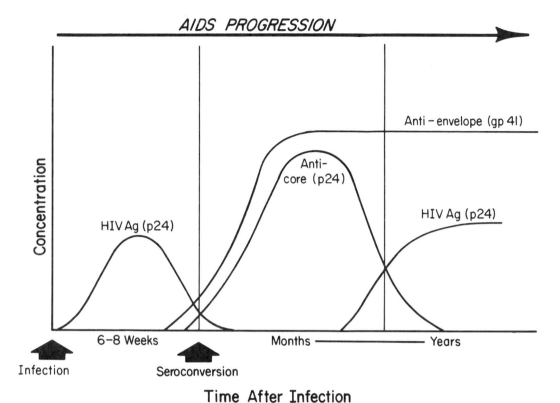

FIGURE 22-3. Antigen and antibody response in AIDS.

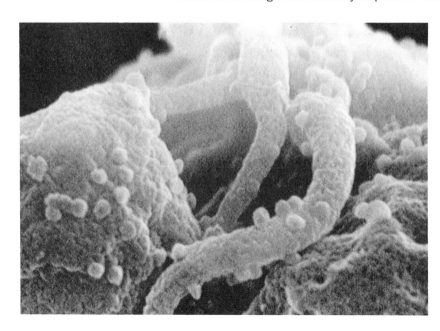

FIGURE 22-4. Scanning electron micrograph of HIV-infected CD4 lymphocytes showing virus budding from the plasma membrane of the lymphocytes. (Courtesy of CDC Archives.)

Effect of HIV on the Immune Response

Detailed information on the normal mechanisms of immune response can be found in earlier chapters (see Chapter 4), and details of the effects of AIDS on the immune response can be found in the literature. AIDS is so devastating primarily because of the destruction of CD4-containing cells and their central role in mediating the immune response. Helper T lymphocytes have a high concentration of CD4 molecules on their surface and are the major targets of HIV virions. The depletion of these cells as a result of HIV infection results in a severe depression of the immune response (Table 22-2). The loss of CD4-positive cells correlates closely with the severity of the clinical course of AIDS.[22] Particularly important are

Table 22-1: Opportunistic Infections and Neoplasms Seen in AIDS

OPPORTUNISTIC INFECTIONS

Bacteria

Mycobacterium avium–intracellulare
Mycobacterium kansasii
Mycobacterium tuberculosis
Streptococcus pneumoniae
Haemophilus influenzae
Salmonella species

Viruses

Cytomegalovirus
Herpes simplex
Herpes zoster
Epstein-Barr virus
Adenovirus

Protozoa

Pneumocystis carinii
Toxoplasma gondii
Cryptosporidium species
Isospora belli

Fungi

Candida albicans
Coccidioides immitis
Histoplasma capsulatum
Cryptococcus neoformans
Aspergillis species

NEOPLASMS

Kaposi's sarcoma
Burkitt-like lymphoma
Undifferentiated non-Hodgkin's lymphoma
  Hodgkin's disease

Central nervous system lymphoma
Peripheral organ lymphoma
Immunoblastic sarcoma
Lymphocytic preleukemia

Table 22-2: Effect of HIV on the Immune Response

EFFECT ON T CELLS	EFFECT ON OTHER IMMUNE CELLS
Depletion of CD4 lymphocytes	Decreased natural killer cell activity
Elevated, normal, or depressed suppressor CD8 lymphocytes	Defective chemotaxis in monocytes and macrophages
Increased susceptibility to opportunistic infections and neoplasms due to decreased T-cell function	Enhanced release of interleukin-1 and cachectin by monocytes
Decreased delayed-type hypersensitivity	
Decreased ability to promote help to B lymphocytes	**OTHER SEROLOGIC ABNORMALITIES**
Decreased production of interleukin-2	Increased circulating α-interferon
	Increased α_1-thymosin
EFFECT ON B CELLS	Increased β_2-microglobulin
Polyclonal hypergammaglobulinemia	Increased serum and urinary neopterin
Elevated circulating immune complexes	
Inability to produce a serologic response to a new antigen or following immunization	
Increased numbers of spontaneous Ig-secreting cells	
Refractory to B-cell activation signals *in vitro*	

the increased viral, protozoal, and fungal infections found in AIDS patients as a direct result of an impaired cell-mediated immune system (see Table 22-1). Cytotoxic–suppressor T cells expressing CD8 do not appear to be infected by HIV.[1] An early immunogenic marker of AIDS is an inverted helper–suppressor (CD4/CD8) cell ratio.

Clinical Features

Epidemiology

As of July 4, 1988, there have been 66,464 reported cases of AIDS in the United States. Adult AIDS victims can be broken down into the following groups: 63% homosexual or bisexual men; 19% heterosexual intravenous (IV) drug abusers; 7% homosexual or bisexual IV drug abusers; 4% heterosexual men and women; 3% recipients of contaminated blood or blood-product transfusions, usually prior to 1985; 1% people with hemophilia or other coagulation disorders; and 3% unknown risk factors.[5] US adult cases broken down by race are as follows: 59% white, 26% black, and 14% hispanic.[5] Of the 1054 pediatric AIDS cases reported, 78% of the infections occurred perinatally and most can be traced to IV drug abuse by the child's mother or father.[5] Nineteen percent of pediatric AIDS cases resulted from blood transfusions or treatment for hemophilia.

HIV has been isolated from a variety of body fluids, cells, and tissues of infected persons: mononuclear cells, plasma, semen, cervical–vaginal secretions, saliva, tears, urine, breast milk, cerebrospinal fluid, lymph nodes, brain, and bone marrow.[23] Transmission of the virus has been documented by one of three routes: sexual transmission (heterosexual, bisexual, or homosexual), parenteral transmission (through blood or blood products or by sharing blood-contaminated drug paraphernalia), and perinatal transmission (transplacental transmission and possibly through breast milk).[23] There are no accounts of AIDS being transmitted by food, water, insects, or casual contact with AIDS victims.[24]

Clinical Manifestations

HIV infection results in a spectrum of disease presentations from an apparently healthy state (asymptomatic infection), to symptomatic infection (ARC), to severe T-cell depletion with complicating opportunistic infections and cancers (AIDS).

HIV infection generally manifests itself initially as a mononucleosis-like illness followed by either asymptomatic infection or chronic lymphadenopathy in HIV-antibody-positive, otherwise healthy individuals.[23] Estimates state that 25% to 50% of persons with subclinical HIV infections progress to full-blown AIDS over a 5-year period.[25] The disease then progresses to symptomatic infection with persistent lymphadenopathy and quantitative T-cell deficiencies (especially a decreased CD4-positive cell count and an inverted CD4/CD8 ratio), but without the typical opportunistic infections and cancers seen in AIDS. This intermediate state is called AIDS-related complex, or ARC. Patients typically present with prolonged constitutional symptoms of fatigue, night sweats, fever, diarrhea, and weight loss (HIV wasting syndrome).[25] ARC can be diagnosed according to CDC criteria if two of the following clinical manifestations plus two laboratory abnormalities are found in a person without explainable etiology: *clinical manifestations*—lymphadenopathy of more than 3

months, fever over 100°F for more than 3 months, more than 10% weight loss, persistent diarrhea, fatigue, or night sweats; *laboratory abnormalities*—CD4 cells less than 400/mm², CD4/CD8 ratio less than 1.0, leukopenia, thrombocytopenia, anemia, elevated serum globulins, anergy to skin tests, reduced blastogenesis, or positive HIV antibody test.[23] The disease then progresses to a syndrome of severe CD4 depletion, resulting in opportunistic infections and cancers suggestive of severe cell-mediated immunity defects in a person with no documented cause for immunodeficiency: AIDS. The reader is urged to consult the CDC guidelines for interpretation of opportunistic infections and cancers in AIDS diagnosis (see also Table 22-1).[26]

Therapy and Vaccine Development

Treatment of HIV infection has largely been limited to the treatment of opportunistic infections and cancers that are complications of AIDS.[27] With increased knowledge of the structure and replicative cycle of HIV, new drugs that inhibit HIV binding to CD4 receptors, inhibit viral replication, or reduce viral budding from cell membranes have been developed. The most promising of these new drugs is 3′azido-3′deoxythymidine, called zidovudine (formerly azidothymidine or AZT). This compound is an inhibitor of reverse transcriptase and is also a DNA chain terminator. Clinical trials have shown that zidovudine has reduced mortality, morbidity, and the number of opportunistic infections in AIDS patients.[28] This drug is orally absorbed and crosses the blood–brain barrier. Side-effects include megaloblastic anemia, neutropenia, nausea, insomnia, and myalgia.[27] Other promising drugs currently in clinical trials that inhibit reverse transcriptase and/or cause DNA chain termination include dideoxycytidine, phosphonoformate, and rifabutin.[29] Another treatment strategy is to produce anti-idiotypic antibodies to the CD4 binding site or to create soluble CD4 (called rCD4) molecules that will block the CD4 binding site and prevent HIV binding to patient cells.[29] α-Interferon, which may reduce viral budding from infected cell surfaces, is also undergoing clinical trials.[29] To date, it has been shown to be of use in the treatment of Kaposi's sarcoma.[30]

Development of an effective AIDS vaccine is problematic for two reasons: the antigenic diversity found among isolates of HIV and the lack of good animal models for vaccine trials. A good HIV vaccine should be able to protect against all viral strains and both viral types. However, the immunogenic envelope proteins of HIV-1 strains and HIV-2 show high degrees of antigenic variation.[31] A good vaccine strategy would be to develop a vaccine composed of single or multiple recombinant virus proteins derived from the more highly conserved shared core proteins of HIV-1 strains and HIV-2.[31] Animal models have been limited to the chimpanzee, which develops viremia followed by antibody production after infection but fails to develop immunodeficiency.[31] Chimpanzees are also rare and expensive, and this has limited animal trials.

Despite problems inherent in developing an AIDS vaccine, many vaccines have been developed and several are in clinical trials. Three types of vaccines have been developed: genetically engineered HIV subunit vaccines (combined with adjuvant or in a virus vector), anti-idiotype vaccines (antibodies against CD4), and killed-virus vaccine.[32] Clinical trials have not been in progress long enough at this time to determine the effectiveness of these vaccines.

Laboratory Diagnosis

General Principles

Since the discovery of the AIDS virus, a variety of methods has been devised to isolate HIV, detect HIV antibodies, and detect HIV antigen in patients' blood and body fluids. Isolation of HIV and methods to detect HIV antigen are primarily used to detect early HIV infection before antibodies develop, to monitor the effectiveness of antiviral drugs, and to detect the progression of asymptomatic to symptomatic AIDS infection by monitoring an increase in p24 antigen. Detection of HIV antigen in patient specimens indicates active HIV infection, whereas detection of antibodies to HIV denotes prior exposure to HIV[21]. HIV antibody tests are of two major classes: screening tests and supplementary tests.

ELISA tests to detect HIV antibodies were first developed to screen the nation's blood supply. AIDS is a clinical diagnosis based on the presence of signs and symptoms of the disease. One may have antibodies to HIV, signifying HIV exposure, and yet be healthy. These antibody-positive, asymptomatic persons harbor active virus and have the potential to transmit the virus to noninfected persons years before developing signs and symptoms of ARC or AIDS. The current Centers for Disease Control recommendations state that HIV-antibody-reactive persons should be regarded as capable of transmitting infection[33] and their blood and mucous secretions should be handled accordingly.

Since false positive and false negative tests occur with the ELISA screening test for a variety of reasons, all "repeatedly reactive" ELISA samples are confirmed by a supplementary test. A reactive supplementary test confirms the presence of HIV antibody and is therefore indicative of past exposure and, presumably, current HIV infection.[21]

Genetic probes for HIV viral RNA or proviral DNA for use in molecular hybridization techniques have recently been developed. The advantage of HIV probes will be to detect HIV genomes directly in cells infected with latent or actively replicating HIV viruses when other serologic markers may be absent.

Detection of HIV-2 infections is currently possible by using ELISA tests for HIV-1 and by modifying current methods to identify HIV-2 antibodies, proteins, and genes. HIV-1 and HIV-2 show genomic similarity in their *gag* and *pol* gene regions (56% and 66% nucleotide sequence homology, respectively).[34] Thus, HIV-2-positive sera may cross-react with HIV-1 core proteins, but probably not with HIV-1 envelope proteins. Because of cross-reactive core proteins, five current HIV-1 ELISA tests have been shown to detect 42% to 92% of HIV-2 infections in blood samples.[35] Tests made more specific for detecting HIV-2 infections are now being devised using HIV-2-derived proteins (especially envelope proteins in ELISA and Western Blot tests) and HIV-2-specific DNA probes.

All tests described in the next section refer to HIV-1 detection. However, the reader should keep in mind that serologic cross-reactions can occur to HIV-2 and that all test methods can be modified to produce specific HIV-2 tests.

Laboratory Methods

HIV Isolation

Isolation of HIV from patients' cells and body fluids is not routinely performed in medical laboratories. This procedure is costly (several hundred dollars), is time-consuming (generally 15 to 30 days), requires adequate safety containment facilities, and may expose personnel to high virus concentrations.[21,36]

Co-cultivation is usually performed using patient and HIV-negative donor peripheral blood monocytes. Monocytes are collected from peripheral blood samples by Ficoll-Hypaque gradients. Donor monocytes are stimulated with phytohemagglutinin for 2 to 4 days before mixing with patient monocytes and interleukin-2. The cell mixture is co-cultivated in tissue culture flasks with added cell culture medium for up to 1 month.[37] Culture fluid is removed on a weekly basis and tested for the presence of HIV by reverse transcriptase assays, antigen indirect immunofluorescence assay, or antigen ELISA testing. Isolation of HIV from patient specimens has two main purposes: to detect HIV antigen in early infection before antibodies form and to monitor antiviral drug therapy (successful therapy results in decreased viral isolation).

Enzyme-Linked Immunosorbent Assay

The enzyme-linked immunosorbent assay (ELISA) test is the most widely used screening test for HIV antibodies. It is simple to perform, relatively inexpensive, and adaptable to screening large numbers of specimens in a short time (<4 hours).

HIV antigens derived from either disrupted virus particles (first-generation assays), recombinant antigens, or chemically synthesized peptides (second-generation assays) are immobilized onto microtiter wells or plastic or metal beads. Patient serum or plasma is then incubated with the fixed antigen and washed. Anti-IgG antibody, conjugated to either horseradish peroxidase, glucose oxidase, or alkaline phosphotase, is then added and allowed to incubate. After a washing step, the appropriate chromogenic enzymatic substrate is added and a color change occurs that is proportional to the amount of human IgG present. Results are read on a spectrophotometer by comparing values obtained from positive and negative controls to those from the test specimen. This results in an absorbance cut-off value above which a reactive test is defined. IgM antibodies can also be detected if the ELISA test is modified to include a mixture of heavy- and light-chain antibodies to human immunoglobulin.

The ELISA test has also been modified into a competitive assay format for detecting HIV antibody. In this test, patient serum or plasma specimens are incubated with enzyme-labeled HIV antibodies in microtiter wells coated with HIV antigens. Patient and enzyme-labeled HIV antibodies then compete for binding sites on the immobilized HIV antigens. The more unbound patient HIV antibody that binds to the antigen, the less labeled HIV antibody binds and the less color development occurs when the substrate is added. Therefore, color development is inversely proportional to the amount of HIV antibodies present in the patient's specimen.

There are several potential sources of error in ELISA testing for HIV antibodies. In addition to technical error, false positives and negative reactions occur. False positive reactions occur in persons with autoimmune diseases (shared-membrane antigens between the HIV virion and the human host cell, *i.e.*, T-cell antigens, HLA antigens, nuclear and cellular antigens), alcoholism, lymphoproliferative diseases, adult T-cell leukemia–lymphoma, and syphilis and in persons with no known risk.[21,38] False negative reactions occur during the incubation stages of AIDS (between the time of infection and the development of detectable antibodies); in the late stages of AIDS, when antibody titers typically decrease; when envelope glycoproteins (*i.e.*, gp41 and gp120) are lost during overstringent purification methods; or when there is insufficient p24 in antigen mixtures as a result of glycoprotein enrichment procedures.[38]

When an ELISA test is "reactive" it is repeated in duplicate to rule out technical error. If the specimen is reactive in two out of three tests, it is termed "repeatedly reactive" and a supplementary test is performed to confirm the positive ELISA result.

Although the sensitivity and specificity of ELISA antibody tests are better than 98% when compared with Western Blot assays,[21] an important concept in ELISA testing is that of the predictive value positive (PVP) of a positive result. The PVP tells the probability of a positive (reactive) test being a true positive. It is dependent upon the prevalence of a disease in a given population. Populations having a low disease prevalence have a low PVP and populations with a high disease prevalence have a high PVP. Therefore, a reactive ELISA test in a high-risk person or population is most likely indicative of true infection, whereas a reactive test result in a low-risk individual or population may indicate a false positive test.[38] For illustration, Reesink *et al* showed that the PVP of a positive ELISA test was 100% in a population of AIDS and ARC patients (a high-prevalence group) but was between 5% and 100% when blood donors (a low-prevalence group) were tested.[39]

ELISA tests have also been modified to detect HIV antigen in serum, plasma, culture fluids, and cerebrospinal fluid. In these tests an antibody sandwich technique is used in which monoclonal or polyclonal anti-HIV antibody is coated to the microwell or bead; a patient specimen is added, incubated, and washed; and rabbit or goat anti-HIV antibody is added. If the patient's sample contains HIV antigen, an antibody–antigen–antibody complex is formed. Enzyme-conjugated antibody to rabbit or goat immunoglobulin is then added, followed by the appropriate substrate in a typical ELISA format. Because antibodies to p24 proteins have higher binding affinities to HIV antigen than other HIV antibodies, these ELISA kits primarily detect free p24 HIV antigens.[40] If the ELISA antigen test is repeatedly reactive, an antibody neutralization assay is performed on the specimen.[21] In this assay the patient specimen is incubated with human antibody to HIV before performing the ELISA antigen test. If HIV antigen is present in the specimen, it will be neutralized by the human antibody and attachment to the ELISA antibody coated microwell or bead will not occur. This results in a reduction in absorbance when compared with a concomitant nonabsorbed patient specimen.

Slide Agglutination Tests

Rapid slide agglutination (SA) tests for detecting the presence of HIV antibodies or antigens have recently been developed. These tests are now being widely used in field work in Africa to detect HIV antibodies in blood products and patients. These screening tests offer distinct advantages over the currently used ELISA antibody tests, because they are simple to perform, they require 5 minutes to 2 hours of technician time, heat inactivation of serum does not affect test results, all materials are portable, results can be read with the naked eye, and no costly equipment is needed.[41,42] In addition, SA tests simultaneously detect both IgG and IgM HIV antibodies.[41]

The principle of SA tests is that of an antigen–antibody reaction made visible on a slide by linking the detector antigens or antibodies to polystyrene or polyvinyl beads[42] or to gelatin carriers.[41] When detector antigens (for HIV antibody tests) or antibodies (for HIV antigen tests) are mixed with the patient serum or plasma on a slide, a visible agglutination reaction is formed if the patient's specimen contains HIV antibody or antigen, respectively.

Western Blot Assay

The Western Blot (WB) assay is the most widely used supplementary test for confirming repeatedly reactive HIV ELISA antibody tests. In this assay HIV virus is disrupted and HIV proteins are separated by molecular weight into discrete bands by electrophoresis onto polyacrylamide gels.[43] The viral proteins are then transferred onto nitrocellulose sheets and cut into strips. Individual strips are incubated overnight with patient serum (HIV antibodies), washed, and incubated with anti–human immunoglobulin conjugated with enzymes or biotin. After addition of the appropriate substrate, color develops to show discrete bands where antigen–antibody reactions have occurred.

The WB assay is cumbersome to perform, is expensive, requires overnight incubation, and is difficult to interpret. Interpretation of positive tests varies between laboratories, depending on which recommendations are followed (i.e., CDC or commercial test kit manufacturers), and individual laboratory experiences. The CDC recommends that test results be called positive when the gp41 band appears alone or when an envelope antibody (gp41, gp120, or gp160) appears in combination with another HIV characteristic band (p15, p18, p24, p31, gp41, p55, p51, p66, gp120, or gp160, CDC personal communication). A newly licensed WB test kit (Biotech/DuPont HIV Western Blot Kit, Wilmington, DE) states that characteristic HIV bands at p24 and p31 plus either gp41 or gp160 must be present for a positive test.

WB tests are negative for HIV antibodies when no bands appear. Indeterminate results occur when there is either isolated reactivity to a single HIV protein or a pattern of reactivity to multiple proteins from the same viral gene product (i.e., polymerase gene products: p31, p51/66 only) appears.[44] When indeterminate results occur, a follow-up patient specimen should be collected in 6 months and the WB assay repeated. In this way, if the patient was in an early stage of HIV infection additional antibody development should have occurred and a more accurate test interpretation can be made.

False positive WB reactions may occur in healthy persons, HTLV-1 or HIV-2 infections, bilirubinemia, connective tissue disease, polyclonal gammopathies, and patients with HLA antibodies.[21]

Indirect Immunofluorescence Assay

The indirect immunofluorescence assay (IFA) test is growing in popularity as a supplemental test for confirming reactive ELISA tests. The antigen is HIV-infected H9 or HUT 78 cells (malignant T-cell lines) dried and acetone fixed to wells of a fluorescence slide.[45] Patient serum or plasma is then applied, followed after washing by an Evans blue counterstain. Results are read on a fluorescence microscope by noting the degree of fluorescence intensity, percentage of fluorescent cells, and localization of the fluorescence to cell surfaces. It is the envelope proteins gp160 and gp120 that are reacting in the IFA antibody test.[21] The advantages to using the IFA rather than WB as a supplemental test are the IFA's comparable sensitivity and specificity, the simplicity of the test, and rapid results (generally less than 2 hours).[21,36] Disadvantages include nonspecific staining, use of expensive fluorescent microscopes, possibly difficult interpretation and necessity for skilled technologists, and fluorescence that fades quickly, so that slides cannot be stored.[21,36]

The IFA test can also be modified to detect HIV antigen in infected cells.[36] In this assay, HIV-infected cells are treated with polyclonal or monoclonal antibody raised against HIV proteins p18 or p24. The assay is then performed similar to the IFA antibody assay.

Radioimmunoassay

Radioimmunoassay (RIA) tests for detecting antibodies to HIV are rarely used in diagnostic laboratories, because of the use of radioactive materials for labeling antibodies. The principle of the RIA antibody test is similar to that of the competitive binding ELISA test. Radioactively labeled (generally with ^{125}I) anti-HIV antibodies compete with unlabeled patient serum (unlabeled antibody) for binding sites on solid-phase, fixed HIV antigen. Radioactivity of bound antibodies is measured in a gamma counter. The amount of HIV antibodies in the patient's specimen is inversely proportional to the number of counts detected.[37]

Radioimmunoprecipitation Assay

The radioimmunoprecipitation assay (RIPA) test is mainly a research technique, because it is expensive, is time-consuming, requires use of radioisotopes, and requires maintenance of infected cell lines.[21] The principle is that HIV-infected cells are exposed to a radioactive isotope, lysed, and centrifuged in an ultracentrifuge to obtain a cell lysate containing radiolabeled viral proteins. Patient serum is preabsorbed with protein A-Sepharose beads, then mixed with the cell lysate. Immunoprecipitates are formed by boiling in buffer, and the immunoprecipitate is separated by electrophoresis on sodium dodecyl sulfate–polyacrylamide gels. Banding patterns similar to those on WB are formed and interpreted.[21]

Gene Probes

Gene probes that detect HIV genes rather than gene products or protein antigens have been developed. They have not yet gained in popularity, because of their low sensitivity in detecting HIV directly in cells and tissues. Both radioactively labeled DNA and RNA probes have been produced that can be used in molecular hybridization tests to detect if proviral HIV DNA or RNA is present in a specimen. Further research is needed to perfect the use of HIV gene probes, but applications of more sensitive versions of these tests might be to detect latent virus or to monitor antiviral drug therapies.[36]

Prevention of HIV Infection in Health Care Workers

Since 1984 there have been 13 cases of AIDS in health care workers with occupational exposure to HIV but without other known risk factors.[46] Five cases involved accidental needle sticks, six cases involved exposure of blood or body fluids to ungloved hands or skin lesions, one case involved a lacerated finger while working, and one case involved unknown exposure. Each day health care workers are exposed to the blood and body fluids of patients during patient care or in the laboratory. Although the risk of transmission of HIV following a needle stick injury with HIV-contaminated blood is less than 1%,[47] the health care worker should take precautions to minimize this risk by appropriate use of protective clothing to minimize direct contact, frequent handwashing, proper use of equipment to prevent exposure to aerosols, and adoption of a policy of universal precautions for all patients (treating all patients and patient specimens as if HIV or hepatitis B infected). The Centers for Disease Control (CDC) has published guidelines of recommended precautions for laboratory workers to help decrease the risk of HIV transmission in health care settings.[46] These recommendations are reprinted here:

The CDC's recommended precautions for laboratory workers

1. Avoid contaminating the outside of containers upon specimen collection. The lid should be tight.

2. Wear gloves when processing patient specimens. Use masks and eyewear if splashing or aerosolization is anticipated. Change gloves and wash hands at the end of processing.

3. Use biological safety cabinets for blending, sonicating, and vigorous mixing.

4. No mouth pipetting.

5. Use precautions when handling needles. No bending, breaking, recapping, or removing of needles from disposable syringes. Place in puncture-resistant containers.

6. Decontaminate work surfaces with a chemical germicide after spills and when work is completed.

7. Dispose of contaminated materials in bags and in accordance with institutional policies for disposal of infective waste.

8. Decontaminate equipment before repair or shipping.

9. Wash hands and remove protective clothing before leaving the laboratory.

Summary

AIDS is the most serious infectious disease threatening humans today. To date, there are no effective vaccines, and antiviral therapies that slow the progress of the disease offer no cure. Extensive research has delineated the structure of the virus, its life cycle, its mode of transmission, and groups at risk of infection. AIDS results in severe immunodeficiency of the host, with T-cell and humoral defenses being affected. Opportunistic infections and cancers are a confounding result of the severe immunosuppression of the host. A variety of methods to isolate HIV virus *in vitro* and to detect HIV antibodies and antigens have been developed and are in use today in research and medical laboratories.

References

1. Ho DD, Pomerantz RJ, Kaplan JC: Pathogenesis of infection with human immune deficiency virus. N Engl J Med 317:278, 1987

2. McDougal JS, Mawle AC, Nicholson JKA: The immunology of AIDS. In Kaslow R, Francis D (eds): The Epidemiology of AIDS. Oxford, Oxford University Press (in press)

3. Shulman J, Blumberg HM, Kozarsky PE, et al: Acquired immunodeficiency syndrome (AIDS): An update for the clinician. Emory Univ J Med 1:157, 1987

4. Centers for Disease Control: Pneumocystis pneumonia—Los Angeles. Surveill Summ 30:250, 1981

5. Heyward WL, Curran JW: The epidemiology of AIDS in the US. Sci Am, Oct 1988, p 72

6. Morgan WM, Curran JW: Acquired immunodeficiency syndrome: Current and future trends. Public Health Rep 101:459, 1986

7. Hardy, AM: Characterization of long term survivors of AIDS. 27th Intersci Conf Antimicrobial Agents and Chemotherapy, American Society for Microbiology, Abstract 98, 1987

8. Clavel F, Mansinho K, Chamaret S, et al: Human immunodeficiency virus type 2 infection associated with AIDS in West Africa. New Engl J Med 316:1180, 1987

9. Barré-Sinoussi F, Chermann JC, Rey F, et al: Isolation of a T-lymphotrophic retrovirus from a patient at risk for acquired immunodeficiency syndrome (AIDS). Science 220:868, 1983

10. Popovic M, Sarngadharan MG, Read E, et al: Detection, isolation, and continuous production of cytopathic retroviruses (HTLV-III) from patients with AIDS and pre-AIDS. Science 224:497, 1984

11. Levy JA, Hoffman AD, Kramer SM, et al: Isolation of lymphocytotrophic retroviruses from San Francisco patients with AIDS. Science 225:840, 1984

12. Ratner L, Haseltine W, Patarca R, et al: Complete nucleotide sequence of the AIDS virus. Nature 313:277, 1985

13. Wain-Hobson S, Sonigo P, Danos O, et al: Nucleotide sequence of the AIDS virus, LAV. Cell 40:9, 1985

14. Aiya SK, Gallo RC: Three novel genes of human T-lymphotrophic virus type III: Immune reactivity of their

products with sera from acquired immune deficiency syndrome patients. Proc Natl Acad Sci USA 83:1553, 1986

15. Fisher AG, Feinberg MB, Josephs SF, et al: The transactivation gene of HTLV-III is essential for virus replication. Nature 320:367, 1986

16. Wong-Staal F, Chanda P, Ghrayeb J: Human immunodeficiency virus: The eighth gene. AIDS Res Hum Retrovirol 3:33, 1987

17. Muesing MA, Smith DH, Capon DJ: Regulation of mRNA accumulation by a human immunodeficiency virus trans-activation protein. Cell 48:691, 1987

18. Luciw PA, Cheng-Mayer C, Levy JA: Mutational analysis of the human immunodeficiency virus: The *orf*-B region down-regulates virus replication. Proc Natl Acad Sci USA 84:1434, 1987

19. Groopman JE, Chen FW, Hope JA, et al: Serological characterization of HTLV-III infection in AIDS and related disorders. J Infect Dis 153:736, 1986

20. Bowen DL, Lane HC, Fauci AS: Immunopathogenesis of the acquired immunodeficiency syndrome. Ann Intern Med 103:704, 1985

21. Jackson JB, Balfour HH Jr: Practical Diagnostic Testing for Human Immunodeficiency Virus. Clin Microbiol Rev 1:124, 1988

22. Zagury D, Bernard J, Leonard R, et al: Long-term cultures of HTLV-III infected cells: A model of cytopathology of T-cell depletion in AIDS. Science 231:850, 1986

23. Redfield RR: The etiology and epidemiology of HTLV-III related disease. Abbott Diagnostics HTLV-III Education Series, 1987

24. Mann JM, Chin J, Piot P, Quinn T: The international epidemiology of AIDS. Sci Am 259:82, 1988

25. Hessol NA, Rutherford GW, O'Malley PM, et al: The natural history of human immunodeficiency virus infection in a cohort of homosexual and bisexual men: A seven year prospective study. Abstract M3.1, Third International Conference on AIDS, Washington, DC, 1987

26. Revision of the CDC Surveillance Case Definition for Acquired Immunodeficiency Syndrome. Surveill Summ 36:15, 1987

27. Weller IA: Treatment of infections and antiviral agents. Brit Med J 295:200, 1987

28. Fischi MA, Richman DD, Grieco MH, et al: The efficacy of azidothymidine (AZT) in the treatment of patients with AIDS and AIDS-Related Complex. N Engl J Med 317:185, 1987

29. Yarchoan R, Mitsuya H, Broder S: AIDS therapies. Sci Am 259:110, 1988

30. Klatzman D, Montagnier L: Approaches to AIDS therapy. Nature 319:10, 1986

31. Seligmann M, Pinching AJ, Roger FS, et al: Immunology of human immunodeficiency virus infection and the acquired immunodeficiency syndrome. Ann Intern Med 107:234, 1987

32. Matthews TJ, Bolognes DP: AIDS vaccines. Sci Am 259:120, 1988

33. Additional recommendations to reduce sexual and drug abuse-related transmission of human T-lymphocyte virus type III (lymphadenopathy-associated virus). Surveill Summ 35:152, 1986

34. Guyader M, Emerman M, Sonigo P, et al: Genome organization and transactivation of the human immunodeficiency virus type 2. Nature 326:662, 1987

35. Denis F, Leonard G, Mounier M, et al: Efficacy of five enzyme immunoassays for antibody to HIV in detecting antibody to HTLV-IV. Lancet 1:324, 1987

36. Khan NC, Hunter E: Detection of human immunodeficiency virus type 1. ACPR, May 1988, p 20

37. Janda WM: Serologic tests for HTLV-III antibodies: Methods and interpretations. Clin Microbiol Newsletter 7:67, 1985

38. Papsidero LD, Montagna RA, Poiesz BJ: Acquired immune deficiency syndrome: Detection of viral exposure and infection. ACPR, p 17, 1986

39. Reesink HW, Lelie PN, Huisman JG, et al: Evaluation of six enzyme immunoassays for antibody against human immunodeficiency virus. Lancet 2:483, 1986

40. Goudsmit J, Lange JMA, Paul DA, et al: Antigenemia and antibody titers to core and envelope antigens in AIDS, AIDS-related complex, and subclinical human immunodeficiency virus infection. J Infect Dis 155:558, 1987

41. Yoshida T, Matsui T, Kobayashi S, et al: Agglutination test for HIV antibody. J Clin Microbiol 25:1433, 1987

42. Riggin CH, Beltz GA, Hung CH, et al: Detection of antibodies to human immunodeficiency virus by latex agglutination with recombinant antigen. J Clin Microbiol 25:1772, 1987

43. Lombardo JM: HIV testing: An overview. ACPR, Nov, p 10, 1987

44. Kleinman S: The significance of indeterminate Western Blots for HIV-1. Update, Ortho Diagnostic Systems, Inc. 2:1, 1988

45. Lennette ET, Karpatkin S, Levy JA: Indirect immunofluorescence assay for antibodies to human immunodeficiency virus. J Clin Microbiol 25:199, 1987

46. Carlson DA: AIDS risks and precautions for laboratory personnel. Med Lab Observ Jan, p 57, 1988

47. CDC: Recommendations for preventing transmission of infection with human T-lymphotrophic virus type III/lymphadenopathy-associated virus in the workplace. Surveill Summ 34:687, 1985

48. CDC: Recommendations for prevention of HIV transmission in health care settings. Surveill Summ 36:1, 1987

CHAPTER 23

Viral Hepatitis

Ann Marie McNamara

Viral hepatitis refers to liver disease caused by four hepatotrophic viruses: hepatitis A (HA); hepatitis B (HB); non-A, non-B hepatitis (NANB); and delta hepatitis (HD). The reader should be aware, however, that hepatitis simply means an inflammation of the liver and is a clinical manifestation of liver disease caused by a variety of bacteria, viruses, fungi, parasites, toxins, autoimmune diseases, radiation, neoplasms, and drugs.[1-3]

This chapter describes current laboratory methods for diagnosing the four viral hepatitis infections and discusses pertinent characteristics of these viruses, including their physical characteristics, epidemiology, clinical manifestations, and patterns of antibody and antigen response to infection.

Hepatitis Testing

General Principles

Detection of specific hepatitis antigens and antibodies from patient serum determines the responsible viral agent, the immune status of the host, and the clinical stage of the infection. Radioimmunoassay (RIA) and enzyme-linked immunosorbent assays (ELISA) are the most widely used diagnostic test methods. ELISA tests are usually preferred, since no radioactive materials are involved, reagents are commercially available, and test kits have a long shelf life.[4] ELISA tests are about as sensitive as RIA, but their specificity is lower.[2] Since false positive results occur in both test formats, only repeatedly reactive specimens should be reported as positive tests. The advantages of RIA are that it is more specific than ELISA and commercial reagents are available. RIA tests have distinct disadvantages in that radioactive materials are involved, expensive equipment is required, and test kits have a short shelf life.[4]

Test methods for detecting hepatitis antigens and antibodies can be grouped into three successive "generations" of tests. Each subsequent generation shows improved test sensitivity when compared to the previous generation. Agar gel diffusion (Ouchterlony double diffusion) is the first-generation test followed by three second-generation tests: counter-immunoelectrophoresis, complement fixation, and reverse passive latex agglutination.[4] All these test formats are outdated and will not be presented here. Third-generation tests include RIA, ELISA, and passive and reverse passive hemagglutination. Because the hemagglutination tests are less sensitive than the RIA and ELISA, they are rarely used in clinical laboratories. Detection of specific antigens and antibodies for diagnosing the hepatitis viruses will be discussed under the sections appropriate to each virus.

Direct detection of hepatitis A virus (HAV) antigens and particles or hepatitis B virus (HBV) particles in patient specimens (liver biopsies, serum, or stools, where appropriate) is limited to electron microscopy and immunofluorescence or immunoperoxidase staining.[2] Generally, these techniques are limited to research, because diagnosis can generally be made serologically.

Radioimmunoassay

Radioimmunoassay (RIA) tests are of two formats: solid-phase radioimmunoassay (sandwich technique) or competitive binding assays.

Solid-phase radioimmunoassays to detect hepatitis antigens are performed by incubating patient sera or plasma (antigen source) with hepatitis antibodies adsorbed to a solid-phase support (plastic tubes or beads).[2] ^{125}I-labeled antibody is then added and allowed to incubate. If antigen is present in the patient specimen, an antibody–antigen-labeled antibody "sandwich" forms. After washing away excess labeled antibody, any bound radioactive material is counted in a gamma counter. The number of counts recovered is proportional to the concentration of antibody in the patient's specimen. The counts per minute (cpm) of the patient's specimen is compared with a positive cutoff value calculated by a mathematical manipulation of the negative control. Specimens with a cpm higher than the cutoff value are considered positive. This assay can be modified to detect hepatitis antibodies by adsorbing antigen to the solid support and adding labeled antigen.

Competitive binding assays to detect viral antigens are performed by incubating patient sera or plasma (antigen source) with radioactively labeled hepatitis antigen.[2] These antigens then compete for binding sites on plastic beads coated with hepatitis antibody. The amount of labeled antigen detected is inversely proportional to the amount of antigen present in the patient specimen. Therefore, a positive test result occurs when the cpm of the patient specimen is less than that of the negative control.

Since false positive reactions can occur, all reactive test results must be repeated. Some causes for false positive tests include inadequate washing steps and cross-contamination of the counting tubes or beads with radioactivity in nonreactive samples caused by faulty technique or contaminated pipette tips.

A confirmatory test is available to rule out false positive tests for hepatitis B surface antigen (HB$_s$Ag). This is a specific antibody neutralization test in which human antibody to hepatitis B surface antigen is incubated with the patient's specimen before testing. If HB$_s$Ag is present in the patient's specimen, it will combine with the added antibody and be unavailable to react in the RIA test. The specimen is considered positive if the neutralized specimen shows a reduction in cpm of at least 50% compared with a concomitantly run nonneutralized specimen.[4]

Enzyme-Linked Immunosorbent Assay

Enzyme-linked immunoabsorbent assay (ELISA) tests can be used to detect hepatitis antigens or antibodies in both solid-phase and competitive binding assays.[4] The principle of these assays is the same as that of the corresponding RIA, except that an enzyme label replaces the radioactive label. Addition of an appropriate chromogenic substrate for the enzyme produces a color change that is measured in a spectrophotometer. Positive samples are determined by comparing the absorbance of the patient's specimen to that of a cutoff value for the negative control. Confirmatory antibody neutralization tests are also available in ELISA format to confirm HB$_s$AG.

False positive tests occur with ELISA testing and all reactive results must be confirmed by retesting or by neutralization. Common sources of false positive ELISA results are inadequate washing, cross-contamination of nonreactive sera with positive sera retained on the pipetting device, contaminating the o–phenylenediamine (OPD) solution with oxidizing agents, contamination of the acid stopping reagent, or contamination of the reaction tray well rim with conjugate or specimen (AUSAB EIA package insert; Abbott Laboratories; North Chicago, IL).

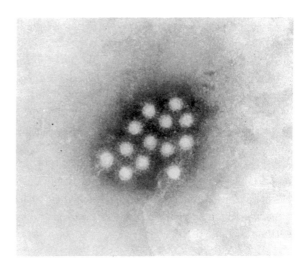

FIGURE 23-1 Electron micrograph of hepatitis A virus. (Courtesy of CDC Archives.)

Hepatitis A

Hepatitis A Virus

Hepatitis A virus (HAV) is a member of the Picornaviridae family of viruses.[5] It is composed of a single serotype and has recently been classified as enterovirus type 72.[2] This virus was first isolated from the stool of acutely ill patients by Feinstone *et al*,[6] in 1973. Electron microscopy (Fig. 23-1) reveals a virion with a mean diameter of 27 nm, icosahedral in shape, and without an envelope.[5] It is both acid stable and ether resistant.[4] Although present in the stool of acutely ill patients, HAV is not detectable in serum. The hosts of the virus are limited to humans, marmosets, chimpanzees, and owl monkeys.[2,4] It has recently been grown in cell culture.[7]

Epidemiology

HAV infections occur worldwide, in both epidemic and endemic forms.[2] In industrialized nations, where standards of living are high, infection is generally seen in adults less than 50 years old.[1] In developing countries, where hygiene is poor, children are most commonly affected.[3] Transmission has been shown to occur most often by the fecal–oral route, although rare parenteral transmission has been documented after transfusion of blood products.[4] Epidemics generally occur from fecal contamination of a single source of food, water, or milk.[2] Hospital outbreaks are rare.[4] Person-to-person spread is responsible in outbreaks linked to day-care centers, mental institutions, and military recruits.[4]

Clinical Manifestations

Hepatitis A infections may be asymptomatic or symptomatic. Symptomatic infections may include a period of jaundice (icteric stage) or not (anicteric). The incubation period of the disease is usually 10 to 50 days,[1] after which clinical illness develops abruptly in symptomatic cases. Clinical findings include fever, anorexia, vomiting, fatigue, and malaise.[1,3] Serum transaminase levels (especially alanine aminotransferase) are elevated and peak before the onset of jaundice. Right upper quadrant pain, dark urine, and pale stools mark the beginning of jaundice. This icteric stage lasts for a few days to a few weeks.[2] Other clinical findings include hyperbilirubenemia and decreased albumin levels.[1] Recovery is generally in 2 to 4 weeks and the mortality rate is approximately 0.1%.[1] Rarely does chronic disease occur. Patients should be placed on enteric precautions, however, as they are considered infectious for approximately 2 weeks following the onset of jaundice.[3] Treatment is based on alleviating the patient's symptoms, as no antiviral drugs are known to be effective. Household contacts should receive immune serum globulin prophylaxis.

Laboratory Diagnosis

Figure 23-2 shows the antibody and antigen markers present in hepatitis A infection. Fecal hepatitis A antigen (HAV-Ag) can be detected by immune electron microscopy, RIA antigen assays, and ELISA antigen assays. These tests are generally not performed, however, as antigen levels are usually declining as symptoms develop. Instead, RIA and ELISA tests are used to detect the presence of specific HAV antibodies in the patient's serum. Patient blood is collected as soon as exposure is known, or at the onset of symptoms, again at 3 or 4 weeks after symptoms appear, and 2 to 3 months after the illness. A fourfold rise in antibody titer to IgM and total (IgG and IgM) antibodies is considered diagnostic. Anti-IgM antibody is present at the onset of symptoms and reaches a maximum titer in 1 to 3 weeks. Anti-HAV total antibodies are present at the onset of symptoms and can remain elevated for years. Patterns of antibody response can be interpreted as follows: both total anti-HAV and IgM anti-HAV signify acute or convalescent infection; total anti-HAV only indicates prior infection, with the patient now immune; and neither antibody present indicates the absence of infection or the incubation phase of the disease.

Hepatitis B

Hepatitis B Virus

Hepatitis B virus (HBV) is a small, enveloped, double-stranded DNA virus belonging to the Hepadnaviridae family[2] (Fig. 23-3). HBV exists in the serum of HBV-infected individuals in three morphologic forms: the infectious 42-nm spherical Dane particle, and two 22-nm-diameter particles existing as spheres or filaments (50 to over 200 nm in length).[5] These latter two forms are considered to be incomplete viral coat proteins consisting of hepatitis B surface antigen (HB_sAg).[4] Since these particles are incomplete virions, they are not considered infectious.

The infectious Dane particle is a complete HBV virion and exhibits a more complicated structure

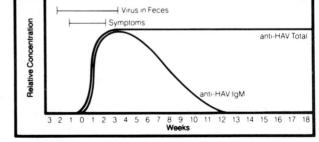

FIGURE 23-2. Antigen and antibody response in hepatitis A infection. (Reproduced with permission from Abbott Laboratories, © 1988 Abbott Laboratories.)

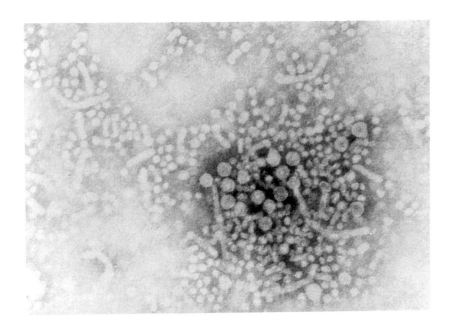

FIGURE 23-3. Electron micrograph of hepatitis B virus. (Courtesy of CDC Archives.)

than the smaller HB$_s$Ag particles. The Dane particle consists of a 22-nm nucleocapsid surrounded by a lipid–protein–carbohydrate envelope containing HB$_s$Ag.[5] HB$_s$Ag was first described in 1964 in the serum of an Australian aborigine and has been previously termed the *Australian antigen*.[5] HB$_s$Ag is a marker of viral replication in liver hepatocytes. The HB$_s$Ag consists of several types of antigenic determinants, including a group-specific determinant *a* and two pairs of mutually exclusive, type-specific determinants located on two independent genetic alleles, the *d* or *y* and *w* or *r* pairs.[5] By combining the group-specific determinant, *a*, with one of each of the two type-specific pairs (*i.e., ayw*), 10 different strains of HBV have been identified.[3] Strain determinations are not routinely performed in the clinical laboratory but may be useful in epidemiologic studies. Antibodies to HB$_s$Ag (anti-HB$_s$) in a patient's serum indicate past infection and subsequent immunity of the patient to HBV.

If the envelope of the Dane particle is removed using detergents, the nucleocapsid remains. This nucleocapsid contains the viral DNA, viral polymerase, and hepatitis B core antigen (HB$_c$Ag). HB$_c$Ag can be detected in liver hepatocytes, but more often serologic diagnosis is determined by the presence of antibodies to HB$_c$Ag (anti-HB$_c$). Anti-HB$_c$ levels are always interpreted relative to finding HB$_s$Ag or anti-HB$_s$ in the patient's serum and signifies either chronic infection or patient immunity.

An antigen found in some HB$_s$Ag-positive sera, either bound to immunoglobulins or free in solution, has been correlated to viral infectivity. This is the HB$_e$Ag antigen, and it is associated with viral replication in the liver.[5] Antibodies to anti-HB$_e$Ag (anti-HB$_e$) usually occur when the patient is recovering from active infection.

Epidemiology

HBV infections were originally called *serum hepatitis*, as opposed to HAV fecal–oral-transmitted *infectious hepatitis*. Serum hepatitis is now a misnomer, since non-A, non-B hepatitis (NANB) and hepatitis delta virus (HDV) are also transmitted by blood and blood products.

HBV can be recovered from the blood and body fluids of infected persons. Infected body fluids include semen, saliva, breast milk, tears, cerebrospinal and ascitic fluids, and urine.[3,4] Transmission occurs either through a parenteral route or through contact of mucous membranes or open wounds with infected body fluids. Parenteral transmission can occur through the use of infected blood or blood products, hemodialysis, intravenous drug use, accidental needle sticks, tattooing, acupuncture, ear piercing, or arthropod-borne vectors.[3,4] Blood banks routinely screen blood and blood products for HB$_s$Ag and infected units are destroyed. Transmission through contact with contaminated body secretions occurs in institutionalized mentally retarded children, sexual partners of infected persons, household contacts, and infants of infected mothers.[3,4] Infections occur worldwide; high-risk groups have been defined as intravenous drug users, homosexual men, hemodialysis patients, and medical and dental personnel. Reservoirs of HBV are chronic carriers of HBV infection.

Clinical Manifestations

Approximately 200,000 new cases of HBV infection occur annually in the United States.[3] Approximately 150,000 patients remain anicteric, 10,000 require hospitalization, 250 die from fulminant hepatitis, and 12,000 to 20,000 become chronic carriers.[3] Clinical symptoms and signs are similar to those found in HAV infections; however, HBV infections tend to have more arthralgia, a more abrupt onset of symptoms, a longer clinical course, and a slower resolution.[1] The infection has an incubation period between 50 and 180 days (mean of 75)[1] and may present as asymptomatic infection, either icteric or nonicteric symptomatic infection, or fulminant hepatitis. Chronic infections can be persistent or active infections. All chronic cases are HB$_s$Ag-positive. Chronic persistent infections are usually benign, but chronic active infections manifest severe liver necrosis and

may develop primary hepatocellular carcinoma.[4] All chronic carriers continue to shed active virus.

Although no antiviral drug is known to be effective against HBV, effective vaccines exist and should be used to immunize high-risk persons. The vaccine consists of purified, formalin-fixed HB$_s$Ag from the sera of HBV carriers[3] or recombinant HB$_s$Ag, and it evokes a protective immune response to HBV when administered. Both commercially available immune serum globulin (ISG) and high-titer anti-HB$_s$ HBV immune serum globulin (HBIG) are used prophylactically following exposure to HBV-contaminated blood and body fluids.

Laboratory Diagnosis

The serologic diagnosis of HBV infections is more complicated than that for HAV infections. Both HBV antibody and antigen markers can be demonstrated in patients' sera using RIA and ELISA techniques. For simplification, the pattern of HBV antigen and antibody response will be divided into responses seen in acute and chronic HBV disease. In acute HBV hepatitis (Fig. 23-4), HB$_s$Ag appears during the incubation period of the infection and is the first detectable serologic marker. HB$_e$Ag develops next and is indicative of the infectivity of the patient. Development of anti-HB$_e$ is the first serologic sign of clinical recovery and decreased patient infectivity. Anti-HB$_c$ is the first antibody to appear in the serum. Anti-HB$_c$ development begins during acute illness and remains high for years. Its presence suggests that the patient is in the later stages of the disease or is immune. This antibody is also a marker of the "core window" period in which neither HB$_s$Ag nor anti-HB$_s$ is found in patient sera. Anti-HB$_c$ is initially IgM and then is replaced by IgG antibodies measured by total anti-HB$_c$. Development of anti-HB$_s$ occurs months to years after infection during the patient's recovery period. The presence of anti-HB$_s$ signals the late stages of disease and the development of immunity.

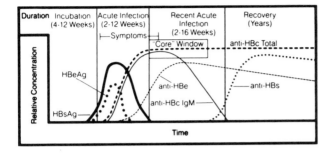

FIGURE 23-4. Antigen and antibody response in acute hepatitis B infection. (Reproduced with permission from Abbott Laboratories, © 1988 Abbott Laboratories.)

In chronic HBV infections (Fig. 23-5), persistent HB$_s$Ag in the serum is the characteristic diagnostic marker. Chronic carriers of HB$_s$Ag have repeatedly demonstrable titers of HB$_s$Ag for 6 months to several years after initial infection. Anti-HB$_c$ and HB$_e$Ag are also present in high titers in chronic hepatitis. A decrease in HB$_e$Ag and a rise in anti-HB$_e$ indicate chronic persistent hepatitis. If no seroconversion to anti-HB$_e$ occurs and high HB$_e$Ag titers persist, the person is highly infectious and is likely to develop serious liver disease.

The clinical stage of HBV infection and the immune status of the host are generally determined by screening for HB$_s$Ag, anti-HB$_s$ and anti-HB$_c$ (both total and IgM), HB$_e$Ag, and anti-HB$_e$.[4] In general, the presence of HB$_s$Ag signifies HBV acute or chronic infection. Patients should then be repeatedly tested for the presence of both HB$_s$Ag and anti-HB$_s$ to detect the recovery stage of HBV illness, when HB$_s$Ag decreases and anti-HB$_s$ increases. If HB$_s$Ag without anti-HB$_s$ persists for more than 6 months, a chronic active or passive case of HBV can be diagnosed. Elevated liver enzymes indicate chronic disease, whereas normal enzyme levels suggest that the patient is a chronic carrier. When anti-HB$_s$ is present in a patient's sera, the patient is immune to HBV infection. Anti-HB$_c$ indicates a chronic carrier state or late infection during the "core window" of acute infection. The presence of HB$_e$Ag indicates infectivity of the patient and viral replication in the liver. Anti-HB$_e$ occurs when the patient is in late disease or recovering.

Non-A, Non-B Hepatitis

Non-A, Non-B Hepatitis Virus

Relatively little is known about the causative agents of non-A, non-B hepatitis (NANB). Several findings suggest that at least two NANB viruses exist: infections seem to be either blood-borne or enteric in na-

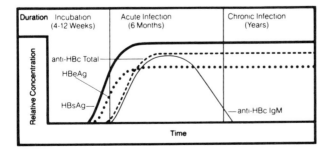

FIGURE 23-5. Antigen and antibody response in chronic hepatitis B infection. (Reproduced with permission from Abbott Laboratories, © 1988 Abbott Laboratories.)

ture, humans have recurrent NANB infections, chimpanzees develop only homologous immunity when infected, and hepatitis infections with two distinct incubation periods (2 to 4 weeks vs. 8 to 12 weeks) occur in chimpanzees.[4] Recent studies have helped to characterize one blood-borne NANBV as an enveloped, single-stranded RNA virus probably belonging to the Togaviridae family.[8] This virus has been termed hepatitis C (HCV).

Epidemiology

NANB infections occur worldwide and are transmitted by either a parenteral or a fecal–oral route. Up to 150,000 cases of parenteral transmission occur in the United States each year, accounting for approximately 95% of the transfusion-related hepatitis cases.[8]

Clinical Manifestations

Cases of NANB hepatitis are usually mild, but a small number can progress to fulminant disease. Anicteric cases occur in up to 50% of patients[4]; however, acute anicteric cases are more likely to progress to chronic hepatitis than icteric cases.[3] Most chronic cases are benign, although some patients develop permanent liver damage. No known antiviral drug is effective against NANB hepatitis, but steroids may be of benefit in chronic cases. Studies have also shown that the incidence of posttransfusion NANB hepatitis is decreased if immune serum globulin is given with blood products.[3]

Laboratory Diagnosis

NANB hepatitis has classically been diagnosed by excluding hepatitis A and B and other causes of hep-

atitis in a patient with hepatitis symptoms and increased liver enzyme levels.

Surrogate testing for detecting blood-borne NANBV in the nation's blood supply has been suggested.[8] The surrogate test indirectly screens for NANBV by measuring first for increased levels of alanine aminotransferase (ALT) and second for antibody to HB_cAg. Units of blood testing positive would be discarded. However, estimates suggest that only 50% of NANB-contaminated donor blood would be detected by this method.[8] A new immunoassay to screen for blood-borne HCV is now in clinical trials.[8] This assay uses a yeast-synthesized blood-borne HCV viral protein for trapping and detecting HCV antibodies. If successful, this new assay should greatly reduce the number of posttransfusion cases of NANB hepatitis.

Delta Hepatitis

Hepatitis Delta Virus

Hepatitis delta virus (HDV) was first described by Rizzetto et al in 1977.[9] Also called the delta antigen, this single-stranded RNA virus is spherical in shape with a diameter of 36 nm.[10] It is a defective hepatotrophic virus in that it requires obligatory helper functions from HBV to ensure its replication and infectivity. One major helper function of HBV is to provide HDV with a protein coat of HB_sAg. This allows the formerly unenveloped, defective particle to function as an infectious agent.[11]

Epidemiology

HDV infection has been shown to occur worldwide. Transmission of HDV is linked to that of its HBV helper virus and occurs by parenteral and transmucosal routes of infection. High-risk populations of HB$_s$Ag are also at risk for HDV infections: intravenous drug users, recipients of blood products, male homosexuals, and mentally retarded individuals.[10,11] Horizontal transmission occurs in households, and infections increase in nonhygienic, crowded living conditions.[11] Mosquitoes have been shown to be a vehicle for transmission of HDV in epidemics.[11]

Clinical Manifestations

HDV infection occurs as either acute or chronic infection in conjunction with concomitant HBV infection. Acute infection can occur in one of two forms: co-infection with acute HBV infection or superinfection of a chronic HBV infection. In cases of acute HDV–HBV co-infection, either both viruses are cleared rapidly or the patient progresses to fulminant hepatitis. There is a higher incidence of fulminant hepatitis and cases of relapse with HDV–HBV co-infection than when HBV is present alone.[11] More than 90% of cases of HDV superinfection of chronic HBV infection progress to chronic HDV infection.[11]

Chronic HDV infection has a poor prognosis for the patient. The severity of liver necrosis, inflammation, and clinical illness are all increased, and cirrhosis often occurs.[11] To date, there are no effective antiviral drugs or immunosuppressive agents for treatment of chronic infections. Vaccination against HBV also provides immunity to HDV because HDV is not infectious and cannot replicate without HBV helper functions.

Laboratory Diagnosis

Since HDV requires helper functions from HBV, only HB$_s$Ag-positive persons need to be tested for HDV infection. The first HDV marker to appear is HDV antigen (HDV-Ag). HDV-Ag is transient in serum (1 to 4 days) and appears prior to symptomatology and elevation of liver enzymes. For this reason HDV-Ag is rarely detected even though RIA, ELISA, and DNA probes exist for its detection. With the decline of HDV-Ag, IgM antibodies to HDV (IgM anti-HDV) appear (seroconversion), followed by low levels of IgG antibodies (IgG anti-HDV) in acute infection. The progression to high levels of IgG anti-HDV in HB$_s$Ag-positive individuals signals the switch to chronic HDV infection. Diagnosis of acute vs. chronic HDV infection should be based on detection of IgM anti-HDV and total anti-HDV (IgM and IgG) in HB$_s$Ag-positive persons using commercially available RIA or ELISA kits.

Summary

The term *hepatitis viruses* refers to four human, hepatotrophic viruses: HAV, HBV, NANBV, and HDV. These viruses have worldwide distribution and are transmitted by parenteral (all four) or fecal–oral (HAV, NANBV) routes of infection. Serologic tests to detect virus-specific antigens or antibodies determine the causative viral agent, the immune status of the host, and the clinical stage of HAV and HBV infections. HDV is a defective hepatotrophic virus requiring helper functions from HBV to allow its replication and infectivity. Diagnosis of HDV infection is made by demonstrating HDV-specific antibodies in HB$_s$Ag-positive persons.

References

1. Fody EP, Johnson DF: The serologic diagnosis of viral hepatitis. J Med Technol 4:54, 1987

2. Hollinger FB, Melnick JL: Viral hepatitis. In Lennette EH (ed): Laboratory Diagnosis of Viral Infections, p 293. New York, Marcel Dekker, 1985

3. Tyrell DLJ, Gill MJ: Hepatitis. In Mandell LA, Ralph ED (eds): Essentials of Infectious Diseases, p 241. Boston, Blackwell Scientific Publications, 1985

4. Rubin SJ: Hepatitis viruses. In Howard BJ, Klass J II, Rubin SJ, et al (eds): Clinical and Pathogenic Microbiology, p 817. St. Louis, CV Mosby, 1987

5. Ginsberg HS: Hepatitis viruses. In Davis BD, Dulbecco R, Eisen HN, et al (eds): Microbiology, p 1218. Philadelphia, Harper and Row, 1980

6. Feinstone SM, Kapikian AZ, Purcell RH: Hepatitis A: Detection by immune electron microscopy of a virus-like antigen associated with acute illness. Science 182:1026, 1973

7. Provost PJ, Giesa P, McAleer WJ, et al: Isolation of hepatitis A virus (in vitro) in cell culture directly from human specimens. Proc Soc Exp Biol Med 167:201, 1987

8. Anonymous: Test for Non-A/Non-B hepatitis. ASM News 54:468, 1988

9. Rizzetto M, Canese MG, Arico S, et al: Immunofluorescence detection of a new antigen-antibody system associated to the hepatitis B virus in the liver and in the serum of HB$_s$Ag carriers. Gut 18:997, 1987

10. Bonino F, Smedile A, Verme G: Hepatitis Delta virus infections. Adv Intern Med 32:345, 1987

11. Govindarajan S: Delta hepatitis: What have we learned in the last decade? Lab Mgt 26:36, 1988

CHAPTER 24

Serology of Miscellaneous Infectious Diseases

Ann C. Albers

Rickettsia

Organisms

Rickettsiae are coccobacilli, gram-negative, obligate intracellular parasites. Highly fastidious bacteria, they are found in nature in arthropods as well as in warm-blooded animals. Because of the extremely infectious nature of these organisms and the difficulty of cultivating them, attempts are rarely made to isolate rickettsiae in the clinical laboratory. Thus, laboratory diagnosis is dependent on a demonstration of antibodies in serum and an increase in titer as disease progresses. Members of the family Rickettsiaceae are currently classified in three genera, *Rickettsia, Rochalimaea,* and *Coxiella.*[1]

Rickettsial diseases of humans are found worldwide; however, in the United States there are three of epidemiologic importance that occur naturally: Rocky Mountain spotted fever (RMSF), murine typhus, and Q fever. Rickettsialpox is also known to exist endemically in cities, but it is a mild disease. Occasionally, other rickettsial diseases are seen, primarily among international travellers. Diseases caused by this group of organisms are classified into five major groups: spotted fevers, typhus fevers, scrub typhus, trench fever, and Q fever.

Diseases

Spotted Fevers

The group of rickettsiae that cause diseases included in the spotted fevers that are endemic to the United States are *R. rickettsii* (Rocky Mountain spotted fever) and *R. akari* (rickettsialpox).

Rocky Mountain spotted fever (tick-borne typhus), although named for the area in which it was first studied, has been reported in all 50 states. The majority of cases (46.9%) reported to Centers for Disease Control (CDC) in 1986 were from the South Atlantic states.[2] Several species of ticks are arthropod hosts of the etiologic agent, *R. rickettsii*. Ticks are most active in spring and summer, accounting for the usual increase of Rocky Mountain spotted fever (RMSF) during this season; however, cases are reported throughout the winter months, so it should not be considered only a seasonal disease. The overall case fatality rate for RMSF is approximately 3%, with the highest mortality (5.8%) observed in adults ≥ 40 years of age. The fatality rate is 1.9% for those <40 years of age.[2] During the 1970s the incidence rate steadily increased, leveling off in 1977 with an average rate for the 8 years from 1977 to 1984 of 0.48 cases per 100,000 population. This febrile disease usually involves many organs and is invariably accompanied by a skin rash, headache, and myalgia. Subclinical cases are known to exist, and it is probable that underreporting of RMSF occurs.

Rickettsialpox infects mites that are ectoparasites of the house mouse. People become infected following the bite of an infected mite. The incubation period is unknown. The disease includes a local erythematous papule that evolves first into vesicular rash, followed by eschar. Frequently, the patient has lymphadenopathy, chills and fever, malaise and myalgia. The rash heals with no scarring; no fatalities have been associated with rickettsialpox.

Typhus Group

Epidemic typhus has been associated with most of the great wars of mankind, becoming epidemic during periods of starvation and crowding. The name *typhus* comes from the Greek *typhos*, meaning "hazy," which describes the mental state of patients with this disease.

Epidemic typhus (louse-borne) is associated with mortality rates of 10% to 40%. Case fatality rates increase with the age of the patient. The incubation period of 10 to 14 days is usually followed by sudden onset of frontal, severe and unremitting headache, fever and chills, and generalized myalgia. A skin rash appears within 4 to 7 days of onset. Untreated, the disease may last up to 3 weeks.

Endemic typhus (flea-borne, also called murine typhus) is usually a mild illness with a mortality rate of less than 2%. The incubation period is 1 to 2 weeks. The disease includes an abrupt onset of fever, headache, malaise, and myalgia followed in 3 to 5 days by a skin rash.

Scrub Typhus

Also known as tsutsugamushi disease (chigger-borne typhus), scrub typhus is transmitted to man by the larval stage (chigger) of infected trombiculid mites. The incubation period is 1 to 3 weeks. Disease onset is abrupt, with chills, fever, and headache, followed in 5 to 8 days by a skin rash. Fatality rates in untreated cases vary from 0 to 50%.

Trench Fever

Caused by *Rochalimaea quintana*, trench fever is transmitted by the body louse. The incubation period is 8 to 18 days. Clinical manifestations are highly variable, ranging from mild to moderately severe febrile disease with relapses.

Q Fever

Caused by *Coxilla burnetti*, Q fever is the only disease in this group that is not transmitted by an arthropod. The disease varies from asymptomatic to multisymptomatic, including pneumonia, prolonged fever, hepatitis, and endocarditis.

Laboratory Assays

Typically, rickettsial antibodies reach detectable levels within 1 week after onset of disease. The maximum titer is usually reached within a few months, and in untreated cases the antibodies are usually detectable for life. Organisms within each of the rickettsial groups have common antigens that cross-react in most serologic tests. The indirect immunofluorescence technique, which involves staining sections of infected skin, is approximately 70% sensitive and 100% specific; however, this test is not generally available.[3] Several serologic procedures for rickettsiae have been described, including agglutination, immunofluorescence (IFA), complement fixation, enzyme-linked immunosorbent assay (ELISA), and Weil-Felix. The sensitivity of serologic tests for RMSF was reported by Kaplan *et al* as follows: 96% for indirect hemagglutination, 94% for indirect fluorescent antibody, 71% for latex agglutination, 70% for OX-19 agglutination, 63% for complement fixation, and 47% for OX-2 agglutination.[4]

Micro-indirect Immunofluorescence Test

The microimmunofluorescence assay is the reference test for rickettsial infections.[5-7] The cross-reactivity among the members of the genus is variable, and it is not possible to differentiate between members of the same group (*e.g.*, RMSF from rickettsialpox, or endemic from epidemic typhus).[8]

Antigens for the rickettsial IFA may be obtained from CDC by state laboratories; alternatively, they can be prepared from cell cultures or infected chicken yolk sacs. Slides are prepared using a template and applying antigen with a pen point, thus allowing multiple antigens to be in a very small area of the slide. To facilitate serum titration, each slide is prepared with several of the multiantigen arrangements. Slides are air-dried and fixed in acetone; after drying, they may be stored indefinitely at $-70°C$. Twofold dilutions, beginning with 1/16, of patient and control sera are made in phosphate-buffered saline (PBS) or PBS with 5% normal yolk sac. The diluted patient and control sera are placed on the multiantigen arrangements, the slides are incubated 30 minutes at 37°C in a moist chamber, rinsed 10 minutes in PBS, and air-dried. Fluorescein-conjugated anti–human IgM or IgG is added to each test and control, incubated 30 minutes at 37°C in a moist chamber, rinsed in PBS, and air-dried. Buffered glycerol is used as a mounting medium for the coverslips and fluorescence is observed with a UV microscope. The IFA titer is the reciprocal of the highest dilution showing fluorescence of morphologically recognizable rickettsiae. A single titer ≥ 64, a fourfold rise in paired sera, or any IgM titer are all considered significant.

Enzyme-Linked Immunosorbent Assay

The ELISA is an indirect test that can be performed using several different soluble rickettsial antigen preparations, including sonic or ether extracts of the organisms.[6,9] Optimal concentrations of antigen, conjugate, and control sera are determined by box titration prior to use in a clinical assay. Microtiter test wells are coated with rickettsial antigen in sodium carbonate buffer (pH 9.6), and control wells are coated with only buffer. Plates are incubated 1 hour at 37°C; subsequently, each well is washed three times with PBS containing tween 20 (to prevent nonspecific binding). Sera diluted in tween-containing PBS are added to both test and control wells and the plates are reincubated and washed as described earlier. Indicator anti–human IgG or IgM linked to alkaline phosphatase (conjugate) is added to each well, the plates are incubated and washed, and the substrate, p-nitrophenylphosphate, is added. The reaction is allowed to continue 45 minutes at 37°C; then it is arrested by the addition of 3 M NaOH. The absorbance of each well is determined at 400 nm. The net value for each dilution is calculated by subtracting the absorbance of the control well from the absorbance of the test well. The absorbance at which the ELISA is considered positive varies with the system used, but in general an absorbance value approximately seven times greater than the negative control is considered positive.

Latex Agglutination Test

The antigen used in the latex agglutination test is prepared by mixing either ether extract or purified antigen from a specific rickettsial group with 0.2 N NaOH and then boiling the suspension for 30 minutes.[10] The antigen is subsequently mixed with the amount of latex beads in 0.01 M glycine-buffered saline (GBS) that has been previously determined by box titration to be optimal for the rickettsial antigen suspension. Patient sera are initially screened at 1/16 dilution in GBS–albumin; positive sera are diluted twofold to the final titer. The test is performed by mixing diluted patient sera with the latex–antigen suspension on a glass slide, rotating the slide by hand for 6 minutes, and incubating the slide for 5 minutes in a moist chamber at 26°C before reading for macroscopic agglutination. The agglutination titer is the reciprocal of the highest dilution of serum resulting in definite agglutination. A fourfold rise in titer or a single titer ≥ 128 is considered diagnostic.[11]

Weil-Felix Test

Antirickettsial antibodies were found to cross-react with certain strains of *Proteus vulgaris*, an observation that led to the widespread use of the Weil-Felix test. This test utilized heat-killed strains of *Proteus* in an agglutination reaction that has since been demonstrated to be neither sensitive nor specific; thus, the Weil-Felix test should not be employed in rickettsial serology.[3,4,12]

Mycoplasma

Organisms

All members of the order Mycoplasmatales lack a cell wall, making the immunology of this group somewhat different from most bacteria. Two genera have been associated with disease in humans, *Mycoplasma* and *Ureaplasma*. First described in pneumonia-like syndrome of cattle, they are currently recognized as a cause of atypical pneumonia and are associated with abortion and pelvic inflammatory disease in humans.[13–15]

Mycoplasma pneumoniae is the etiologic agent in most cases of atypical pneumonia and has been im-plicated in upper respiratory disease as well. Atypical pneumonia comprises 10% to 20% of all pneumonia cases, an incidence rate of 1 to 2 per 1000.[16,17]

These organisms are difficult to cultivate in the routine clinical laboratory; thus, laboratory diagnosis of these infections is frequently by immunologic procedures.

Laboratory Assays

Cultivation of mycoplasma is difficult and time-consuming. Most laboratories have limited success in isolation of these organisms. There are several kinds of serologic assays to identify antibodies that develop against *M. pneumoniae*, but, with the exception of the DNA probe, none are commercially available.

Cold Agglutinins

Principle. Autoantibodies that agglutinate human erythrocytes at temperatures less than 37°C are called cold agglutinins.[18] Cold agglutinins, which are IgM antibodies to the I antigen of human erythrocytes, appear during the first or second week of *M. pneumoniae* disease and disappear by the sixth week in 34% to 68% of patients that are culture positive.[18,19] These autoantibodies are not unique to infection with *M. pneumoniae* but are found in several other diseases, including infectious mononucleosis, rubella, influenza, trypanosomiasis, blood dyscrasias, liver diseases, allergies, and hemolytic anemias.[20]

Procedure. The blood sample should be kept at body temperature (*i.e.*, 37°C) until the serum is removed from the clot. Serial dilutions of patient serum are mixed with a 5% suspension of human group O erythrocytes, incubated 1 hour at 4°C, and read for hemagglutination, as evidenced by a lawn of RBCs (which does not dislodge with gentle shaking) on the bottom of the tube. This hemagglutination is reversed (*i.e.*, it disappears when the tubes are warmed to 37°C for 15 to 30 minutes).

Results. The titer is the highest dilution that has agglutination at 4°C that is reversed at 37°C.

Interpretation. A convalescent titer of >32, or a fourfold rise between acute and convalescent sera, is considered significant. Because only about half of patients with *M. pneumoniae* infection produce these antibodies, the test for cold agglutinins is only a screening test. Additionally, there are a number of other infections and diseases in which cold agglutinins are also produced.

Complement Fixation

The complement fixation (CF) test is usually sent to state labs to be performed. The test uses either whole cell antigen or, preferably, lipid antigen (a mixture of glycolipids from the unit membrane), which binds the organisms.[21] False positives are seen subsequent to bacterial meningitis.[22] The CF antibodies develop during the second or third week of illness and persist for 6 to 12 months.[19]

DNA Probes[17]

Principle. When complementary strands of DNA are mixed together, they will hybridize along the complementary sequences of the nucleotide bases. DNA probes are small pieces of DNA that are complementary for target cellular nucleic acids, either ribonucleic (RNA) or deoxyribonucleic acid (DNA). The target nucleic acid in the organism must be made available to the probe for hybridization to occur; subsequently, the extent of the hybridization is measured. DNA probes can be used on direct patient specimens or on the isolated organism.

Procedure. The only DNA probe currently on the market for identification of *M. pneumoniae* is Gen-Probe. This DNA probe is to ribosomal RNA (rRNA). The ^{125}I-labeled probe is contained in a reagent that has lysing agents, nuclease inhibitors, and agents that promote hybridization. After hybridization has occurred, hybridized probes are separated from unhybridized probes by a magnet and counts of the hybridized probes are obtained in a γ counter.

Results. A ratio of the counts per minute of the sample to the counts per minute of the negative control is calculated for each specimen.

Interpretation. A ratio of ≥3 is considered positive. The test will detect 5×10^4 colony-forming units/mL of specimen.

Legionella

Organisms

Legionellae are ubiquitous environmental bacteria. They have been isolated from a variety of environmental sources, including soil and ground water, as well as water supplies within homes, offices, and institutions. These organisms are opportunistic pathogens, causing disease primarily in compromised patients. They are aerobic, fastidious, non-spore-forming, gram-negative rods. Currently, there are 22 species recognized, including more than 40 subgroups.[23]

Many community and nosocomial epidemics have been documented, invariably involving immunocompromised patients. People who are infected with these organisms, including those on immunosuppressive therapy, produce antibodies. A fourfold or greater rise in antibody titer is consistent with infection, albeit there may be no clinical disease.

The humoral antibody response is to several groups of immunogens (*i.e.*, antigens common to all members of the genus *Legionella*, serogroup- and serotype-specific antigens, and antigens common to gram-negative bacteria).[24]

Demonstrable antibodies appear in the serum within 1 to 6 weeks of infection and reach peak titer by 3 months.[25,26] Seroconversion is demonstrable in two thirds of patients with legionellosis within 3 weeks and in the remaining one third within 6 weeks of disease onset.[27] Antibodies are detectable for years following legionellosis; it was demonstrated that 94% of survivors of legionnaires disease from the 1976 American Legion Convention in Philadelphia had significant levels of IgG or IgM 24 months after the disease.[28]

Patients with legionellosis produce antibodies of three immunoglobulin classes: IgG, IgM, and IgA.[29] No class of antibodies is more specific in diagnosing legionellosis than any other. IgA is not synthesized in as large a quantity nor is it detectable for as long as IgG and IgM.[30] There is no consistent evidence for earlier synthesis of IgM; thus, the presence of IgM is not evidence of a recent infection.[31] The extent of antibody production is a function of the patient, not the infecting strain or the severity of disease; there is no correlation between severity of disease and magnitude of the titer.[40]

Laboratory Assays

The sensitivity of culture for legionellae is significantly less than 100%; thus, demonstration of anti-*Legionella* antibodies is a valuable augmentation to culturing. The sensitivity of the indirect immunofluorescence assay (IFA) is high only when multiple convalescent sera are collected, up to and including 6 weeks after infection. For retrospective and epidemiologic identification of legionellosis, the IFA is the assay of choice. The IFA for legionellae was first described in 1977 by McDade *et al* and was modified by Wilkinson *et al* in 1979.[33,34]

Legionella Indirect Fluorescent Antibody Test

Principle. The *Legionella* indirect fluorescent assay is a procedure for the detection of anti-*Legionella* antibodies in serum. This is a sandwich technique in which patient serum is added to a known antigen or antigens and subsequently this antigen–antibody complex is overlaid with fluorescent labeled anti–human globulin. The first antigen–antibody complex is thus rendered fluorescent by the second antigen–antibody reaction, which will occur only if the patient serum has antibody to the test antigen.

Procedure. Using a transfer pipet, heat-killed antigens of Legionellae are applied to a six-well Fluoro-glide-coated (Chemplast, Inc., Wayne, NJ 07470) slide, leaving approximately 500 organisms per high-power field (450×). The slides are air-dried 30 minutes, fixed in acetone 15 minutes, and air-dried. Appropriate dilutions of patient sera and known positive controls are allowed to react with the antigens 30 minutes in a moist chamber. The slides are then washed 10 minutes in phosphate-buffered saline (PBS), rinsed in distilled water, and blotted dry. Each well is subsequently flooded with fluorescein-conjugated polyvalent anti–human immunoglobulins, incubated for 30 minutes in a moist chamber, washed in PBS, rinsed in distilled water, and blotted dry. Buffered glycerol, *p*H 9.0, is used as a mounting medium and fluorescence is recorded for each dilution.

Interpretation. The recommended criterion for seropositivity is seroconversion (*i.e.*, fourfold rise in titer to ≥128, or a single titer of ≥256).[34] The test has been validated using *L. pneumophila* serogroup 1 only; Wilkinson *et al* demonstrated 78% to 91% sensitivity, 99% specificity, and 98% reproducibility.[30] It is known that seroconversion in patients with legionellosis caused by other species and serogroups is similar to seroconversion observed in *L. pneumophila* serogroup 1 infections, but the test has not been validated for legionellosis caused by other serogroups of *L. pneumophila* or for other species of *Legionella*.[35]

References

Rickettsia

1. Moulder JW: The Rickettsias. In Buchanan RE, Gibbons NE (eds): Bergey's Manual of Determinative Bacteriology, 8th ed, p 882. Baltimore, Williams & Wilkins, 1974

2. Centers for Disease Control: Rocky Mountain Spotted Fever—United States, 1986. Surveill Summ 36:314, 1987

3. Walker DH, Burday MS, Folds JD: Laboratory diagnosis of Rocky Mountain spotted fever. South Med J 73:1443, 1980

4. Kaplan JE, Schonberger LB: The sensitivity of various serologic tests in the diagnosis of Rocky Mountain spotted fever. Am J Trop Med Hyg 35:840, 1986

5. Phillip RN, Casper EA, Ormsbee RA, et al: Microimmunofluorescence test for the serological study of Rocky Mountain spotted fever and typhus. J Clin Microbiol 3:51, 1976

6. Eisemann CS, Osterman JV: *Rickettsiae*. In Rose NR, Friedman H, Fahey JL (eds): Manual of Clinical Laboratory Immunology, 3rd ed, p 593. Washington, DC, American Society for Microbiology, 1986

7. Robinson DM, Browm G, Gan E, et al: Adaptation of a microimmunofluorescence test to the study of human *Rickettsia tsutsugamushi* antibody. Am J Trop Med Hyg 25:900, 1976

8. Newhouse NF, Sheppard CC, Tedus MD, et al: A comparison of the complement fixation, indirect fluorescent antibody, and microagglutination tests for the serological diagnosis of rickettsial diseases. Am J Trop Med Hyg 28:387, 1979

9. Halle S, Dasch GA, Weiss E: Sensitive enzyme-linked immunosorbent assay for detection of antibodies against typhus Rickettsiae, *Rickettsia prowazekii* and *Rickettsia typhi*. J Clin Microbiol 6:101, 1977

10. Hechemy KE, Anacker RL, Phillip RN, et al: Detection of Rocky Mountain spotted fever antibodies by a latex agglutination test. J Clin Microbiol 12:144, 1980

11. Hechemy KE, Michaelson EE, Anacker RL, et al: Evaluation of latex–*Rickettsia rickettsii* test for Rocky Mountain spotted fever in 11 laboratories. J Clin Microbiol 18:938, 1983

12. Hechemy KE, Stevens RW, Sasowski S, et al: Discrepancies in Weil-Felix and microimmunofluorescence test results for Rocky Mountain spotted fever. J Clin Microbiol 9:292, 1979

Mycoplasma

13. Fernwald GW: Pathogenicity of *Mycoplasma pneumoniae* disease. Zbl Bakt Hyg I Abt Orig A 245:139, 1979

14. Quinn PA, Shewchuk AB, Shuber J, et al: Serologic evidence of *Ureaplasma urealyticum* infection in women with spontaneous pregnancy loss. Am J Obstet Gynecol 145:245, 1983

15. Moeller BR, Taylor-Robinson D, Furr PM: Serologic evidence implication of *Mycoplasma genitalium* in pelvic inflammatory disease. Lancet 2:1102–1103, 1984

16. Kenny GE: Serology of mycoplasmal infections. In Rose NR, Friedman H, Fahey JL (eds): Manual of Clinical Laboratory Immunology, 3rd ed, p 440. Washington, DC, American Society for Microbiology, 1986

17. Kohne DE: Application of DNA probe tests to the diagnosis of infectious disease. Am Clin Prod Rev, Nov, p 20, 1986

18. Schmidt NJ, Lennette EH, Dennis J, et al: On the nature of complement fixing antibodies to *Mycoplasma pneumoniae*. J Immunol 91:95, 1966

19. Weissfeld AS, Howard BJ, Almazan RD, et al: Miscellaneous pathogenic organisms. In Howard BJ (ed): Clinical and Pathogenic Microbiology, p 455. St. Louis, CV Mosby, 1987

20. Embree JE, Embil JA: Mycoplasmas in Disease of Humans. Can Med Assoc J 123:105, 1980

21. Kenny GE, Newton RM: Close serological relationship between glycolipids of *Mycoplasma pneumoniae* and glycoproteins of spinach. NY Acad Sci 225:54, 1973

22. Kleemola M, Kayhty H: Increase in titers of antibodies to *Mycoplasma pneumoniae* in patients with purulent meningitis. J Infect Dis 146:284, 1983

Legionella

23. Benson RF, Thacker WL, Wilkinson HW, et al: *Legionella pneumophila* serogroup 14 isolated from patients with fatal pneumonia. J Clin Microbiol 26:382, 1988

24. Wilkinson HW, Reingold AL, Brake BJ, et al: Reactivity of serum from patients with suspected legionellosis against 29 antigens of *Legionellaceae* and *Legionella*-like organisms by indirect immunofluorescence assay. J Infect Dis 147:23, 1983

25. Gump DW, Frank RO, Winn WC, et al: Legionnaires' disease in patients with associated serious disease. Ann Intern Med 90:538, 1979

26. Kallings I, Nordstrom K: The pattern of immunoglobulins with special reference to IgM in legionnaires' disease patients during a 2 year follow-up period. Zbl Bakt Hyg I Abt Orig A 225:27, 1983

27. Kirby BD, Snyder KM, Meyer RD, et al: Legion-

naires' disease: Clinical features of 24 cases. Ann Intern Med 89:297, 1978

28.   Lattimer GL, Rhodes LV III, Salventi JS, et al: The Philadelphia epidemic of legionnaires' disease: Clinical, pulmonary, and serologic findings two years later. Ann Intern Med 90:522, 1979

29.   Wilkinson HW, Farshy CE, Fikes BJ, et al: Measure of Immunoglobulins G-, M-, and A-specific titers against *Legionella pneumophila* and inhibition of titers against nonspecific, gram-negative bacterial antigens in the indirect immunofluorescence test for legionellosis. J Clin Microbiol 10:685, 1979

30.   Wilkinson HW, Cruce DD, Broome CV: Validation of *Legionella pneumophila* indirect immunofluorescence assay with epidemic sera. J Clin Microbiol 13:139, 1981

31.   Nagington J, Wreghitt JO'H, Macrea AD: The antibody response in legionnaires' disease. J Hyg (Camb) 83:377, 1979

32.   Blackmon JW, Chandler FW, Cherry WB, et al: Legionellosis. Am J Pathol 103:429, 1981

33.   McDade JE, Shepard CC, Fraser DW, et al: Legionnaires' disease. Isolation of a bacterium and demonstration of its role in other respiratory disease. N Engl J Med 297:1197, 1977

34.   Wilkinson HW, Fikes BJ, Cruce DD: Indirect Immunofluorescence test for serodiagnosis of legionnaires' disease: Evidence for serogroup diversity of legionnaires disease bacterial antigens and for multiple specificity of human antibodies. J Clin Microbiol 9:379, 1979

35.   Wilkinson HW: Serodiagnosis of *Legionella pneumophila*. In Rose NR, Friedman H, Fahey JL (eds): Manual of Clinical Laboratory Immunology, 3rd ed, p 395. Washington, DC, American Society for Microbiology, 1986

25

Hypergammaglobulinemia

T. B. Datiles
R. L. Humphrey

Cellular Basis

B lymphocytes that are appropriately stimulated by an antigen are transformed into plasma cells that synthesize and secrete immunoglobulin (Ig; Fig. 25-1). These Ig bind to the stimulating antigens and help the body eliminate them or neutralize their harmful properties. Different types of Ig are recognized and are classified by their structure into five different classes—IgG, IgA, IgM, IgD, and IgE. The secreted Ig is found in the blood and other body fluids and can be characterized by immunologic methods. Throughout life an individual is continuously exposed to diverse antigens, thereby stimulating the production of a mixture of antibodies composed of different isotypes and idiotypes. Normally, in an adult, IgG constitutes 70% of serum Ig; IgA 10% to 15%; and IgM, 10%. IgD and IgE are present in very small, often undetectable quantities (Fig. 25-2).[1] The in-

creased production of these Ig is termed hypergammaglobulinemia and can be polyclonal or monoclonal, depending on the pathophysiology of the process.

Polyclonal Hypergammaglobulinemia

Exposure to a complex antigen (Ag) transforms many clones of B cells to produce many different Ig; hence, there is a polyclonal response. Each clone will synthesize an antibody with a different specificity, corresponding to the different epitopes on the complex antigen (Fig. 25-3). The antibody response may be composed of one or more classes and subclasses and both light-chain types. Polyclonal hypergammaglobulinemia (gammopathy) results when this normal interplay between Ag and Ig response is either unregulated or exaggerated. Polyclonal gammo-

ANTIGEN

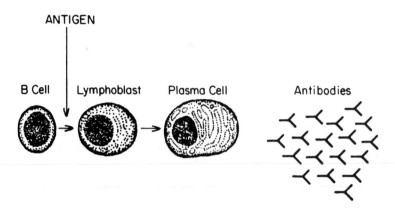

FIGURE 25-1. An antigen (Ag) interacts with a B cell and triggers its transformation into a lymphoblast, which then multiplies by cell division and differentiates into a plasma cell. The plasma cell synthesizes and secretes Ig, which binds to the triggering Ag, inactivates it, and helps the body in its clearance.

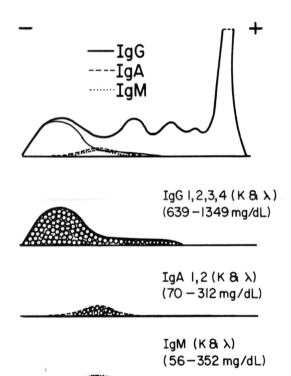

FIGURE 25-2. Serum protein electrophoretogram (SPE) with normal Ig (IgG, IgA, IgM) migrating from the α_2-region through the γ-region. The major portion of the γ-region is contributed by IgG (solid line). The relative electrophoretic mobility and concentration are indicated by the areas under the respective curves. A diagrammatic representation of the plasma cells producing these classes and their relative numbers is given by the lower curves. The normal range in mg/dL for each of these classes is also shown.

pathy can be observed in a variety of clinical situations (*e.g.*, acute and chronic infections, AIDS, sarcoidosis, connective tissue disorders, and liver diseases; Fig. 25-4B).[1]

Monoclonal Hypergammaglobulinemia

In contrast to the usual antigenic transformation of many B cells in a polyclonal response, an autonomous, antigen-independent, "malignant" transformation of a clone of B cells results in the production of one immunoglobulin restricted to one heavy chain and one light chain (Fig. 25-5).[2] Since all these monoclonal Ig molecules have the same structure, they have the same constant domains (isotype) and variable domains (idiotype that includes the antigen combining site), although the complementary anti-

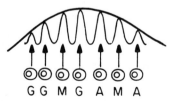

FIGURE 25-3. Diagrammatic representation of many cell clones responding to the constant exposure to many different antigens resulting in the normal heterogeneity of the immunoglobulins.

A

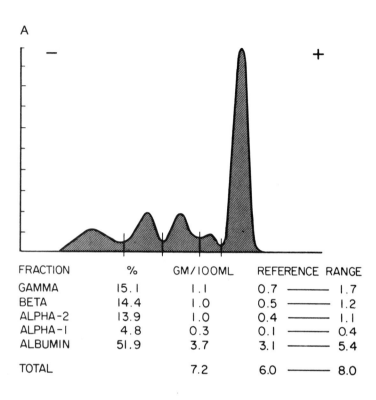

FRACTION	%	GM/100ML	REFERENCE RANGE
GAMMA	15.1	1.1	0.7 ——— 1.7
BETA	14.4	1.0	0.5 ——— 1.2
ALPHA-2	13.9	1.0	0.4 ——— 1.1
ALPHA-1	4.8	0.3	0.1 ——— 0.4
ALBUMIN	51.9	3.7	3.1 ——— 5.4
TOTAL		7.2	6.0 ——— 8.0

B

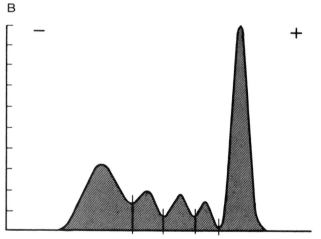

FRACTION	%	GM/100ML	REFERENCE RANGE
GAMMA	32.9	2.3+	0.7 ——— 1.7
BETA	10.7	0.7	0.5 ——— 1.2
ALPHA-2	8.8	0.6	0.4 ——— 1.1
ALPHA-1	5.2	0.4	0.1 ——— 0.4
ALBUMIN	42.5	2.9-	3.1 ——— 5.4
TOTAL		6.9	6.0 ——— 8.0

FIGURE 25-4. (*A*) Normal SPE pattern. (*B*) In contrast with the normal pattern, polyclonal gammopathy is characterized by a broad-based, diffuse increase in the γ-region.

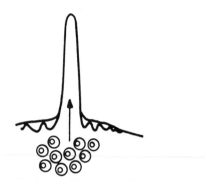

FIGURE 25-5. Diagrammatic representation of a monoclonal proliferation of a single B-cell clone.

gen is usually not known.[3] The protein produced during the expansion of this single clone is homogeneous and is called a monoclonal immunoglobulin or an M component (MC; Fig. 25-6). The general terms for the various growth disorders of plasma cells that result in a monoclonal immunoglobulin are plasma cell dyscrasias or monoclonal gammopathies.[4,5]

Monoclonal Ig may be found in malignant, benign, or transient disorders. The malignant processes include multiple myeloma, Waldenstrom's macroglobulinemia, the heavy-chain diseases, and primary amyloidosis. Sometimes a monoclonal protein is detected in other lymphoreticular neoplasms (leukemia and lymphomas) and is associated with malignant epithelial tumors (lungs, gastrointestinal tract, and genitourinary tract) and other diseases (polycythemia vera and renal tubular acidosis). Occasionally, elderly patients demonstrate a monoclonal protein in the absence of a progressive disease; this process is called benign monoclonal gammopathy or monoclonal gammopathy of unknown significance (MGUS).[6]

Laboratory Evaluation

Serum Protein Electrophoresis

Electrophoresis separates charged molecules, such as serum proteins, in an electrical field.[7] The serum protein is applied to a solid support medium (cellulose

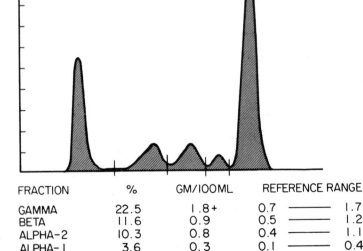

FRACTION	%	GM/100ML	REFERENCE RANGE	
GAMMA	22.5	1.8+	0.7 ————	1.7
BETA	11.6	0.9	0.5 ————	1.2
ALPHA-2	10.3	0.8	0.4 ————	1.1
ALPHA-1	3.6	0.3	0.1 ————	0.4
ALBUMIN	52.0	4.2	3.1 ————	5.4
TOTAL		8.1+	6.0 ————	8.0

FIGURE 25-6. In contrast with the normal pattern (Fig. 25-4A) and with polyclonal hypergammaglobulinemia (Fig. 25-4B), monoclonal gammopathy results in a single, sharply defined, narrow-based peak or "spike," illustrated here in the γ-region. Note the disappearance of the normal polyclonal immunoglobulins.

acetate or agarose gel); in the standard buffer at pH 8.6, most of the serum proteins will have a net negative charge. Albumin, α_1 globulins, α_2 globulins, and β globulins will migrate toward the positive pole (anode), whereas most γ globulins will migrate toward the negative pole (cathode). After electrophoresis, the separated proteins are fixed and stained and the membrane is cleared so that the protein bands can be quantitated by densitometry (see Figs. 25-2 and 25-4A). Serum protein electrophoresis (SPE) can be performed with diluted or undiluted serum, depending on the procedure used; urine and cerebrospinal fluid have a lower protein concentration and therefore require concentration—commonly, 100-fold prior to electrophoresis. There are a number of ways to concentrate dilute solutions of proteins. A commonly used method is to pass the fluid through a membrane with a pore size such that water and salt can easily pass but larger molecules (e.g., proteins) are retained and concentrated.

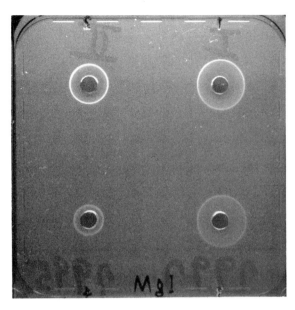

FIGURE 25-7. Radial immunodiffusion (RID). The diameter of the precipitin ring is directly proportional to the Ig concentration.

Quantitative Immunoglobulin Measurement

Immunoglobulin measurement can be performed in a liquid phase (e.g., rate nephelometry) or semisolid phase (radial immunodiffusion [RID]). Nephelometry measures light scattering resulting from immune complex formation. For example, patient IgG reacts with the commercially available anti-IgG; the IgG–anti-IgG complex scatters light, which can be detected electronically. The amount of relative light scatter is directly proportional to the Ig present in the patient's sample. (Nephelometry is discussed in Chapter 16.)

Radial immunodiffusion is a precipitation reaction in which soluble patient Ig reacts with anti-Ig in the semisolid agar, and, at the zone of equivalence, a precipitin ring forms. The diameter of the precipitin ring is directly proportional to the concentration of patient Ig (Fig. 25-7).

Immunoelectrophoresis

Immunoelectrophoresis (IEP) is a method to identify and characterize Ig through the antigenic determinants on their heavy and light chains. IEP consists of two phases: electrophoresis and immunodiffusion. In the electrophoresis phase, proteins are applied to the agarose gel and separated in an electrical field. Then the troughs are filled with specific antisera (anti-IgG, -IgA, -IgM, -κ and -λ) and allowed to incubate overnight. Separated serum proteins and the antisera diffuse toward each other through the agar, and when the monospecific antiserum binds to its antigen, an Ig–anti-Ig complex precipitates and forms an arc. Unprecipitated proteins are removed by a washing step. The shape and position of the precipitin arcs are interpreted by comparing them with the arcs formed by the control, a normal serum (Figs. 25-8A, 25-8B, and 25-9).[5]

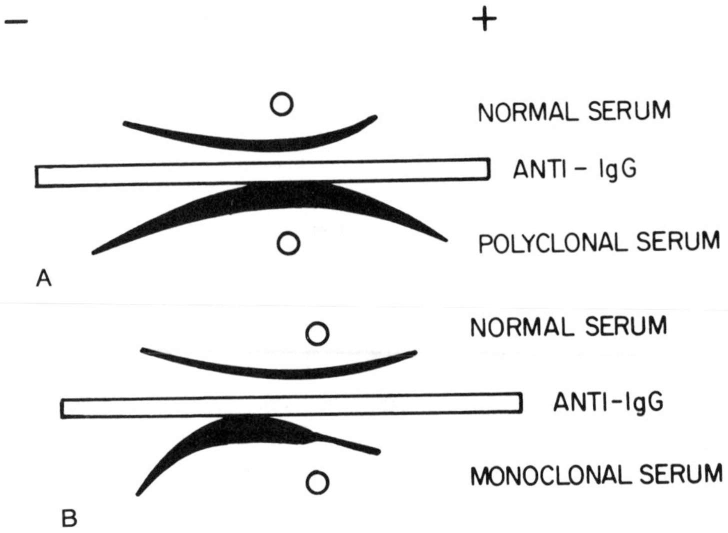

−   +

FIGURE 25-8. (A) Serum immunoelectrophoresis (SIEP) pattern of normal serum
IgG compared with a polyclonal increase
of serum IgG. Polyclonal increase causes
the arc to bow toward the trough. (B) SIEP
pattern of normal serum IgG compared
with a monoclonal increase of serum IgG.
The monoclonal arc shows both restricted
mobility and increased concentration as
compared with normal serum.

NORMAL SERUM

ANTI − IgG

POLYCLONAL SERUM

NORMAL SERUM

ANTI−IgG

MONOCLONAL SERUM

Immunofixation Electrophoresis

Immunofixation electrophoresis (IFE), a more sensitive method than IEP, has recently begun to supplant
IEP.[7] IFE also is composed of two phases: electrophoresis, to separate the proteins, and fixation, to
precipitate the proteins. Serum is applied to the agarose gel and the proteins are separated during electrophoresis. Specific proteins are then fixed by over-
laying specific antiserum on the area of separated
proteins; the antiserum fixes the selected specific
protein by precipitation. Unprecipitated proteins are
removed by washing. The precipitated protein then
can be stained; the resulting bands are compared
with a normal serum control. Particular attention is
paid to the diffuse or restricted nature of the band,
permitting characterization of the bands as polyclonal or monoclonal in nature. A diffuse band recognized by the specific antiserum suggests a heterogeneous group of proteins (i.e., a polyclonal
hypergammaglobulinemia; Fig. 25-10). If the band's
electrophoretic mobility, all of which migrates in a
narrow area, is restricted, it suggests a monoclonal
protein (Fig. 25-11).

Recent efforts to combine high-resolution electrophoresis with immunofixation and immunoglobulin

quantitation have resulted in the detection of low
concentration abnormalities that would have been
overlooked with prior, less sensitive screening techniques. It has also been suggested that quantitation
of the κ and λ light chains in serum may prove to be
very helpful in the detection of immunoglobulin abnormalities.[8]

Clinical Correlation

Polyclonal Hypergammaglobulinemia

Infectious Diseases

Chronic antigenic stimulation, which occurs in a variety of clinical conditions, such as chronic infection,
sarcoidosis, and connective tissue disease (autoimmune disorders), usually causes polyclonal hypergammaglobulinemia (Figs. 25-3, 25-4B, 25-8A, and
25-10). Serum protein electrophoresis shows a
broad-based, diffuse (heterogeneous) increase of the
protein in the γ region (Fig. 25-4B). Quantitative Ig
measurement will show an increased concentration
of one or more Ig classes. On occasion, the γ region
becomes very accentuated and may either obscure or
mimic a monoclonal Ig (M component). The poly-

clonal nature of the abnormality can be confirmed by considering other laboratory findings (*e.g.*, the quantitative measurement of the Ig classes and the use of IEP/IFE).[5,7,8]

Inflammatory Processes

During tissue destruction and acute inflammation, the concentration of acute-phase reactants increases, which leads to an increase in the α_2 region of serum protein electrophoresis (Fig. 25-12) and, to a lesser extent, an increase in α_1 and a decrease in albumin. With persistence of the inflammatory process, the electrophoretic pattern can overlap with and share features with the pattern seen with chronic antigenic stimulation (Fig. 25-4*B*).

Liver Disease

The electrophoretic pattern seen in chronic liver disease also is characterized by a polyclonal increase in the γ region. In addition, there often is a polyclonal increase in IgA, which results in a bridging or obliteration of the space usually present between the β and γ regions. Additional features often include a stair-step-like decrease from the γ to β to α_2 to α_1 regions and a reduction in the albumin concentration (Fig. 25-13). This pattern overlaps with and is a variation of that seen with chronic antigenic stimulation (compare Figs. 25-4*B* and 25-13). However, the following four characteristics often help to establish chronic liver disease: (1) decreased albumin; (2) stair-step decrease ranging from γ region to α_1 region; (3) bridging between the β and γ regions; and (4) polyclonal increase in the γ region.

Monoclonal Hypergammaglobulinemia

Multiple Myeloma

Multiple myeloma is a lymphoproliferative disease that results from the uncontrolled proliferation of a single clone of plasma cells and produces excess homogeneous immunoglobulin or immunoglobulin

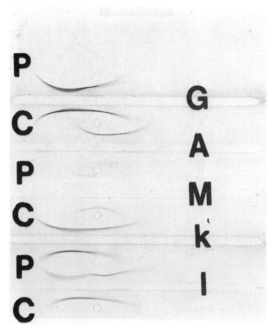

FIGURE 25-9. SIEP comparing normal serum and that from a patient with an IgG λ monoclonal gammopathy. Patient (P) and normal control (C) serum alternate on the gel. After the electrophoretic separation, the troughs in the agar gel were filled with anti-IgG (G), anti-IgA (A), anti-IgM (M), anti-κ, and anti-λ antisera. Note the marked increase and restricted electrophoretic mobility of the patient arcs seen with anti-IgG (G) and anti-λ antisera. In addition, IgA and IgM are markedly reduced.

fragment.[4,5] Traditionally, multiple myeloma is subclassified according to the heavy-chain class and light-chain type of the monoclonal protein (Table 25-1). IgG myeloma is the most common form, accounting for 50% of all myeloma; IgA accounts for 25%. IgD myeloma rarely occurs (less than 1%), and IgE is extremely rare. In some instances the malignant plasma cells have lost the ability to synthesize the heavy chain and can only produce the light chain (see Table 25-1, line 5).[9] This accounts for about 24% of the cases (light-chain myeloma), leaving about 1% of the cases in which neither the heavy nor the light chain is produced (nonsecretory myeloma). In addi-

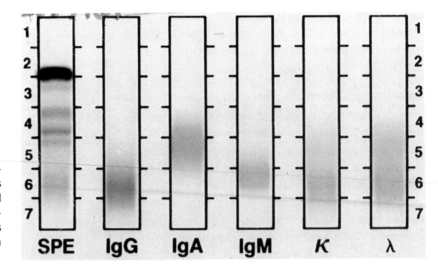

FIGURE 25-10. Serum immunofixation electrophoresis (SIFE) revealing a polyclonal hypergammaglobulinemia involving all three major classes of Ig(G, A, and M) and both light-chain types (κ and λ).

tion to the 24% of cases that produce only light chain, about one third of IgG and IgA producers have a relative overproduction of light chain (unbalanced synthesis) compared with the heavy chain. This free or unattached light chain circulates in the blood, and because of its low molecular weight (20,000 d), it is easily filtered by the glomeruli. Thus, free light chain can be found in the urine, where it is called Bence Jones protein (see Table 25-1, lines 2, 4, and 5). The ratio of κ to λ light chain involvement is 2:1 in IgG myeloma and light-chain myeloma, whereas the ratio is closer to 1:1 in IgA myeloma.

The incidence of multiple myeloma is approximately 3 per 100,000 in the general population, with onset at a median age of approximately 60 years. Though the pathogenesis in man is unknown, epide-

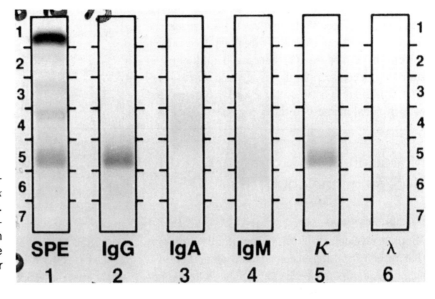

FIGURE 25-11. SIFE of a patient's serum with an IgG κ monoclonal gammopathy. Note the restricted electrophoretic mobility of the band seen in IgG and κ lanes and the marked reductions of the other Ig.

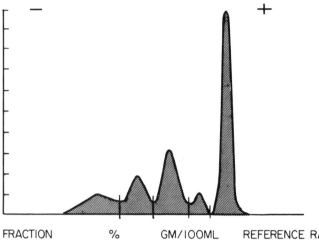

FRACTION	%	GM/100ML	REFERENCE RANGE	
GAMMA	14.9	0.8	0.7	1.7
BETA	15.4	0.8	0.5	1.2
ALPHA-2	23.1	1.2+	0.4	1.1
ALPHA-1	5.2	0.3	0.1	0.4
ALBUMIN	41.5	2.2-	3.1	5.4
TOTAL		5.3-	6.0	8.0

FIGURE 25-12. Acute inflammation pattern-SPE shows a moderate increase of proteins in α_2; slight increase in α_1; and slight decrease in albumin regions. Compare with Figs. 25-4A and 25-4B.

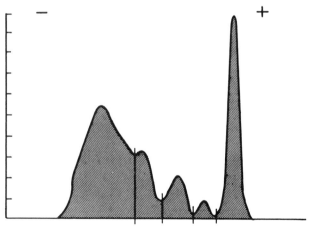

FRACTION	%	GM/100ML	REFERENCE RANGE	
GAMMA	51.9	2.6+	0.7	1.7
BETA	12.3	0.6	0.5	1.2
ALPHA-2	8.0	0.4	0.4	1.1
ALPHA-1	2.3	0.1	0.1	0.4
ALBUMIN	25.5	1.3	3.1	5.4
TOTAL		5.1-	6.0	8.0

FIGURE 25-13. Liver disease pattern-SPE shows decreased albumin; stair-step decrease from γ to α_1; bridging between β- and γ-regions; and polyclonal increase in the γ-region. Compare with Figs. 25A and 25-4B.

Table 25-1: Classification of Multiple Myeloma Based on Heavy- and Light-Chain Production

Serum M-Component "Spike"	Urine M-Component "Spike"	Approximate % of Multiple Myeloma Patients
IgG	None*	33
IgG	Yes†	17[ǁ]
IgA	None*	16
IgA	Yes†	9[ǁ]
None‡	Yes†	24[ǁ]
None**	None**	1[ǁ]
		100

* Synthesis of H + L chains is "balanced."
† Overproduction of L chain.
‡ Ability to produce H chain is lost.
** Neither H nor L chain is produced. This is called nonsecretory myeloma.
ǁ Approximately 50% of myeloma patients (17 + 9 + 24) will have free L chain found in the urine (Bence Jones protein).

miologic studies show increased incidence of myeloma following low-dose radiation exposure. The prevalence is the same for men and women. For unknown reasons, the incidence is somewhat greater in blacks and the onset is somewhat earlier.

The clinical findings include weakness, anorexia, and weight loss, suggesting a chronic, progressive, systemic illness. As the disease advances, bone involvement with skeletal destruction (Fig. 25-14) and pain, anemia, renal insufficiency, various neurologic deficits, and recurrent bacterial infections often occur.

Laboratory findings in multiple myeloma include the demonstration and characterization of the monoclonal Ig. As seen in Table 25-1, half the patients with multiple myeloma (rows 1 to 4) show a peak, or "spike," of variable size in the γ or β region on SPE (see Fig. 25-6). The Ig class of the monoclonal pro-

tein is markedly increased, whereas the normal, uninvolved Ig classes are commonly decreased. Serum IEP shows an abnormal position, density, or shape of a precipitin arc restricted to one heavy-chain class and one light-chain type (Figs. 25-8*B* and 25-9). The precipitin arc of the heavy chain will be identical to that of the light chain, since both antisera are detecting different antigens on the same molecule. Similarly, the serum IFE will identify a band of restricted electrophoretic mobility with the anti–heavy-chain antisera that is identical to that revealed by the light-chain antisera (see Fig. 25-11). When there is "unbalanced synthesis" (see Table 25-1, rows 2, 4, and 5), the free light chain can be demonstrated in the urine by protein electrophoresis (Fig. 25-15). The free light chain also can be identified and typed by IEP or IFE (Fig. 25-16).

Light-chain myeloma is the production of a monoclonal light chain without a corresponding heavy chain (see Table 25-1, row 5).[9] SPE usually shows a markedly reduced γ region (Fig. 25-17) without a spike or band, because the free light chain is rapidly cleared from the blood by glomerular filtration into the urine. Occasionally, the monoclonal light chain

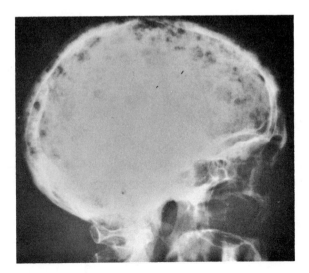

FIGURE 25-14. Skull x-ray showing osteolytic "punched-out" lesions.

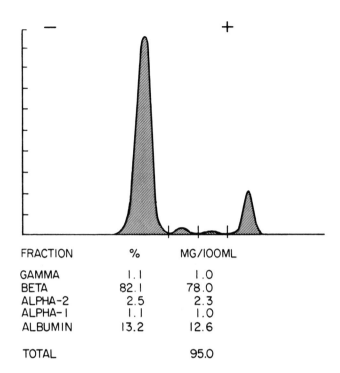

FRACTION	%	MG/IOOML
GAMMA	1.1	1.0
BETA	82.1	78.0
ALPHA-2	2.5	2.3
ALPHA-1	1.1	1.0
ALBUMIN	13.2	12.6
TOTAL		95.0

FIGURE 25-15. Excess product proteinuria-UPE shows a markedly increased band in the β-region.

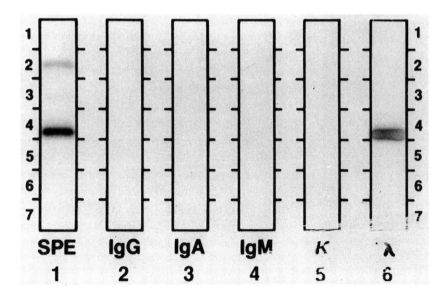

FIGURE 25-16. UIFE revealing the presence of a markedly increased band of restricted electrophoretic mobility in the λ-lane.

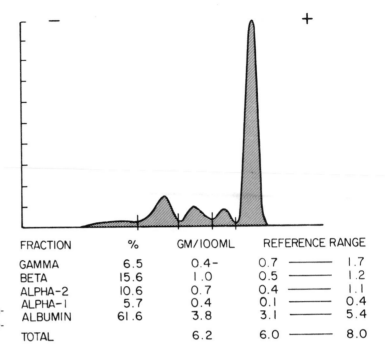

FRACTION	%	GM/100ML	REFERENCE RANGE
GAMMA	6.5	0.4-	0.7 ———— 1.7
BETA	15.6	1.0	0.5 ———— 1.2
ALPHA-2	10.6	0.7	0.4 ———— 1.1
ALPHA-1	5.7	0.4	0.1 ———— 0.4
ALBUMIN	61.6	3.8	3.1 ———— 5.4
TOTAL		6.2	6.0 ———— 8.0

FIGURE 25-17. Hypogammaglobulinemia-SPE shows marked reduction of the γ-region.

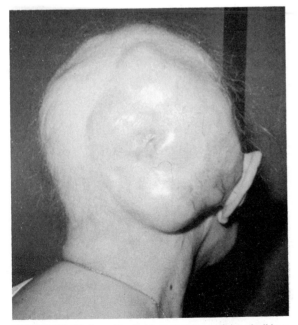

FIGURE 25-18. Localized plasmacytoma of the skull in a patient with far-advanced multiple myeloma.

can be detected by serum IEP or IFE, because they are more sensitive than SPE. Taken altogether, free light chains can be found in the urine by protein electrophoresis and can be identified by urine IEP or IFE in approximately 50% of myeloma patients (see Table 25-1, rows 2, 4, and 5; footnote ‖).

Multiple myeloma is a malignant tumor of plasma cells. The plasma cells typically are present in the bone marrow and less commonly in other tissues; rarely, localized tumor masses develop (plasmacytoma) (Fig. 25-18). A typical plasma cell infiltrate of the bone marrow is shown in Figure 25-19. Osteolytic lesions are associated with bone pain and fractures and appear as "punched-out" areas when evaluated by x-ray. The skull is commonly affected, as shown in Figure 25-14. Treatment of multiple myeloma includes local radiation therapy of myelomatous tumors and chemotherapy to reduce the plasmacytosis of the bone marrow. Alkylating agents (such as melphalan and cyclophosphamide) are com-

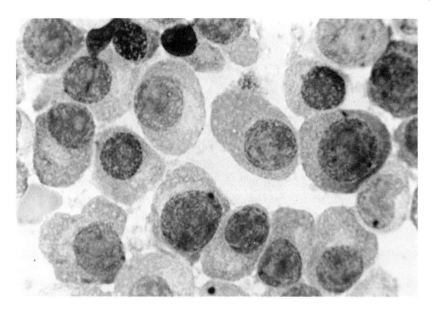

FIGURE 25-19. Oil immersion micrograph of a bone marrow smear stained with Wright's stain taken from a patient with multiple myeloma. The malignant plasma cells are characterized by abundant cytoplasm and eccentrically placed nuclei. They have a granular-appearing cytoplasm that represents the dilated endoplasmic reticulum due to the active synthesis of the monoclonal Ig. A zone of reduced staining is often seen next to the nucleus, the perinuclear clear zone.

monly used and work by interfering with cell replication. Responding patients have a median survival expectancy of about 3 to 4 years, whereas unresponsive patients have a median survival of 12 to 18 months.

Waldenström's Macroglobulinemia

Waldenström's macroglobulinemia is a relatively rare disorder characterized by an uncontrolled proliferation of a single clone of plasma cells that synthesize a homogeneous IgM. It represents one form of several related lymphoproliferative disorders characterized by their production of a monoclonal IgM.[10] It is usually observed in individuals over age 50, with incidence peaking in the sixth decade. The frequency in men is almost twice that in women.

Clinical findings include weakness, ease of fatigue, headache, and weight loss. As the disorder progresses, the features associated with the hyperviscosity syndrome develop. These features can mimic abnormalities of the cardiovascular (congestive heart failure), neurologic (headache, dizziness), ocular (partial or total loss of visual acuity), and hematopoietic systems (bleeding, anemia).

Laboratory findings include a spike in the β or γ region on SPE. IgM is increased, whereas IgG and IgA usually are decreased. Serum IEP and IFE demonstrate a monoclonal IgMκ or IgMλ protein. In the presence of hyperviscosity, the relative serum viscosity is elevated. The relative serum viscosity is the comparison of the time it takes for a standard volume of saline to pass through a capillary tube compared with the time required for the patient's serum to do the same. The relative serum viscosity is an indication of the resistance of the serum to flow and, when markedly increased, results in the symptoms of the hyperviscosity syndrome. The threshold for symptoms will differ among patients but often occurs when the relative viscosity is greater than 3.0 (normal 1.4 to 1.8). The hyperviscosity syndrome in Waldenström's macroglobulinemia is caused by the excess monoclonal IgM, because it is a very large molecule (close to 1 million in molecular weight) and quite asymmetric in shape.[11]

The diagnosis of Waldenström's macroglobulinemia centers on the presence of the monoclonal IgM and the abnormal accumulation of plasmacytoid lymphocytes in bone marrow and other tissues. Kyle[10] has arbitrarily set the level of the monoclonal IgM as $\geq$3000 mg/dL in order to discriminate between Waldenström's macroglobulinemia and the other related lymphoproliferative disorders characterized by the presence of a monoclonal IgM.

When defined in this way, the median survival expectancy is about 6 years. When it occurs, death is related to infection, bone marrow failure, or uncontrolled hyperviscosity. Initial treatment centers on the rapid control of the hyperviscosity by the removal of the monoclonal IgM from the serum by plasmapheresis. Longer-term control of the production of the IgM often is achieved by chemotherapy with alkylating agents, such as chlorambucil or cyclophosphamide. When successful, the plasmapheresis requirement can often be reduced or eliminated.

Heavy-Chain Diseases

The heavy-chain diseases are rare lymphoproliferative disorders characterized by the presence of fragments of the heavy (H) chains without light chain. The H chains of α, γ, and μ classes have been involved and serve as a convenient way to classify those disorders.[12] Although the clinical syndromes differ, the proteins are characterized by major deletions in the variable (VH) and first constant portions (CH$_1$) of the Ig molecule that preclude the attachment of the light chains.

α-Heavy-chain disease is the most common, occurring predominantly among young Arabs and non-Ashkenazi Jews in the Middle East. The disease is characterized by abdominal pain and severe malabsorption due to lymphoid and plasma cell infiltration of the small intestines and mesenteric lymph nodes.

γ-Heavy-chain disease is characterized by fever, recurrent infection (especially pneumonia), peculiar edema and erythema of the palate and uvula, generalized lymphadenopathy, and hepatosplenomegaly. The survival is variable, from a few weeks to more than 5 years after onset of symptoms. Recurrent infection and progressive plasma cell proliferation are frequent problems.

μ-Heavy-chain disease is characterized by hepatosplenomegaly and retroperitoneal adenopathy with less prominent peripheral adenopathy. The lymphocytoid-plasma cells are characterized by vacuolated cytoplasm and frequently circulate in high numbers, causing this disease to mimic chronic lymphocytic leukemia.

Although these syndromes vary in their clinical expression, in the laboratory they are characterized by finding a band of restricted electrophoretic mobility that is identical in both serum and urine. This band will be identified by antisera directed against the involved heavy chain but will not react with anti–light-chain antisera. The band is present in both the serum and the urine because the large deletion (VH and CH$_1$) reduces the molecular size of the remaining fragment (about 40,000 d) to the point where it can be filtered by the glomeruli into the urine. Confirmation of the diagnosis rests on the measurement of the molecular weight of the heavy-chain fragment and biochemical proof of the absence of the light chain.

Primary Amyloidosis

Primary amyloidosis is a rare disorder occurring in less than 1% of autopsies in general hospitals. It is characterized by the accumulation of a complex extracellular proteinaceous substance that is dominated by a fibrillar component visualized by electron microscopy.[13]

Amyloidosis is diagnosed by the histologic examination of a biopsy of an involved tissue, such as tongue, gingiva, nerve, muscle, skin, bone marrow, rectum, kidney, or heart. Congo red staining of affected tissues when examined under polarized light reveals the characteristic apple green to yellow birefringence. The course of the disease varies with the organs most involved.

In the primary form of the disease, the fibril has been shown to be related to immunoglobulin, usually the variable end of light chain. It derives from abnormal plasma cells that are usually present in the bone marrow but not in sufficient numbers or with the skeletal destruction seen in multiple myeloma. However, amyloid deposition can complicate myeloma as well as the other plasma cell disorders. Other forms of amyloidosis exist with biochemical structure unrelated to immunoglobulin. The secondary form occurs after prolonged infection (*e.g.*, tuberculosis, osteomyelitis) or in association with chronic inflammatory processes such as rheumatoid arthritis. There are also a number of inherited forms of amyloidosis.[4,13]

In the laboratory, primary amyloidosis can often be suspected because of the frequently associated abnormalities of the serum immunoglobulins. Many cases are characterized by hypogammaglobulinemia (see Fig. 25-17), often involving more than one of the major Ig classes. Frequently, a low-concentration monoclonal gammopathy is detected in the serum with associated free light chains found in the urine. On occasion, the abnormalities are subtle and not easy to detect. This can be especially true when there is kidney damage by the amyloidosis leading to substantial proteinuria that may obscure the low concentration of the monoclonal free light chain in the urine. Under these circumstances, IFE often proves to be of enormous help in detecting and identifying the abnormal proteins.

Monoclonal Gammopathy of Unknown Significance (MGUS)

Sometimes a monoclonal protein in serum or urine is present without other manifestations of a plasma cell disorder. The frequency of this finding increases with age and has been estimated at about 10% in persons greater than 60 years of age.[14] Some patients may demonstrate progression over time, but many do not. It is important to distinguish between early detection of a malignant, progressive process and MGUS, which can behave in a benign fashion for years. Unfortunately, there is no easy, reliable way to predict whether or when a given patient will progress. The amount, class, or type of the monoclonal gammopathy or the presence of Bence Jones protein also fails to predict which patient's disease process will progress. All people with monoclonal gammopathy

should be monitored indefinitely for the possible emergence of malignant behavior.

References

1. Stites DP, Stobo JD, Wells JV (eds): Basic and Clinical Immunology, 6th ed. East Norwalk, Appleton and Lange, 1987
2. Farhangi M, Merlini G: The clinical implications of monoclonal immunoglobulins. Semin Oncol 13:366, 1986
3. Duggan DB, Schattner A: Unusual manifestations of monoclonal gammopathies, autoimmune and idiopathic syndromes. Am J Med 81:864, 1986
4. Humphrey RL, Owens AH Jr: The Plasma Cell Dyscrasias. In Harvey AM, Johns RJ, McKusick VA, et al (eds): Principles and Practice of Medicine, 22nd ed, p 429. East Norwalk, Appleton and Lange, 1988
5. Kyle RA: Classification and diagnosis of monoclonal gammopathies. In Rose NR, Friedman H, Fahey JL (eds): Manual of Clinical Laboratory Immunology, 3rd ed, p 152. Washington, DC, American Society for Microbiology, 1986
6. Kyle RA: Monoclonal gammopathy of undetermined significance: Natural history in 241 cases. Am J Med 64:814, 1978
7. Keren DF: High-resolution electrophoresis and immunofixation, techniques and interpretation. Boston, Butterworths, 1987
8. Keren DF, Warren JS, Lowe JB: Strategy to diagnose monoclonal gammopathies in serum, high-resolution electrophoresis, immunofixation and κ/λ quantification. Clin Chem 34:2196, 1988
9. Solomon A: Clinical implications of monoclonal light chains. Semin Oncol 13:341, 1986
10. Kyle RA, Garton JP: The spectrum of IgM monoclonal gammopathy in 430 cases. Mayo Clin Proc 62:719, 1987
11. Bloch KJ, Maki DG: Hyperviscosity syndromes associated with immunoglobulin abnormalities. Semin Hematol 10:113, 1973
12. Franklin EC: The heavy chain diseases. Harvey Lect 78:1, 1984
13. Glenner GG: Amyloid deposits and amyloidosis: The beta-fibrilloses. N Engl J Med 302:1283, 1333, 1980
14. Crawford J, Eye MK, Cohen HJ: Evaluation of monoclonal gammopathies in the "well" elderly. Am J Med 82:39, 1987

CHAPTER 26

Lymphoid Malignancy

Suio-Ling Chen

With the current understanding of the intricate cellular interplay in regulation of lymphocyte differentiation and activation, it is hardly suprising that the control of such a complex system can go awry. The lymphoproliferative diseases can be envisioned as the clonal expansion of the cells of the immune system that underwent malignant transformation at a particular maturational or activation stage. Thus, accumulation of malignant lymphocytes with a similar degree of maturation occurs. This phenomenon is known as maturational arrest. These neoplastic lymphocytes maintain most, if not all, of the biological properties of their normal counterparts in addition to their malignant properties, such as tumor formation, invasiveness, and metastatic capability. Therefore, the biological properties of normal lymphocytes are exceedingly useful for the diagnosis and classification of lymphoproliferative diseases. For example, B-cell neoplasms usually express B-cell markers, such as surface immunoglobulin, and home to B-cell domains in a lymphoid organ.

Lymphoproliferative diseases are subdivided into two categories: leukemia and lymphoma. Diseases arising from the lymph nodes are lymphomas, which are categorized into Hodgkin's and non-Hodgkin's lymphoma. Leukemias are diseases originating in the bone marrow with a peripheral blood phase. There is, however, overlap between lymphoma and leukemia. Occasionally, lymphoma may develop into a leukemic phase, or a leukemia may have lymph node manifestation.

Lymphocyte Markers

Currently, the lymphocyte marker analysis is utilized in conjunction with morphologic observations for the diagnosis of lymphoid malignancy. The multiparameter analysis tends to offer increased sensitivity and reproducibility. Since the phenotypes of most malignant lymphoid cells reflect their corresponding normal counterparts, none of the markers presently used in a clinical laboratory are specific for the neo-

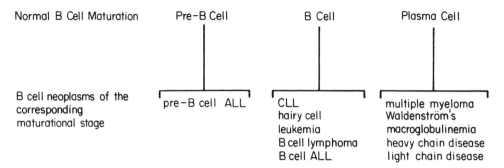

FIGURE 26-1. Maturational arrest seen in B-cell neoplasms.

plastic lymphocytes. Nevertheless, some insight as to the maturation state of the malignant cell is obtained by the marker study. (Refer to Chapter 3 for a discussion of lymphocyte markers.)

Immunoglobulin analysis is one of the most specific markers for the B-cell malignancy (Fig. 26-1). Malignant B cells express the characteristic immunoglobulin corresponding to the maturational stage. Thus, a B-cell neoplasm with small resting B-cell morphology expresses surface immunoglobulin with little or no cytoplasmic immunoglobulin, whereas malignant plasma cells contain cytoplasmic immunoglobulin without expressing surface immunoglobulin. Between the two extremes are the neoplasms that are arrested at various stages of maturation with malignant cells that express varying amount of surface and/or cytoplasmic immunoglobulin. Furthermore, because the clonal expansion of a single transformed B cell is an inherent part of the malignant process, the expression of restricted light chain is a strong indicator of malignancy. Therefore, a polyclonal B-cell proliferation in response to antigenic stimuli can be distinguished from neoplastic B-cell proliferation with confidence because the B cells in the former condition express the normal ratio of light chains, whereas the latter condition has B cells that have restricted light chain (*i.e.*, either κ or λ light chain).

The common acute lymphoblastic leukemia associated antigen (CALLA) was originally defined by an antibody produced by rabbits that were immunized with non-T, non-B lymphoblastic leukemic cells. CALLA is a 100-kd glycoprotein and is designated as CD10.[1,2] It is a useful marker because approximately 75% of non-T, non-B acute lymphoblastic leukemias (ALL) and 40% of lymphoblastic lymphomas express this marker. Furthermore, it is also present on some follicular lymphoma cells.[3–5] A small percentage of bone marrow cells is also positive for CALLA; presumably, these are lymphohematopoietic precursor cells.[6]

Terminal deoxynucleotidyl transferase (TdT) is a nuclear enzyme that catalyzes the addition of deoxynucleotide triphosphate to the 3′-hydroxyl end of oligo- and polydeoxynucleotides without template instruction.[7] TdT is present in thymocytes and a small percentage of bone marrow cells (<5%) but is absent from mature lymphocytes.[8] Except for B-ALL and Burkitt's lymphoma, TdT is identified in all cases of ALL. Frequently, TdT-positive leukemic cells appear during the blast crisis of chronic myelogenic leukemia (CML). Therapeutic significance is implied for TdT positivity because a patient who has positive TdT cells during blast crisis is most likely to respond to combination chemotherapy consisting of vincristine and prednisone. Conversely, a negative TdT finding is associated with a poor prognosis.[9] TdT is also observed in T-lymphoblastic lymphoma.[3]

Expression of functional receptors by both T and B cells (*i.e.*, T-cell antigen receptor heterodimer and

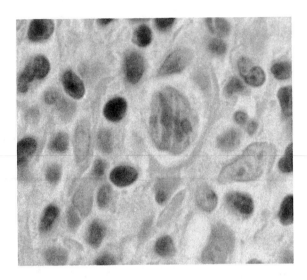

FIGURE 26-2. Hodgkin's cell, 1000×. (Courtesy of Dr. JJ Marty.)

B-cell surface immunoglobulin) requires sequential gene arrangement during cell maturation. Study of clonal rearrangement of these genes is most likely to be an extremely sensitive tool to identify and characterize lymphoid malignancy in the future.

Lymphoma

Hodgkin's Disease

The hallmark of Hodgkin's lymphoma is the giant binucleated Reed-Sternberg cells and their mononuclear variants (Fig. 26-2). The origin of these neoplastic cells remains controversial. Presently, Hodgkin's lymphoma is classified by histologic findings. A standardized histopathologic classification recommended in 1965 includes lymphocyte predominant, nodular sclerosing, mixed cellularity, and lymphocyte depletion.[10] Most investigators believe that strong host immune response is associated with a favorable prognosis, and this appears to be sup-

ported by clinical observation. Thus, the lymphocyte-predominant type tends to occur in younger patients who have limited disease at the time of diagnosis and have a favorable prognosis. Conversely, the lymphocyte-depleted type tends to be associated with widespread disease and a poor prognosis.

Cell-mediated immune response is frequently compromised in patients with Hodgkin's disease. For example, skin anergy is a common finding.[11]

Non-Hodgkin's Lymphoma

Non-Hodgkin's lymphoma is a heterogeneous group of neoplasms whose classification has long been controversial. For the past 5 to 10 years, the histopathologic classification proposed by Rappaport has been widely accepted for the diagnosis of this malignancy.[12] As the modern concept of the immune system emerges, new classifications are proposed in which both lymphoid morphology and physiology are acknowledged. Recently, a working formulation was proposed as a result of the study led by the National Cancer Institute.[3] In this formulation the prognosis as determined by survival is correlated with morphology and immunology of the tumors. Three major groups are proposed: low-grade, intermediate-grade, and high-grade. Each of these is associated with favorable, intermediate, and unfavorable prognosis, respectively.

Low-Grade Lymphoma

Malignant Lymphoma: Small Lymphocytic Cell. In general, small lymphocytic (SL) malignant lymphoma has diffuse lymph node architecture. The cells are round and the size varies from small to medium. Mitotic activity is scant or absent. The presence of plasmacytoid lymphocyte may be associated with monoclonal gammopathy. The tissue manifestation of chronic lymphocytic leukemia may present with similar morphology. This is mainly a B-cell

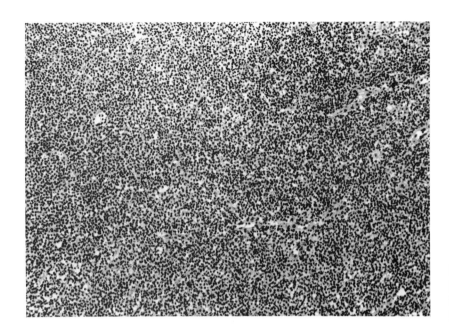

FIGURE 26-3. Follicular lymphoma with predominantly small cleaved cells, 100×. (Courtesy of Dr. JJ Marty.)

neoplasm with the malignant cells expressing surface immunoglobulin, Fc receptors, complement receptors, and MHC class II molecules.

Malignant Lymphoma: Follicular, Predominantly Small Cleaved Cells. In follicular, predominantly small cleaved cells (FSC) lymphoma, the involved lymph node is usually replaced by follicles that are relatively uniform in size and shape (Fig. 26-3). The cells are predominantly small with a cleaved nucleus (indentation of the nuclear membrane). The neoplastic B cells express surface immunoglobulin, CALLA, and MHC class II molecules.

Malignant Lymphoma: Follicular, Mixed Small Cleaved and Large Cells. The lymph node architecture in follicular, mixed small cleaved and large cells (FM) lymphoma is similar to that in FSC except that the cells in the follicles are a mixture of small cleaved and large cells. The small cleaved cells are surface immunoglobulin positive, whereas the large cells tend to be surface immunoglobulin negative but may be cytoplasmic immunoglobulin positive. Both small cleaved cells and large cells are positive for MHC class II molecules and CALLA.

Intermediate-Grade Lymphoma

Malignant Lymphoma: Follicular, Predominantly Large Cells. The lymph node architecture in follicular, predominantly large cell (FL) lymphoma is similar to that in FM; however, the predominant cells are large and noncleaved. There are numerous mitotic figures. Most cases have neoplastic cells that express surface immunoglobulin, MHC class II molecules, and CALLA.

Malignant Lymphoma: Diffuse, Small Cleaved Cells and Diffuse, Mixed Small and Large Cells. Diffuse, small cleaved cells (DSC; Fig. 26-4) and diffuse, mixed small and large cells (DM) lymphoma represent diffuse counterparts of FSC and FM, respectively. The neoplastic cells express surface immunoglobulin and MHC class II molecules. However, unlike their follicular counterparts, the cells do not usually express CALLA.

Malignant Lymphoma: Diffuse, Large Cells. In diffuse, large cell lymphoma (DL) the normal lymph node architecture is entirely replaced by a diffuse proliferation of malignant cells. The cell population may be composed of large cleaved and noncleaved

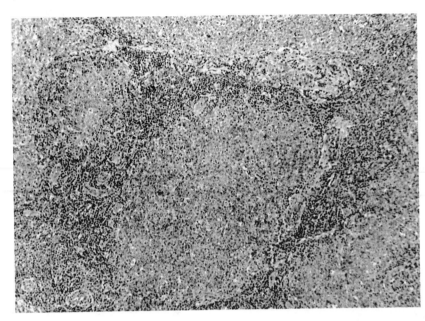

FIGURE 26-4. Small-cell lymphoma with diffuse lymph node architecture, 100×. (Courtesy of Dr. JJ Marty.)

cells. The large cleaved cells may have minimal cytoplasm and inconspicuous nucleoli, whereas large noncleaved cells possess a rim of cytoplasm and one or more prominent nucleoli. The malignant cells of the majority of cases express surface immunoglobulin and MHC class II molecules.

High-Grade Lymphoma

Malignant Lymphoma: Large-Cell, Immunoblastic. Large-cell immunoblastic lymphoma (IBL) is divided into three categories: plasmacytoid, clear cell, and polymorphous immunoblastic lymphoma. The cells of the plasmacytoid variant possess eccentric nuclei with abundant cytoplasmic immunoglobulin. The clear-cell type and polymorphous variant appear to be of T-cell lineage.

Malignant Lymphoma: Lymphoblastic. In lymphoblastic lymphoma (LBL) the lymph node is typically associated with diffuse effacement of normal architecture. A "starry-sky" pattern due to evenly distributed macrophages may be prominent. The neoplastic cells may have convoluted nuclei with scanty cytoplasm. There are invariably numerous mitotic figures. The neoplastic cells also form rosettes with sheep red blood cells and react with monoclonal antibody against T cells. Approximately one third of childhood and 5% of adult non-Hodgkin's lymphomas are identified as LBL. The disease is more prevalent in males and often is associated with a mediastinal mass. In some cases, the disease may evolve into a leukemic phase that is frequently indistinguishable from T-cell acute lymphoblastic leukemia.

Malignant Lymphoma: Small, Noncleaved Cell. Small, noncleaved cell (SNC) malignant lymphoma includes Burkitt's lymphoma and other high-grade undifferentiated non-Burkitt's lymphomas. Most cases of African Burkitt's lymphoma are endemic and associated with Epstein-Barr virus; however, most American Burkitt's lymphomas are not associated with Epstein-Barr virus. Furthermore, cells of African Burkitt's lymphoma express Fc receptors, receptor for complement (C3b), and receptors for Epstein-Barr virus. Conversely, none of the preceding markers are expressed by the malignant cells of American Burkitt's lymphoma. The Burkitt's lymphoma cells usually do not express CALLA, though some express surface IgM, suggesting some degree of differentiation.

Cutaneous T-Cell Lymphoma

Cutaneous lymphoma is also known as mycosis fungoides whose leukemic phase is referred to as Sézary cell leukemia. The clinical feature of this disease is the skin lesion that varies from limited plaques to generalized plaques, tumors, and generalized erythroderma. In the skin the malignant cells are referred to as mycosis fungoides cells; in the peripheral blood they are called Sézary cells. Both cell types form rosettes with sheep red blood cells or are CD2 positive. In most reported cases the malignant T cells are CD4 positive and are able to help antibody synthesis by B cells *in vitro*.[13-15]

Leukemia
Chronic Lymphocytic Leukemia

Chronic lymphocytic leukemia (CLL) is primarily a disease due to clonal expansion of B cells in older patients. The patients usually present with an elevated peripheral white blood cell count and bone marrow involvement. The malignant B cells have the morphology of a small resting lymphocyte. They express weak surface immunoglobulin that is invariably restricted to one light chain, either κ or λ. Complement receptors, Fc receptors, and MHC class II molecules are also expressed by the malignant cells. Approximately 5% of CLL are reported to be of T-cell type.[16,17]

Hairy Cell Leukemia

Hairy cell leukemia, or leukemic reticuloendotheliosis, is characterized by infiltration of bone marrow and spleen by the leukemic cells without peripheral lymphadenopathy. The disease occurs in patients from 20 to over 80 years of age, with male predominance (4:1 male-to-female ratio). The majority of patients initially present with pancytopenia, with decreased granulocytes and increased lymphocytes. The malignant cells usually have irregular or "hairy" cytoplasmic projections (hairy cells).[18] Monoclonal surface immunoglobulin (restricted light chain) is frequently identified on the surface of hairy cells. Therefore, hairy cell leukemia is most consistent with a B-cell malignancy.[19] These cells also contain cytoplasmic acid phosphatase, which is tartrate resistant.[20]

Acute Lymphoblastic Leukemia

Acute lymphoblastic leukemia (ALL) is characterized by the presence of increased blast cells in the bone marrow that frequently disseminate to the peripheral blood. Although their rate of proliferation is often slower than that of normal blast cells in the bone marrow, the leukemic blast cells maintain their ability to divide for a long period of time, resulting in their accumulation in the reticuloendothelial tissues.[21] They are also able to invade other organ systems, including spleen, liver, lymph node, meninges, testes, kidney, and skin.

ALL consists of a heterogeneous group of diseases that is divided into three major types: T-cell ALL; B-cell ALL; and non-T, non-B ALL. The non-T, non-B ALL is further classified into common ALL (cALL), which is CALLA positive, and "null-cell" ALL, which is CALLA negative. The preceding grouping predicts the prognosis in terms of survival; thus, cALL has the most favorable prognosis, followed by null-cell ALL, T-cell ALL, and B-cell ALL. The markers that are frequently utilized in a clinical laboratory for typing ALLs are listed in Table 26-1.

T-Cell ALL

T-cell ALL represents approximately 15% to 25% of all ALL cases. The characteristic clinical features include high blast cell count, predominance in older

Table 26-1: Cell Markers Frequently Used for ALL Typing

	HLA-DR	CALLA	IgG R	Cμ	SIg	TdT	CD2
Common ALL	+	+	+	−	−	+	−
Null ALL	+	−	+	−	−	+	−
Pre–B ALL	+	+	+	+	−	+	−
B-cell ALL	+	+	+	−	+	−	−
T-cell ALL	−	+/−	−	−	−	+	+/−

CALLA: Common acute lymphoblastic leukemia associated antigen.
IgG R: Receptor for IgG.
Cμ: Cytoplasmic IgM heavy chain.
SIg: Surface immunoglobulin.
TdT: Terminal deoxynucleotidyl transferase.
CD2: Sheep red blood cell receptor.

male patients, and presence of mediastinal mass. The leukemic cells form rosettes with sheep red blood cells, are CD2 positive, but lack MHC class II molecules. They also contain the cytoplasmic enzyme TdT. Approximately 10% to 25% of T-cell ALL cases express CALLA.

B-Cell ALL

B-cell ALL represents less than 3% of ALL cases. B-cell ALL in children is probably a leukemic phase of Burkitt's lymphoma. The leukemic cells express surface immunoglobulin, Fc receptor, and complement receptors (C3d and C3b), indicating that the malignant cells derive from the follicular center. Pre–B-cell ALL is a unique malignancy in which the neoplastic B cells are arrested at the maturational stage in which only the heavy-chain gene rearrangement has occurred. Therefore, the cells are able to synthesize only IgM heavy chain (μ chain) but not light chain. These malignant cells are identified by the presence of cytoplasmic μ chains. They also express CALLA, TdT, and MHC class II molecules.

Non-T, Non-B ALL

Non-T, non-B ALL does not express any conventional T- or B-cell markers. Based on the expression of CALLA, these are divided into two groups: Common ALL (cALL) is CALLA positive, whereas null-cell ALL is CALLA negative. However, both groups express MHC class II molecule, Fc receptor, and nuclear TdT. Approximately 70% of ALL are cALL. The clinical features of cALL include a younger patient population and markedly elevated leukocyte count. The disease is not usually associated with mediastinal mass, lymphadenopathy, or hepatosplenomegaly. Null-cell ALL is CALLA negative, with a prognosis next to that of cALL.

Plasma Cell Dyscrasias

Plasma cell dyscrasias include multiple myeloma, Walsenstrom's macroglobulinemia, heavy-chain diseases, and light-chain diseases. These are discussed in Chapter 25.

References

1. Greaves MF, Brown G, Rapson NT, et al: Antisera to acute lymphoblastic leukemia cells. Clin Immunol Immunopathol 4:67, 1975

2. Foon KA, Todd RF: Review: Immunologic classification of leukemia and lymphoma. Blood 68:1, 1986

3. The non-Hodgkin's lymphoma pathologic classification project: National Cancer Institute sponsored study of classification of non-Hodgkin's lymphomas: Summary and description of a working formulation for clinical usage. Cancer 49:2112, 1982

4. Hoffman-Fizer G, Knapp W, Thierfelder S: Anatomical distribution of CALL antigen-expressing cells in normal tissue and in lymphoma. Leuk Res 6:761, 1982

5. Stein H, Gerdes J, Lemke H, et al: The normal and malignant germinal center. Clin Haematol 11:531, 1982

6. Greaves M, Delia D, Janossy G, et al: Acute lymphoblastic leukemia associated antigen. IV Expression on non-leukemic lymphoid cells. Leuk Res 4:15, 1980

7. Bollum FJ: Terminal deoxynucleotidyl transferase. In Boyer PD (ed): The Enzyme, Vol 10, p 145. Orlando, FL, Academic Press, 1974

8. Greenwood MF, Coleman MS, Hutton JJ, et al: Terminal deoxynucleotidyl transferase distribution in neoplastic and hematopoietic cells. J Clin Invest 59:889, 1977

9. Marks SM, Baltimore D, McCaffrey R: Terminal transferase as a prediction of initial responsiveness to vincristine and prednisone in blastic chronic myelogenous leukemia. N Engl J Med 298:812, 1978

10. Thomas MG: Hodgkin's disease. In Jaffe ES (ed): Surgical Pathology of the Lymph Nodes and Related Organs, p 86. Philadelphia, WB Saunders, 1985

11. Kaplan HS: Review: Hodgkin's disease: Biology, treatment, and prognosis. Blood 57:813, 1981

12. Rappaport H: Tumors of the hematopoietic system. In Atlas of Tumor Pathology, section 3, fascicle 8. Washington, DC, US Armed Forces Institute of Pathology, 1966

13. Edelson RL: Cutaneous T cell lymphoma: Mycosis fungoides, Sézary syndrome, and other variants. J Am Acad Dermatol 2:89, 1980

14. Harris TJ, Bhan AK, Murphy E, et al: Lymphomatoid papulosis and lymphomatoid granulomatosis: T cell subset populations. Refined microscopic morphology and direct immunofluorescence observations. Clin Res 29:579, 1981

15. McMillan EM, Wasik R, Beeman K, et al: In situ immunologic phenotyping of mycosis fungoides. J Am Acad Dermatol 6:888, 1982

16. Van Der Reigden HJ, Van Der Gaag R, Pinkster J, et al: Chronic lymphocytic leukemia: Immunologic markers and functional properties of the leukemic cells. Cancer 50:2826, 1982

17. Huhn D, Theil E, Rodt H, et al: Subtype of T-cell chronic lymphocytic leukemia. Cancer 51:1434, 1983

18. Golomb HM: Hairy cell leukemia: Lesson learned in twenty-five years. J Clin Oncol 1:652, 1983

19. Golomb HM, Davis S, Wilson C, et al: Surface immunoglobulin in hairy cells of 55 patients with hairy cell leukemia. Am J Hematol 12:397, 1982

20. Variakojis D, Vardiman JW, Golomb HM: Cytochemistry of hairy cells. Cancer 45:72, 1980

21. Shumacker HR, Garven DF, Triplett DA: Acute Leukemia. In: Introduction to Laboratory Hematology and Hematopathology, p 109. New York, Alan R Liss, 1984

CHAPTER 27

Allergy

Catherine Sheehan

The wide spectrum of allergic conditions includes allergic rhinitis (hay fever), extrinsic asthma, urticaria (hives), anaphylaxis, and atopic dermatitis.[1] The term *allergy* refers to a harmful reaction experienced by some people to commonly encountered environmental antigens. Why are some people allergic to ragweed, cats, pollen, milk, penicillin, or bee stings? The answer rests in part with the overproduction of IgE in response to one or more exogenous antigens. Exogenous antigens are called allergens when they provoke an overproduction of IgE. Allergic patients will produce an abnormally large amount of specific IgE when exposed to very small quantities of an antigen. This abnormal response, called atopy, is frequently inherited. If both parents are atopic for hay fever or asthma, there is a 75% chance that the child will be atopic. If one parent is affected, there is a 50% chance that the child will develop symptoms.[2] Atopic disease is very common, affecting approximately 10% of the population. Seasonal allergic rhinitis (hayfever) is the most common form of allergy.[1]

Overview of Immediate Hypersensitivity

All of us can and do synthesize IgE. Allergic individuals simply produce too much IgE, resulting in immediate hypersensitivity. Allergens stimulate B lymphocytes to undergo blastogenesis, transforming them into plasma cells capable of producing and secreting IgE. The IgE produced is complementary for the allergen that induced its production. The lymphoid cells capable of producing IgE are located in the tissue that lines the respiratory, genitourinary, and gastrointestinal tracts and can react with allergens from the external environment. IgE is homocytotropic, which means it binds to basophils and mast cells in the individual that produced the IgE. The binding occurs by way of the Fc(ϵ) receptor on the basophil or mast cell membrane of the host. Subsequently, when the sensitizing allergen is encountered, the membrane-bound IgE recognizes the allergen. If the allergen cross-links two membrane-bound IgE molecules, the cell becomes activated (see Fig. 6-3).

Activated mast cells release preformed chemical mediators stored in their granules and synthesize other mediators. The principal preformed mediators are histamine and eosinophil chemotactic factor (ECF). Histamine, a bioactive amine, is responsible for bronchoconstriction, increased mucus production, pruritus, vasopermeability, and vasodilation. Early symptoms of immediate hypersensitivity are caused by the action of released histamine. ECF attracts eosinophils to the area of activated mast cells; eosinophils contain chemicals, such as histaminase, that inactivate mediators released from mast cells and modulate immediate hypersensitivity. Increased numbers of eosinophils in the blood, eosinophilia, is a common laboratory finding in 10% to 20% of people who are experiencing allergic episodes.[2]

Mediators synthesized after initial mast cell stimulation are leukotrienes, prostaglandin D_2, and platelet-activating factor. The leukotrienes (LTC_4, LTD_4, and LTE_4) are generated by mast cells and basophils from membrane-derived arachidonic acid by way of the lipoxygenase pathway. They are potent bronchial smooth muscle constrictors and stimulate mucus production and secretion. Prostaglandin D_2 is produced in mast cells and is derived from arachidonic acid through the cyclo-oxygenase pathway in mast cells. It causes a wheal and flare reaction (hives) similar to that caused by histamine.[3] Platelet-activating factor is a phosphorylcholine derivative that is chemotactic for neutrophils, aggregates platelets, increases vascular permeability, and constricts the bronchial smooth muscle.[3,4]

Types of Immediate Hypersensitivity Reactions

Immediate hypersensitivity reactions occur most commonly in tissues rich in mast cells: skin, nasal membranes, tongue, lungs, and gastrointestinal tract.[3] Inhaled allergens, such as animal danders, dust, pollen, and molds, are responsible for allergic rhinitis. Attacks occur only when the allergen is present. For some this is seasonal (when certain pollens are available), and for others, it is perennial (when an offending allergen, such as house dust, is always available). If the immediate hypersensitivity reaction is localized in the nasal mucosa and conjunctiva, symptoms include rhinorrhea (runny nose), itching eyes and nose, sneezing, and nasal congestion. Elevated levels of eosinophils are present in nasal secretions and blood. Serum IgE may or may not be elevated.

If the immediate hypersensitivity reaction is localized in the bronchus, allergic (intrinsic) asthma results. Symptoms of bronchial involvement are tightness of chest, shortness of breath, and wheezing. Inhaled allergens may directly combine with IgE on bronchial mast cells, whereas ingested or injected allergens circulate to the lung, then combine with the mast cells. In either case, stimulation of the mast cells releases histamine and leukotrienes to contract the bronchial smooth muscle. Frequently, serum IgE is elevated.

Atopic dermatitis is commonly associated with allergic rhinitis, intrinsic asthma, eosinophilia, and very high levels of serum IgE. Skin testing does not generate useful information about the allergen. Patients with atopic dermatitis often have dry skin and pruritus (itching). Allergens, such as pollen, house dust, animal dander, milk, and grains, may be responsible for atopic dermatitis.

Food allergies or allergic gastroenteropathy is the least common form of atopy. Ingested food allergens can stimulate the local production of IgE, which can bind to mast cells in the gut. Local degranulation of mast cells and release of stored mediators promotes the food allergy. Signs and symptoms include nausea, vomiting, cramps, abdominal pain, and diarrhea —usually within 2 hours of allergen ingestion. Gastrointestinal loss of protein and blood may lead to anemia and hypoproteinemia. In infants the disease is transient; in adults it is uncommon.

Anaphylaxis is the sytemic form of immediate hypersensitivity. It can affect more than one organ and is potentially life-threatening when the allergic reaction causes shock or edema of the upper respiratory tract. Most often the precipitating allergen is food (peanuts, seafood, or egg albumin), insect venom (honeybee, wasp, or hornet stings), or drugs (vaccines, penicillin, and sulfonamides). Increased vascular permeability can result in leakage of plasma from the blood into extravascular tissue, resulting in decreased blood volume; the resultant decreased cardiac output may contribute to hypoxemia and acidemia leading to respiratory failure.[5]

Clinical and Laboratory Evaluation of Immediate Hypersensitivity

Skin Testing

Patient history and physical examination may suggest that an allergy is present. If atopic allergy is suspected, skin testing with many different allergens may identify the allergen responsible for the symptoms. Three skin testing techniques can demonstrate increased numbers of IgE-coated mast cells: scratch testing, prick testing (epicutaneous scratch), and intradermal testing. In each method, when the allergen is recognized by the IgE on the surface of mast cells in the skin, histamine is released within minutes, causing the characteristic wheal (localized edema from increased vascular permeability) and flare (vasodilatation) with pruritus. The scratch test is performed by scratching the volar surface of the forearms or the back, then applying an allergen to the scratch. The prick test is accomplished by applying a drop of allergen to the skin surface then pricking the skin directly underneath the drop. After 15 to 30 minutes, the areas are observed for the presence of wheal and erythema. If the results of the prick or scratch tests are equivocal, the intradermal test should be performed. In the intradermal test a small volume of allergen is injected into the epidermis of the upper arm or forearm, resulting in the formation of a mound of fluid 3 to 4 mm in diameter. After 20 minutes the area is observed for the wheal and erythema.

Total Serum IgE Levels

Another approach to assess atopic allergic individuals is to measure serum IgE *in vitro*. The concentration of total serum IgE in nonatopic individuals is low and varies with age. During the first year of life, total serum IgE concentration is less than 10 IU/mL. The level rises during childhood, peaks in adolescence, and declines after age 65.[6] In the majority of nonatopic North American adults, the serum IgE level ranges from 30 to 80 IU/mL; the mean adult level is 40 IU/mL.[6,7] Variation in the serum IgE concentration between individuals of the same age exists, including an overlap in serum IgE levels between atopic and nonatopic individuals. Generally, when the level of total IgE is greater than 100 IU/mL (95th percentile), IgE-mediated disease is present. Total serum IgE concentration may predict the risk of developing allergic disease in asymptomatic infants where there is a family history of allergy.[6,8]

Methods to detect total IgE include competitive radioimmunosorbent test (RIST), noncompetitive RIST, double-antibody radioimmunoassay (RIA), and sandwich enzyme-linked immunosorbent assay (ELISA) and are shown in Fig. 27-1. Competitive or indirect RIST is a competitive RIA based on the simultaneous incubation of radiolabeled IgE and reference or unknown IgE with an anti-IgE bound to a solid phase. The greater the concentration of the reference or unknown IgE, the fewer radiolabeled

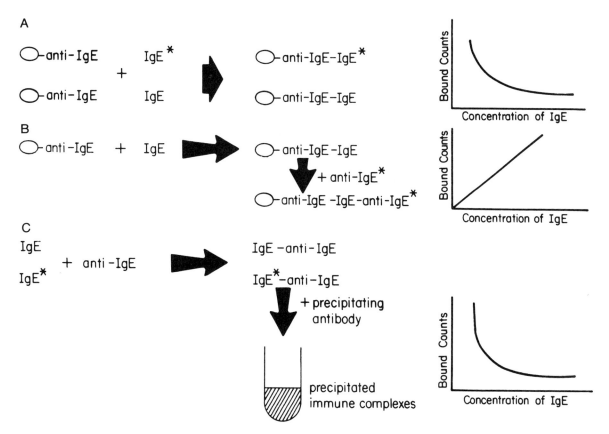

FIGURE 27-1. Methods to detect total serum IgE. (*A*) Competitive radioimmunosorbent test. Labeled IgE* and unlabeled IgE compete for the solid phase anti-IgE. (*B*) Noncompetitive or indirect radioimmunosorbent test. Immobilized anti-IgE captures IgE; radiolabeled anti-IgE is added and detects the bound IgE. (*C*) Double antibody RIA. Labeled IgE* and unlabeled IgE compete for soluble anti-IgE antibody; subsequently, a precipitating antibody is added to precipitate bound IgE*.

IgE that bind to the solid phase. There is a corresponding decrease in measured counts per minute (CPM).

Direct or noncompetitive RIST is a sandwich-type RIA in which solid-phase anti-IgE is incubated with reference or unknown IgE; the bound IgE then reacts with radiolabeled anti-human IgE. The greater the concentration of the reference or unknown IgE, the greater the concentration of radiolabeled anti-human IgE that binds, which is indicated by higher CPM.

The double antibody RIA or radioimmuno-precipitation test involves the liquid-phase incubation of reference or unknown IgE and radiolabeled IgE with anti–human IgE. Resulting complexes are precipitated by adding a second, precipitating antibody. The greater the concentration of reference or unknown IgE, the fewer radiolabeled IgE present in the precipitate. At one time the double-antibody method was preferred because of its sensitivity and reproducibility. Currently, ease of performance and commercial availability favors the use of direct RIST.[9]

Modifications in testing procedures have included the development of enzyme-labeled assays in which enzyme activity is monitored by measuring the change in absorbance resulting from a change in concentration of substrate or product.[10,11]

Total serum IgE is reported in international units (IU) per milliliter; 1 IU is equivalent to 2.4 ng of IgE protein.[9,12,13] Standardization of total IgE immunoassay against a reference preparation is necessary to assure the accuracy and comparability of interlaboratory assay results. In 1981 the second International Reference Preparation (75/502) of human serum IgE became available from the World Health Organization. A U.S. Reference Preparation is available from the National Institutes of Health and contains 900 IU/mL of IgE.[14] A trilevel Canadian IgE Reference Preparation is available through the Canadian Society for Allergy and Clinical Immunology.[13]

Total IgE is generally, though not always, elevated in atopic individuals. In children, an elevated serum IgE concentration suggests the likelihood of developing an allergic disease—especially if one or both parents have allergic disease. A normal IgE concentration, however, does not exclude the possibility of allergic disease in infancy or later in life. In older children or adults, some patients with atopic disease have elevated serum IgE levels; others do not. Again, low serum levels do not exclude the presence of IgE-mediated hypersensitivity. IgE may also be elevated in diseases other than allergy, such as Wiskott-Aldrich syndrome, Hyper-IgE syndrome, and parasitic infections.

Quantitation of Allergen-Specific IgE

The radioallergosorbent test (RAST) is the serologic quantitation of IgE antibodies directed against specific allergens.[15] This *in vitro* test yields information similar to skin testing. In fact, RAST testing may be preferred when skin testing is difficult to perform (in a young child) or interpret (when a second skin condition exists), when skin testing is negative, or when medication interference is suspected.[9] This test is a sandwich-type immunoassay in which the solid phase is coated with allergen. After incubation with reference or unknown sera, the specific allergen will capture IgE. Radiolabeled anti–human IgE is added to detect the bound IgE. The greater the amount of allergen-specific IgE bound, the greater the CPM of bound labeled IgE. When enzyme-labeled anti–human IgE replaces the radiolabeled antibody, the change in absorbance is measured.

There are two classifications to score and evaluate results of the RAST method. In the first, the average patient counts per minute are compared with the average counts per minute of the reference sera. The reference serum is a standardized pool of human serum containing a high content of IgE directed against specific allergens such as birch tree or perennial ryegrass. The greater the content of IgE, the greater the counts per minute that are measured. A standard curve establishes the relationship between the concentration of several reference sera and the CPM or absorbance; from this the IgE concentration in patient or control sera is assigned. The patient results are graded from 0 to 4, indicating an increasing amount of specific IgE.

The second classification is a modification of the RAST scoring system. The patient counts are expressed as a percentage of the time control or positive control. The time control is the time required for the IgE standard (with a concentration of 25 U/mL) to record 25,000 counts; all specimens will then be counted for that period of time. The reading of the negative serum control is the second point to be plotted. A straight line is drawn between the readings of the negative control and the 25 IU/mL standard. The line is divided into five sections, defining classes from 0 to 5; the higher the class, the greater the level of allergen-specific IgE that is present.[10,11] The time control minimizes variation in allergen, an-

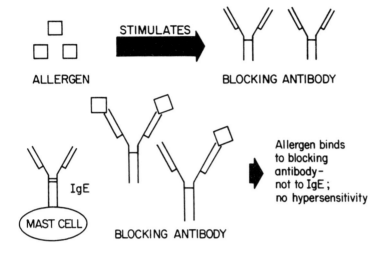

FIGURE 27-2. Principle of immunotherapy. Injections of the offending allergen stimulate the production of blocking antibodies. When the allergen is encountered later, it will be neutralized by the blocking antibody and will not bind the IgE-sensitized mast cells.

tibody affinity, and radioactive decay rates, so that more reliable results are generated.[16] Procedural modifications for better low-end sensitivity include longer incubation time with the labeled anti–human IgE and transferring the solid phase to a clean tube prior to quantitation.

New methodologies continue to emerge. The FAST (fluoroallergosorbent test) is a fluorescent enzyme immunoassay test in which total or specific IgE can be quantitated. FAST is a sandwich immunoassay in which the allergen is bound to the solid-phase membrane in the bottom of microtitration wells; following incubation with patient or reference serum, an enzyme-labeled anti–human IgE is added. The fluorescence is measured.[17] The MAST[R] (MAST[R] Immunosystems, Mountain View, CA) chemiluminescent assay (CLA) is a sandwich CLA in which a solid-phase cellulose thread is impregnated with a battery of allergens; after incubation with patient or reference serum, enzyme-labeled anti–human IgE is added.[18,19] The enzyme label reacts with photoreagents to produce light. When the light is exposed to photographic film, a permanent record, an immunograph, is produced. Most recently, enzyme immunoassay dipstick methods have been introduced as screening tests for total IgE and for some common allergens. The short time required to perform the tests and the visual endpoint are advantages of these screening tests.

Treatment

Treatment includes allergen avoidance, drug therapy, and immunotherapy. Ideally, once an allergen is defined, it should be avoided. Food and drug allergies can be best managed this way. Controlling household dust, avoiding household pets, and preventing mold are ways of controlling allergens.[1]

Drug therapy is directed at controlling allergic symptoms. Antihistamines antagonize the effect of histamine by competing for the histamine H_1 receptors on target cells. Increased vascular permeability, vasodilatation, itching, bronchial smooth muscle contraction, and gastrointestinal mucosal smooth muscle contraction can be blocked by antihistamine therapy. Antihistamine therapy is useful in allergic rhinitis. Cromolyn (disodium cromoglycate) protects asthmatic patients by preventing the release of mediators from mast cells. When it is administered prior to exposure to the allergen, bronchial spasm can be prevented. Asthma is often treated with theophylline, a methylxanthine that relaxes bronchial smooth muscle.

Immunotherapy or hyposensitization is the planned introduction of an allergen into a patient to reduce the IgE allergic response (Fig. 27-2). Allergic rhinitis, extrinsic asthma, and insect venom anaphylaxis may respond to this therapy. The allergen is injected weekly in gradually increasing doses. After an initial increase in circulating specific IgE, there is a decline. More importantly, allergen-specific IgG blocking antibody appears in the serum. This IgG binds to the allergen and prevents the allergen from stimulating mast cells, thus preventing the allergic reaction. The maximum tolerated dose or the maintenance dose is then administered less frequently, every 2 to 6 weeks, to maintain sufficient IgG blocking antibody to alleviate the symptoms.

References

1. Terr AI: Allergic diseases. In Stites DP, Stobo JD, Wells JV (eds): Basic and Clinical Immunology, 6th ed, p 435. East Norwalk, Appleton and Lange, 1987

2. Frick OL: Immediate hypersensitivity. In Stites DP, Stobo JD, Wells JV (eds): Basic and Clinical Immunology, 6th ed, p 197. East Norwalk, Appleton and Lange, 1987

3. Serafin WE, Austin KF: Mediators of immediate hypersensitivity reactions. N Engl J Med 317:30, 1987

4. Parker CW: Allergic Mediators. In Korenblat PE, Wedner HJ (eds): Allergy: Theory and Practice. Orlando, Grune and Stratton, 1984

5. Shatz GS: Anaphylaxis. In Korenblat PE, Wedner HJ (eds): Allergy: Theory and Practice. Orlando, Grune and Stratton, 1984

6. Halpern GM: Markers in human allergic disease. J Clin Immunoassay 6:131, 1983

7. Barbee RA, Halonen M, Lebowitz M, et al: Distribution of IgE in a community population sample: Correlations with age, sex and allergen skin test reactivity. J Allergy Clin Immunol 68:106, 1981

8. Orgel HA: Genetic and development aspects of IgE. Ped Clin North Am 22(1):17, 1975

9. Adkinson NF Jr: Measurement of total serum immunoglobulin E and allergen-specific immunoglobulin E antibody. In Rose NR, Friedman H, Fahey JL (eds): Manual of Clinical Laboratory Immunology, 3rd ed, p 664. Washington, DC, American Society for Microbiology, 1986

10. Hamilton RG, Adkinson NF Jr: Clinical laboratory methods for the assessment and management of human allergic diseases. Clin Lab Med 6(1):117, 1986

11. Hamilton RG, Adkinson NF Jr: Serological methods in the diagnosis and management of human allergic disease. CRC Critical Reviews in Clinical Laboratory Sciences 21(1):1, 1984

12. Homburger HA: Current status of laboratory tests for allergic disease. In Rippey JH, Nakamura RM (eds): Diagnostic Immunology: Technology Assessment and Quality Assurance, p 195. Skokie, College of American Pathologists, 1983

13. Mandy FF, Perelmutter L: Laboratory measurement of total human serum IgE. J Clin Immunoassay 6:140, 1983

14. Evans R: A U.S. reference for human immunoglobulin E. J Allerg Clin Immunol 68:79, 1981

15. Wide C, Bennich H, Johansson SGO: Diagnosis of allergy by an in-vitro test for allergen antibodies. Lancet 2:1105, 1967

16. Ali M, Nalebuff DJ, Fadal RG, et al: Allergy testing: From *in vivo* to *in vitro*. Diag Med, May/June:3, 1982

17. Rodriquez GE: A new IgE fluorescent allergosorbent test (FAST). Clinical Immunology Newsletter 9:81, 1988

18. Miller SP, Marinkovich VA, Riege DH, et al: Application of the MAST™ immunodiagnostic system to the determination of allergen-specific IgE. Clin Chem 30:1467, 1984

19. Brown CR, Higgins KW, Fazer K, et al: Simultaneous determination of total IgE and allergen-specific IgE in serum by the MAST chemiluminescent assay system. Clin Chem 31:1500, 1985

CHAPTER 28

Immune Deficiency

T. B. Datiles
R. L. Humphrey

Deficiency of the immune system had been considered rare until the emergence of acquired immune deficiency syndrome (AIDS). At the current rate, more than 350 new cases of AIDS are being reported each week. Apart from AIDS, the most common deficiencies of cellular and/or humoral immunity are secondary to some underlying abnormality or disease process. For example, immune deficiency (ID) states are observed in acquired lymphoreticular tissue diseases (*e.g.*, myeloma, lymphoma) or occur after prolonged treatment with cytotoxic and immunosuppressive drugs. The hereditary or primary immunodeficiency states are quite rare.

Despite their rarity, careful study of these conditions provides important insights into the organization and function of the normal immune system. A schematic diagram of the organization of the immune system is provided by Figure 28-1, which depicts the development and differentiation of the immune system into two main compartments, the cellular immune system and the humoral immune system. In the cellular arm the main effector agent is the T cell; in the humoral arm it is the antibody molecule.

The ID state is caused by an impairment of various host defense mechanisms, resulting in decreased resistance to infectious agents (*e.g.*, bacteria, viruses, fungi, parasites). This impairment includes abnormalities of stem cells, thymus, gut-associated lymphoid tissue (GALT), T and B lymphocytes and phagocytes; impairment of the complement system and other amplifying systems (*e.g.*, production of interleukin-1 or -2 and MIF); or impairment of general health status (*e.g.*, starvation, diabetes, uremia).

Primary ID are grouped according to whether the defect is chiefly humoral or cellular or whether there are a combination of defects. Figure 28-1 indicates the presumed locus of the defect for a number of the prototype immune deficiency states. Table 28-1 outlines some of the commonly used tests that help to

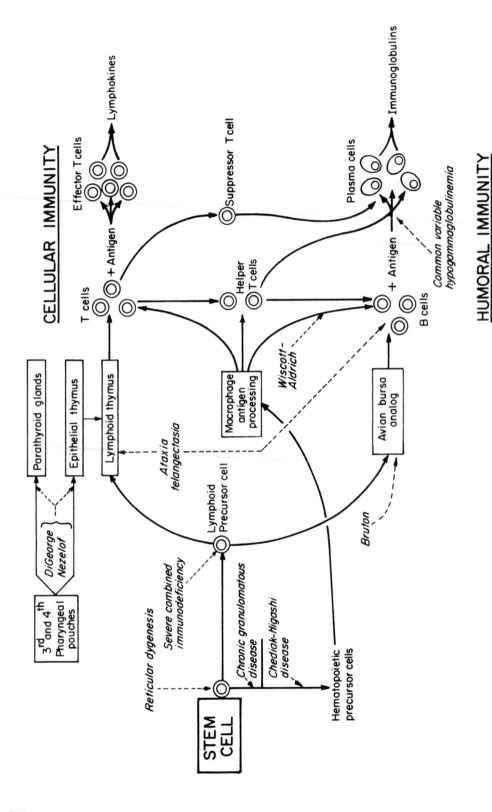

FIGURE 28-1. Diagrammatic representation of the ontogeny and organization of the mammalian immune system, emphasizing its two main functional divisions, cellular immunity and humoral immunity. The dashed lines indicate the presumed locus of the defects responsible for some of the prototype immune deficiency states discussed in the text.

Table 28-1: Laboratory Evaluation of Immunocompetence

Test	Comment
HUMORAL IMMUNITY	
Immunoglobulin survey (serum protein electrophoresis, Ig quantitation, immunofixation electrophoresis, IgG subclass levels)	General assessment of B-cell function
Isohemagglutinin titer (anti-A, anti-B)	General indicator of IgM production
Titers before and after immunization with a specific vaccine (tetanus toxoid, pneumovax, typhoid–paratyphoid)	Demonstrates the *in vivo* ability to respond to a known antigen (tests both the afferent and efferent loops of B-cell function)
B-cell enumeration by surface Ig (SIg) or flow cytometry	Measures the number of circulating B-cells (normally 10% to 20% of the total peripheral blood lymphocytes)
Biopsy of bone marrow, lymph node, or gut	Assessment of the presence and/or location of lymphocytes (germinal centers, plasma cells)
CELL-MEDIATED IMMUNITY	
Peripheral lymphocyte count and morphology	General assessment of T-cell presence (normally 80% to 90% of total blood lymphocytes)
T-cell enumeration by nonimmune rosetting or flow cytometry (CD3)	Measures the total number of T cells in the peripheral blood (normally, >1200 cells/μL)
Enumeration of T-cell subsets (CD4, CD8)	The T_H/T_S ratio is usually 2:1
Measurement of lymphokine production (MIF, IL-2)	Assessment of the T-cell ability to secrete lymphokines
Response to phytohemagglutinin or mixed lymphocyte culture	Evaluation of the T-cell ability to undergo blastogenesis
Delayed hypersensitivity skin testing to recall antigens (PPD, histoplasmin, trichophyton, *Candida*, mumps, streptokinase–streptodornase)	Assessment of the *in vivo* function of T cells to a previously encountered antigen (tests the efferent loop of T-cell function)
Dinitrochlorobenzene skin (DNCB) sensitization	Assessment of the *in vivo* function of T cells to respond to a newly encountered antigen (tests both the afferent and efferent loops of T-cell function)
Biopsy of lymph node	Assessment of the presence of T cells in thymus-dependent areas

define the immune deficiencies that might be present in a given patient. Table 28-2 outlines the patterns of lymphocyte markers seen in the prototype immune deficiency states described in the following sections.

Humoral ID or agammaglobulinemia is characterized by recurrent bacterial infection. Patients are chronically ill. Children usually have retarded growth. Tonsils and lymph nodes are small and serum immunoglobulin levels are low or absent.

Cellular ID is characterized by severe viral or fungal infections. Patients are chronically ill and growth may be retarded. Tonsils and lymph nodes

Table 28-2: Lymphocytes in Immunodeficiency Diseases

	T-Cell Markers				B-Cell Markers
	CD3	CD4	CD8	CD4/8	SIg
I. Primary immunodeficiency					
A. Humoral					
1. Bruton's X-linked agammaglobulinemia	N-↑	↓-N	N	N	0-↓↓
2. Selective IgA deficiency	N	↓-N	N-↑	20% ↑ 10% ↓	N
3. Common variable ID	↓-N	↓-N-↑	↓-N-↑	25% ↓ 15% ↑	↓↓-N
B. Cellular					
1. DiGeorge syndrome	0-↓↓	↓↓	↓↓	N	↑
2. Nezelof's syndrome	↓↓	↓	↓	N	N
C. Combined humoral and cellular					
1. Severe					
a. SCID (autosomal recessive)	0-↓↓	↓↓	↓↓	N	N-↑
b. SCID (general hematopoietic hypoplasia)	0-↓↓	↓↓	↓↓	N	↓↓
2. Partial					
a. Wiskott-Aldrich	↓	↓	↓	N	N
b. Ataxia-telangiectasia	↓	↓	N-↑	↓	N
II. Secondary immunodeficiency					
1. Viral diseases					
a. AIDS	N-↓	↓↓	N-↑	↓↓	N-↓

0 = absent
N = normal

are small and thymus is absent. Disseminated vaccinia occurs when there is vaccination against smallpox. Similar dissemination may occur if other live vaccines, such as bacillus Calmette-Guérin (BCG) or polio, are used. Graft-versus-host reaction may develop if live immunocompetent cells are transferred by blood or platelet transfusion. Early infant deaths or similarly affected siblings are observed in the family history.

The combined IDs are subdivided into severe or partial combined ID. The severe combined ID (SCID) is characterized by severe deficiency of both T and B lymphocytes, which may be due to underlying defects in stem cells. Survival is limited to a few days after birth to a few months and is characterized by recurrent, severe, and overwhelming infections.

In the following sections some of the more common and well-understood examples of these disorders will be described as prototypes to illustrate the major features of this group of diseases. More than 70 ID syndromes have been described, some involving only a few patients. This emphasizes the complex web of cells and their interactions in the normal immune system and illustrates that there are a great many ways in which the system can become impaired. These complex relationships are suggested in Figure 28-1, which is necessarily a schematic oversimplification. A number of comprehensive reviews are available for further study.[1-6]

Primary Immune Deficiency

Humoral Immune Deficiency

Bruton's X-Linked Agammaglobulinemia

X-linked agammaglobulinemia, a congenital inherited disorder, was first reported in a male infant by Bruton in 1952. When maternal immunoglobulins (Ig) disappear at about 6 months of age, the deficiency of all classes of Ig becomes apparent, and recurrent, life-threatening pyogenic infections are observed. Pyogenic organisms most often involved are *Streptococcus pneumoniae* and *Haemophilus influenzae*, and the recurrent infections are pneumonia, sinusitis, bronchitis, otitis, furunculosis, meningitis, and septicemia. Fungal infections are usually not a significant problem. *Pneumocystis carinii* pneumonia rarely occurs unless neutropenia is present.

Infections with viruses usually do not cause severe complications, the exceptions being viral hepatitis and enterovirus infections, which can be fulminant and even fatal. Fatal central nervous system infections have occurred with echoviruses.

Live virus vaccines are usually handled normally. Paralysis has occurred in several patients after polio vaccination, possibly due to mutation of this vaccine from an enterovirus to a more neurotropic form.

Serum concentrations of IgG, IgA, and IgM are markedly reduced and functional levels of antibody are absent. Antigenic stimulation by bacterial infections or by injected soluble or particulate antigens produces no demonstrable antibody response.

T-cell subset percentages are usually normal, though the total number of T cells is usually increased. The thymus is histologically normal; however, B cells are markedly decreased or absent. The defect seems to be a block in pre–B-cell differentiation to B cells, because the normal number of pre–B cells is found in the bone marrow. The lymph nodes, adenoids, and tonsils are small and hypoplastic and lack germinal centers. Plasma cells are completely absent from lymph nodes, Peyer's patches, appendix, and bone marrow.

Treatment consists of prompt use of appropriate antimicrobials and chronic administration of γ globulin. The prophylactic use of antibiotics is not advisable, because it is not likely to prevent most infections and may result in colonization with antibiotic-resistant bacteria. Long-term results are fairly good, but these patients often develop chronic lung disease because of destruction of lung parenchyma by repeated infections. They are also prone to develop leukemia and lymphoma.

Selective IgA Deficiency

The incidence of isolated IgA deficiency in the general population is about one case per 500 to 700. A recent study done with Tennessee blood donors demonstrated a ratio of IgA deficiency to normals of 1:333. Markedly reduced or total absence of serum and secretory IgA (<10 mg/dL) is the hallmark of this disorder. The mode of inheritance varies among families. In some families it seems to be a recessive trait; others have a dominant form of transmission. Equal occurrence in male and female suggests autosomal inheritance. Selective IgA deficiency can be caused by some drugs (e.g., phenytoin sodium and penicillamine); however, the disorder is corrected when these drugs are stopped.

Most of these individuals are asymptomatic, but some individuals suffer from recurrent infections. These infections commonly occur in the respiratory, gastrointestinal, and urogenital tracts. This deficiency is associated with other syndromes, such as allergies, autoimmune disorders, various malignancies, malabsorption, and mental retardation.

A serious difficulty for some patients is the presence of anti-IgA antibodies (the incidence of which is as high as 44% in some series), which can lead to gastrointestinal symptoms after milk ingestion. These anti-IgA antibodies may interfere with the laboratory measurement of IgA. Patients with such antibodies may face a serious complication (e.g., anaphylaxis) when blood or plasma that contains IgA is administered. Similarly, if IgA is administered in a blood product, antibodies may develop so that life-threatening anaphylaxis may result later when another blood product is administered. Patients with IgA deficiency should be warned to avoid exposure to IgA and hence avoid being immunized against this immunoglobulin.

Sinopulmonary hygiene and specific antibiotic therapy are currently the only available treatment. No commercial source of IgA is available for administration; in addition, there would be serious reservations about its use, because anaphylaxis may result

and the IgA would not be transported to the mucous membrane surface, where its presence and function are needed.

A study of 11 IgA-deficient individuals suggests a B-cell maturation arrest, because their IgA-bearing B cells failed to mature into IgA-secreting plasma cells.[7]

The normal production and maturation of B cells destined to produce IgA depend heavily on helper T-cell activity. Helper-to-suppressor ratios (and function?) are abnormal in bone marrow transplantation patients (especially allogeneic transplants), and it is observed that this class of immunoglobulin is low or absent for prolonged periods in the posttransplant patient. This relationship may also suggest that subtle abnormalities in T-cell function may contribute to the IgA deficiency state.

Common Variable Immunodeficiency (Acquired Agammaglobulinemia)

Immunodeficiency may occur in adults with a history of previous good health. The presumption is that their immune system was previously normal and that it is therefore an acquired disorder. Clinically, this ID is similar to the X-linked agammaglobulinemia, as shown by marked decrease in serum Ig concentration and similar infections caused by *S. pneumoniae* and *H. influenzae*. The main differences are the adult onset, less severe infections, almost equal sex distribution, normal-sized or enlarged tonsils and lymph nodes, and splenomegaly.

Other conditions that may develop are collagen vascular disorders (rheumatoid arthritis, dermatomyositis), malabsorption (*Giardia lamblia* is common in this disorder, though rare in X-linked agammaglobulinemia), hemolytic anemia, pernicious anemia, bronchiectasis, gastric carcinoma, lymphoreticular malignancy, and cholelithiasis. Recurrent infections of paranasal sinuses and middle ear and bacterial conjunctivitis are also common. Though bacterial infection responds well to antibiotic treatment, the frequent recurrence of infections constitutes a problem.

Some patients lack B cells altogether. In most patients, the lymphocytes do not transform into plasma cells to produce Ig. Even *in vitro* the B cell is unable to differentiate into a plasma cell when challenged by a potent polyclonal B-cell activator such as pokeweed mitogen.

Normal levels of the T-cell subsets are usually found, but their functioning may be reduced in some patients. Recent studies indicate that for some patients, the defect is overactive suppressor T cells, and this observation may lead to new ways to treat or control the disorder.

Chronic administration of γ globulin and specific antibiotics and supportive care during acute infections are the current standards of therapy. Approximately 8% of these patients develop malignancy, including leukemia, lymphomas, and epithelial cell tumors.

Cellular Immune Deficiency

Thymic Hypoplasia (DiGeorge Syndrome)

The predominant feature of DiGeorge syndrome is the appearance of hypocalcemic tetany shortly after birth as a result of the failure of the parathyroids and thymus to develop normally from the third and fourth pharyngeal pouches during embryonic development. This disorder occurs in both males and females. Familial cases and chromosome abnormalities are rare. There are often a number of associated physical abnormalities, including hyperteliorism (wide-set eyes), anti–mongoloid slant of the eyes, low-set and notched ears, micrognathia (small jaw), a short philtrum of the upper lip, mandibular hypoplasia, and cardiac and aortic arch anomalies (tetralogy of Fallot).

The thymus is absent, and T lymphocytes are absent from the blood and the thymus-dependent areas of the lymph nodes and spleen. However, humoral-mediated immunity develops normally. Characteristically, these patients are very susceptible to infections with opportunistic pathogens (*e.g.*, fungi, virus, *Pneumocystis carinii*) and are prone to develop graft versus host disease (GVHD) from the lymphocytes transferred by the transfusion of nonirradiated blood products.

Serum Ig levels are usually normal, though IgA may be decreased and IgE may be increased. Total B-cell percentage is increased, and total T-cell percentage is decreased; however, the ratio of helper T cells to suppressor T cells is normal. T-cell function may be normal. Delayed hypersensitivity skin test reactions may be absent or reduced, and delayed hypersensitivity to sensitizing antigens, such as dinitrochlorobenzene, fails to stimulate patients with DiGeorge syndrome.

Correction has been achieved by means of early (14 weeks gestational age) fetal thymus transplants with the beneficial effect mediated by thymosin produced by the epithelial cells in the transplanted thymus. Bone marrow transplantation has also been helpful in correcting this disorder.[8]

Nezelof's Syndrome (Cellular Immunodeficiency with Normal or Increased Immunoglobulins)

Characteristic of Nezelof's syndrome is the profound T-cell dysfunction with abnormal immunoglobulin synthesis. Children with this disease usually have chronic pulmonary infection, failure to thrive, oral or cutaneous candidiasis, chronic diarrhea, recurrent skin infection, gram-negative sepsis, urinary tract infection, and severe progressive varicella. Patients usually have lymphopenia, diminished lymphoid tissue, abnormal thymus architecture, normal numbers of B cells, and the presence of normal or elevated serum concentrations of most of the five classes of Ig's. Frequently, IgA is deficient and IgD and IgE levels are elevated. Unresponsiveness to delayed hypersensitivity skin tests and decreased to absent lymphocyte response to mitogens and allogeneic cells have been noted in the cellular immune function studies.

Because of the presence of normal Ig levels, the following features may be useful to differentiate Nezelof's syndrome from acquired immunodeficiency syndrome (AIDS): (1) There is a marked decrease of total T cells and T-cell subset with a normal ratio of helper (T_H) to suppressor (T_S) T cells as compared with AIDS, where there is an inverse T_H/T_S ratio due to a marked decrease of T_H cells. (2) There is a paracortical lymphocyte reduction and hypoplastic peripheral lymphoid tissue as compared with lymphadenopathy in AIDS. The thymus is small and has little corticomedullary differentiation and no Hassall's corpuscles, yet thymic epithelium is present, which contrasts with patients with AIDS, who show marked atrophy of thymic epithelium. Except for appropriate supportive measures, including antibiotics, no treatment has been curative except for one patient, who had an HLA-matched bone marrow transplant from a sibling.

Combined Humoral and Cellular Immune Deficiency

Severe Combined Immune Deficiency

Severe combined immune deficiency (SCID) was first described in 1958; however, later characterization showed this to be a collection of IDs showing a diversity of genetic, enzymatic, dermatologic, and immunologic features. Basically, these disorders are characterized by a failure to develop lymphoid stem cells, which results in an absence of both the cellular and humoral components of the immune response. This syndrome is the most severe of the recognized immunodeficiencies, and survival for more than a few months is unlikely, because of recurrent severe infections.

Successful treatment with correction of all these abnormalities has been achieved using histocompatible bone marrow transplantation from sibling donors.[9]

Autosomal Recessive SCID (Swiss-Type Lymphopenic Agammaglobulinemia) With or Without Adenosine Deaminase Deficiency. In 1958 Swiss workers reported the first SCID syndrome. These infants initially appear to grow normally, but extreme wasting develops after diarrhea and infections (*e.g.*, otitis, pneumonia, sepsis, dermatitis) begin. Death is caused by infections with opportunistic organisms (*e.g.*, *Candida albicans*, *P. carinii*, varicella, measles, and cytomegalovirus [CMV]) and by dissemination of live organisms used for vaccination (*e.g.*, BCG and vaccinia).

These infants have a markedly decreased percentage of T cells (but rarely have inverted helper–suppressor ratio as compared with AIDS patients, and this observation can help in the diagnosis), but many have increased B-cell percentages. However, both T and B cells are largely nonfunctional. Immunologic findings include profound lymphopenia, delayed hypersensitivity anergy, and failure to reject transplants, thereby increasing their risk for GVHD from maternal lymphocytes acquired *in utero* or inadvertently transferred by blood transfusions. Serum Ig concentrations are extremely low, and antibody is not formed after immunization.[10]

Natural killer (NK) function is absent in most SCID patients; however, a recent study reported a new phenotype in two SCID infants who had large granular lymphocytes with NK cell phenotype and function, further confirming the heterogeneity in these disorders at a cellular level. (NK cells are similar to T cells morphologically and mature in the thymus gland; however, they appear to be capable of mediating a cytotoxic reaction without the need of prior antigen sensitization).[11]

In SCID patients the thymus is atrophic with absent Hassall's corpuscles but with normal-appearing thymic epithelium. This latter observation may help to differentiate SCID from AIDS, because thymic epithelium is markedly atrophic in AIDS patients.

The best treatment is to reconstitute the lymphoid cell populations by a histocompatible bone marrow transplant. The ideal donor is an HLA-matched sibling with tissue compatibility confirmed by the microcytotoxicity test and the mixed lymphocyte reaction.

Approximately 40% of the autosomal recessive form of SCID has been observed to have adenosine deaminase (ADA) deficiency. ADA deficiency causes abnormal purine metabolism leading to combined T- and B-cell immunodeficiency. The presence of rib-cage abnormalities similar to a rachitic rosary and multiple skeletal abnormalities (chondro-osseous dysplasia) are characteristic. Some patients may have some Hassall's corpuscles in their thymus, which may represent early thymic differentiation that is very different from other types of SCID.

Enzyme replacement therapy has been attempted by the administration of irradiated packed normal erythrocytes, or polyethylene glycol-modified bovine ADA. Bone marrow transplantation has also been used. The prospect for gene insertion therapy is very attractive, since this would provide the missing enzyme without the complications of immune reactions to foreign ADA or the risk of graft versus host disease.

X-Linked Recessive SCID. X-linked recessive SCID is clinically, immunologically, and histopathologically indistinguishable from the autosomal recessive form described earlier and seems to be the most common form of SCID in the United States. The fact that different genetic loci can be involved and yet lead to very similar syndromes reveals that the immune system is dependent upon and under the control and regulation of many different genes, any one of which, if defective, can have profound consequences. This heterogeneity also suggests that the different mechanisms involved may require elucidation before individualized treatment strategies can be devised.

SCID with Hematopoietic Hypoplasia. Characteristic of SCID with hematopoietic hypoplasia (re-ticular dysgenesis) is the severe deficiency of both T and B lymphocytes and the failure to develop granulocytes. Most of the few reported cases have died of overwhelming infection within the first 3 months of life. One patient has been treated with a bone marrow transplant and has achieved complete immunologic reconstitution. The thymus gland is small, weighing <1 g; Hassall's corpuscles are absent; and thymocytes are rarely observed. It is thought to be inherited as an autosomal recessive.

A total failure of stem cells is not entirely satisfactory as an explanation for the defect, because heterogeneity among these patients has been observed, with a few cases having very low numbers of normal-appearing granulocytes and one patient having a normal percentage of nonfunctional T cells in cord blood.

Bone marrow transplantation would be the treatment of choice but would almost require prenatal diagnosis of the affected child to accomplish the procedure promptly after birth.

Partial Combined Immune Deficiency

Wiskott-Aldrich Syndrome. Patients with Wiskott-Aldrich syndrome, an X-linked recessive disorder, are characterized by the presence of eczema, thrombocytopenic purpura, and increased susceptibility to infection. Clinically, the eczema is similar to infantile atopic dermatitis. Petechiae, prolonged oozing from the umbilicus or circumcision, or bloody diarrhea may call attention to the thrombocytopenia. Normal megakaryocytes are found in the bone marrow, suggesting the presence of an intrinsic defect in the platelets. In the early phases of the disorder, recurrent infections, such as pneumonia, meningitis, otitis, and sepsis, occur with the pyogenic encapsulated bacteria at fault. Later on, as cellular immune function declines, infection with *P. carinii* and the herpes viruses becomes more of a problem. Death results from infection and bleeding. There is also a 12% incidence of malignancy. Survival beyond the teens is rare.

There are multiple immune defects. Humoral response to polysaccharide antigens is impaired. Anamnestic responses are poor or absent. Dysgammaglobulinemia with decreased IgM, elevated IgA and IgE, and normal or low levels of IgG is often seen. Ig synthesis is actually increased, with hypercatabolism of IgG, IgA, IgM, and albumin. This explains the high degree of variation in Ig concentration seen in different patients as well as within a single patient when measured over time. There is a low percentage of total T, helper T, and suppressor T cells, but the helper–suppressor ratio is usually normal.

Some patients with uncontrollable bleeding have been helped by splenectomy. Long-term survival has been possible with carefully maintained antibiotic therapy. Antibody replacement therapy by intravenous administration of γ globulin has been useful. Both platelet and immunologic abnormalities have been successfully treated by HLA-identical sibling bone marrow transplants.

Ataxia-Telangiectasia. The characteristics of ataxia-telangiectasia, an autosomal recessive disorder, include ataxia, telangiectasia, recurrent sinopulmonary infections, high incidence of malignancy, and variable defects of humoral and cellular immunity. Ataxia is often not noticed until the child begins to walk. From then on, it is progressive, with the child often confined to a wheelchair by 10 to 12 years of age. Telangiectasia is observed by 3 to 6 years of age and progresses slowly. Chronic sinopulmonary infection is observed in about 80% of patients. Malignancy is most often of the lymphoreticular type, but a high incidence of adenocarcinomas has been reported in patients' normal relatives. Patients show a selective absence of serum and secretory IgA, which in 50% to 80% of cases may be due to hypercatabolism of IgA. The serum concentration of IgA2 and IgG4 may be decreased in some patients. In others IgE is absent, and serum IgM may be of the low-molecular-weight (monomeric) type. Cellular immunity

is impaired. The total number of T cells and the helper cell percentage are low, but normal or high percentages of suppressor cells are observed.

Ig synthesis studies show defects in B cells and helper T cells. The thymus is hypoplastic, with poor organization and a deficiency of Hassall's corpuscles. To date, treatment attempts have been unsatisfactory.

Secondary Immune Deficiency

The secondary immunodeficiency states occur in previously healthy individuals, who are therefore considered to have had a normal immune system. They result from some underlying illness and may be more or less reversible, depending upon how completely the underlying illness can be controlled. Almost any severe illness can lead to an impairment in immune function. Examples would include diabetes, uremia, starvation, cystic fibrosis, burns, rheumatic heart disease, indwelling catheters and other foreign bodies, splenectomy, viral infections, prematurity, and so on. A few selected examples will be described later to illustrate some of the disorders involved.

Transient Hypogammaglobulinemia of Infancy

Transient hypogammaglobulinemia is an uncommon disorder occurring in about 0.1% of newborns. The disorder is characterized by an abnormal prolongation and accentuation of the decline in serum Ig concentrations normally seen during the first 3 to 7 months of life. By 6 to 11 months of age, all cases are able to synthesize normal amounts of antibodies to human type A and B erythrocytes and to diphtheria and tetanus toxoids. This occurs well before the Ig concentrations themselves become normal. Normal percentages of the different lymphoid cell subpopulations are observed along with normal responses to mitogens.

These patients can be divided into two groups. One group has no significant health problems during infancy; the other group has recurrent infections. The majority of the patients in the first group later developed normal serum Ig levels. However, the second group's serum Ig levels remained below the normal range, although significantly higher than during infancy. Follow-up studies showed that these patients did not have any subsequent serious infection even though none received Ig replacement therapy. Gammaglobulin replacement therapy is not indicated in this condition, as the passively administered immunoglobulin could suppress the patient's own antibody formation. Other than careful management of recurrent infections, no other specific therapy is required. Careful differentiation from the other, more serious immune deficiency states is required so that the parents can be reassured that the infant will outgrow the problem with no lasting consequences.

Malignancy

A number of cancers (if not most of them) clearly show a suppressive effect upon normal immune function. Defects in T-cell function are well known in Hodgkin's disease, and functional impairment of antibody formation is seen with many lymphomas, CLL, and multiple myeloma. More subtle defects can be elicited (*e.g.*, a failure to respond to DNCB skin testing) in many patients with a variety of metastatic cancers (*e.g.*, melanoma, breast, colon). The converse is also true; suppression of the immune system can lead both to an abnormal incidence of cancer and to unusual types of cancer (*e.g.*, Kaposi's sarcoma in

AIDS patients, CNS lymphomas in renal transplant patients).

These considerations clearly reveal the interdependency and interaction of the immune system and malignancies and have led to the postulation that there is constant surveillance by the immune system, which eliminates newly developed malignant cells. A primary or secondary immune defect or other special circumstance is needed for the cancer cell to evade this immune elimination, and of course when it does and a newly developed cancer is established, the immune system is no longer functional in eliminating the tumor. Efforts to overcome this and enhance the specific immune elimination of the cancer cells (*e.g.*, interferon, IL-2, LAK cells) are currently areas of intense interest and active research out of which it is hoped new forms of cancer therapy will emerge.

Viral Disease

It is widely appreciated that a variety of viral illnesses can impair the proper functioning of the immune system. AIDS can be thought of as representing a more recently recognized and severe form of this immune suppression, and a great deal has already been learned about the molecular biology of this interaction.[12]

Older observations of bacterial infections (*e.g.*, pneumonia) following on the heels of the influenza epidemics are still valid, although the availability of modern antibiotics has served to ameliorate much of the resulting mortality, if not the morbidity, of this association. The exact molecular nature of the viral-induced impairment of the immune system is not well understood but may share some features with the more dramatic effects of the HIV virus in AIDS patients. Viruses such as those that cause the common cold, the herpes family of viruses, CMV, EBV, and so on, also affect host defense mechanisms and are, of course, more prevalent and dangerous when host resistance is impaired (*e.g.*, chemotherapy, immunosuppressive therapy, stress). It is likely that the knowledge gained in the current intensive investigations of AIDS will have a dramatic impact on our understanding of these viral, host, and immune system interactions.

Bone Marrow Transplantation and Graft Versus Host Disease

Although in some ways the use of bone marrow transplantation is an attempt to re-create the immune system, there are a number of ways in which the transplanted immune system does not follow normal ontogeny. The immune system as it normally develops in the developing fetus has some very special features. It occurs under the influence of the thymus and the mammalian equivalent of the bursa, and during this development it is protected from antigen encounter. Ratios of the various cellular elements are maintained as the immune system matures and regulation occurs that eliminates autoimmune reactions. Altogether, the protected environment in which the fetus develops provides a very elegant system for keeping the development of the immune system on target and in balance.

Bone marrow transplantation re-creates few, if any, of these features of the normal immune system development. The donor cell population is only a minor sample of the whole immune system as represented by its presence in the bone marrow. The cells are not naive; that is, antigen abounds in the donor and a whole new universe of antigen is encountered in the recipient. There is no active thymus present in the recipient, and the bursal equivalent is also probably much different from that of the fetus. It is remarkable that the immune system reconstitution proceeds as well as it does under these very altered circumstances. Recovery of the immunoglobulins,

especially IgG and IgM, occurs, but may take several months, and regulation is not precise. Frequent monoclonal immunoglobulins are observed, including Bence Jones proteinuria, but their presence has not yet proceeded to a plasma cell malignancy. They are usually transient, being replaced by more normal polyclonal immunoglobulins. IgA recovery tends to be very delayed, and very low levels of IgA can be observed for up to several years. T-cell function is also impaired and may persist for prolonged periods.

These abnormalities account for the pattern and frequency of posttransplant infections, with CMV and the herpes viruses predominating. In addition, the minor differences between the graft and the host may very well set up a chronic rejection reaction of the host by the transplanted immunocompetent cells. When severe, the gut (diarrhea), the skin (exfoliation), and the liver (hepatitis) can be severely and fatally affected. Minor degrees of rejection also occur, which can also be associated with significant morbidity. Better means of suppression of these reactions have been developed (*e.g.*, cyclosporin), but this in turn also leads to host defense impairment as well as other host side-effects.

Despite these drawbacks, a great deal has been learned about immune system functioning and its manipulation that makes this the treatment of choice for a number of otherwise fatal diseases (*e.g.*, aplastic anemia, relapsing acute leukemia), and the technology is sure to be improved in the future, extending it to other disease processes.

References

1. Stiehm ER, Fulginiti VA (eds): Immunologic Disorders in Infants and Children, 2nd ed. Philadelphia, WB Saunders, 1980

2. Rosen FS, Cooper MD, Wedgwood RJ: The primary immunodeficiencies. N Engl J Med 311:235, 1984

3. Primary immunodeficiency diseases: Report of a World Health Organization scientific group. Clin Immunol Immunopathol 40:166, 1986

4. Buckley RH: Immunodeficiency diseases. JAMA 258:20, 1987

5. Humphrey RL: Immunodeficiency diseases. In Harvey AM, Johns RJ, McKusick VA, et al (eds): Principles and Practice of Medicine, 22nd ed, p 482. East Norwalk, Appleton and Lange, 1988

6. Waldmann TA: Immunodeficiency diseases: Primary and acquired. In Santer M (ed): Immunological Diseases, 4th ed, p 411. Boston, Little, Brown, 1988

7. Conley ME, Cooper MD: Immature IgA B cells in IgA deficient patients. N Engl J Med 305:495, 1981

8. Buckley RH, Schiff SE, Sampson HA, et al: Development of immunity in human severe primary T cell deficiency following haploidentical bone marrow stem cell transplantation. J Immunol 136:2398, 1986

9. Bortin MM, Rimm AA: Severe combined immunodeficiency disease: Characterization of the disease and results of transplantation. JAMA 238:591, 1977

10. Buckley RH: Studies of patients with severe cellular and humoral immunodeficiency diseases using monoclonal antibodies. In Haynes BF, Eisenbarth GS (eds): Monoclonal Antibodies: Probes for the Studies of Autoimmunity and Immunodeficiency, p 83. San Diego, Academic Press, 1983

11. Herberman RB: Natural killer cells. In Dixon FJ, Fisher DW (eds): The Biology of Immunologic Disease, p 75. Sunderland, MA, Sinauer Assoc, 1983

12. Bowen DL, Lane HC, Fauci AS: Immunologic abnormalities in the acquired immunodeficiency syndrome. Prog Allergy 37:207, 1986

CHAPTER 29

Autoimmunity

Catherine Sheehan

Autoimmunity is a general term to describe an immune response generated by the body against its own cells or organs. The basis of protective immunity is specific and nonspecific immune mechanisms that recognize and eliminate foreign configurations from a host. Under normal circumstances, the host tolerates self-antigens because an immune reaction directed against itself would injure the host, an undesired effect. Therefore, detrimental or abnormal autoimmunity represents a failure to tolerate self-antigens.

The general mechanisms of harmful autoimmunity include

1. Interaction of antibodies with cell surface components (*e.g.*, in myasthenia gravis, antibodies bind to acetylcholine receptors).

2. Formation of autoantigen–autoantibody complexes in fluids with or without deposition in tissue (*e.g.*, immune complex mediated glomerulonephritis in systemic lupus erythematosus).

3. Sensitization of T cells (*e.g.*, the lymphocyte infiltrate associated with Hashimoto's thyroiditis).

These autoimmune mechanisms may be primary (an immunologic abnormality without other underlying abnormalities) or secondary (the immune abnormality resulting from another abnormality).

Recent evidence suggests that some autoimmunity is beneficial, even necessary, to the host. Two beneficial mechanisms utilize the ability of immune cells and antibodies to recognize self-antigens. First, to initiate an immune response, a major histocompatibility complex (MHC) molecule must accompany an antigen. MHC class II molecules and antigens must be coexpressed on an antigen-presenting cell to activate helper T cells, and MHC class I molecules and antigen are needed to activate cytotoxic T cells. Second, regulation of an immune response occurs by an idiotype–anti-idiotype interaction. In 1974 Jerne proposed an idiotype network based on the ability of B lymphocytes to recognize the idiotype (composed of antigenic determinants within the antigen binding site in the variable region) of an antibody molecule and to produce an anti-idiotype antibody.[1] This anti-idiotype antibody can then modulate the activity of B cells and T cells.

Theories to Explain Harmful Autoimmune Reactions

At the beginning of the century Paul Ehrlich described the central immunologic concept of tolerance in his dictum "horror autotoxicus."[2] When, in experiments, he introduced soluble autologous constituents into the host, no immune reaction was detected. By unknown mechanisms, autologous antigens were tolerated. Apparently, the host was incapable of mounting an immune response to itself. Yet autoimmunity is a real phenomenon representing an abnormal response to autologous antigens and needed an explanation.

Theories proposed to explain the mechanism of autoimmune disease include (1) the forbidden-clone theory, (2) the sequestered-antigen theory, and (3) the immunologic deficiency theory (Table 19-1).[3] The forbidden-clone theory was originally postulated by Burnet. In Burnet's model, antibodies on the surface of immune cells served as receptors for specific antigens. When the specific antigen is present, the corresponding cell is stimulated to eliminate the specific antigen. Stimulated cells proliferated, establishing a clone of identical cells. Some cells of the clone became antibody-secreting cells; others became memory cells. Thus, clonal selection and expansion was a normal response to foreign antigens. To explain tolerance to autologous antigens, Burnet postulated that during fetal development, when immune cells were exposed to autologous antigens, the specific cell was eliminated and the subsequent clone did not develop. The mature host was then unresponsive to the specific self-antigens and would tolerate these autologous antigens. An error in this process, failure to

Table 29-1: Theories to Explain Harmful Autoimmune Reactions

Forbidden-clone theory

Clonal anergy

Sequestered-antigen theory

Immunologic deficiency theory

eliminate a lymphocyte directed against a self-antigen, would allow the expression of immune products against self: autoimmunity. Refinement of this model led to the concept of clonal anergy: During fetal development, clones encountering fetal antigens would not be eliminated but would be unresponsive to low doses of the antigen. Thus, the ability to respond to higher doses of antigens later in life would be preserved.

According to the sequestered-antigen theory, some antigens in the body are hidden from cells of the immune system, and since the immune system never encounters these antigens, tolerance results. If there is damage to these organs, sequestered antigens are exposed, and an autoimmune reaction can occur. This theory explains some autoimmune reactions, such as the development of antibodies against spermatozoa following vasectomy and against the lens after eye injury. In these cases, the autoimmune response is usually short-lived and disappears prior to development of clinical symptoms.[4]

The immunologic deficiency theory relates the increased frequency of autoantibodies and increased immune system deficiency to increasing age. Normally, suppressor T lymphocytes prevent expression of antibody and cellular reactions by suppressing the activity of B lymphocytes and T lymphocytes. When there is a decline in the activity of the suppressor T-lymphocyte population, response to an antigen can continue uncontrolled and can result in an autoimmune response.

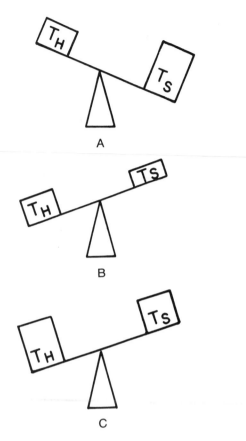

FIGURE 29-1. Autoimmunity: immunologic deficiency. (A) No overt autoimmune reaction occurs when suppressor T cells (T$_S$) dominate over helper T cells (T$_H$), preventing the expression of a harmful autoimmune response. (B) An overt autoimmune reaction may occur when hypoactive T$_S$ cells fail to turn off a T$_H$ reaction to an autologous antigen. (C) An overt autoimmune reaction may occur when hyperactive T$_H$ cells dominate and encourage an inappropriate response.

The immunologic deficiency theory has evolved to reflect current understanding of immunoregulation.[5] Control of the immune response requires both T and B lymphocytes: Both can respond to antigens and communicate with each other. Immunocytes must recognize an antigen and then coordinate a response by intercellular signals. As shown in Figure 29-1, the balanced interaction between helper T cells and sup-

pressor T cells determines whether an immune response will occur and to what extent. The helper T cells encourage other T cells and B cells to react to the antigen, whereas suppressor T cells discourage other T cells and B cells from reacting. Hyperactive helper T cells can encourage an inappropriate autoimmune response, and hypoactive suppressor T cells may fail to turn off a response. Either mechanism of impaired function results in the impaired regulation of an immune response and can produce an autoimmune reaction shown by a variety of antibodies to common autoantigens.

Lack of appropriate immune regulation occurs by another mechanism and contributes to some autoimmune diseases.[6,7] As shown in Figure 29-2, the idiotype of an antibody is an area within the variable domain that is immunogenic and can stimulate the production of an antibody, an anti-idiotype antibody. When the anti-idiotype antibodies and the idiotype are produced by the same host, the anti-idiotype antibody is called an auto-anti-idiotype. Auto-anti-idiotypes are believed to be important in regulating a normal immune response by interacting with the idiotypic area of the antibody. When an anti-idiotype behaves as an autoantibody, autoimmunity can result. The best example is Graves' disease, an autoimmune disease of the thyroid gland. In the normal regulation of thyroid function, thyroid stimulating hormone (TSH or thyrotropin) binds to a TSH receptor on thyroid follicle cells, which stimulates thyroid hormone production and release; these hormones negatively feed back to the anterior pituitary and decrease the TSH level reaching the thyroid. In Graves' disease, an autoantibody combines with the TSH receptor and stimulates thyroid cells to produce and release thyroid hormones. Since it is an antibody, not TSH, that stimulates the thyroid, this pathologic process is outside of the normal thyrotropin control mechanism. In fact, there is no control. Experimentally, TSH antibodies can be used to produce anti-TSH antibodies that are anti-idiotype antibodies. The anti-idiotype antibody stimulates thyroid cells in tis-

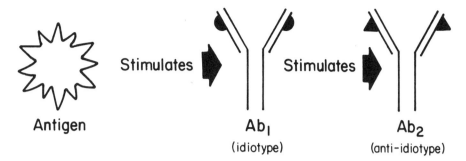

FIGURE 29-2. Idiotype network. The antigen stimulates the production of a specific antibody (Ab_1) or the idiotype. The variable region of Ab_1 is immunogenic and stimulates the production of a second antibody (Ab_2) or the anti-idiotype. When Ab_1 and Ab_2 are produced in the same individual, Ab_2 is an auto-anti-idiotype. Some anti-idiotype antibodies mimic the antigen and stimulate the production of more idiotype antibody.

sue culture, mimicking the metabolic events in spontaneous Graves' disease. This experimental evidence suggests that the autoantibody in Graves' disease is an anti-idiotype antibody.[5]

Organ Versus Non–organ Specificity

The spectrum of autoimmune diseases ranges, as listed in Table 29-2, from organ specific to non–organ, non–species specific. In organ-specific autoimmune diseases autoantibody and cellular reactions take place in only one organ, for instance in the thyroid gland in Hashimoto's thyroiditis. At the other end of the spectrum are those autoimmune diseases in which multiple antibodies affect multiple organs; systemic lupus erythematosus is the prototypic non–organ-specific autoimmune disease. Other autoimmune diseases, such as primary biliary cirrhosis, occur primarily in one organ but exhibit multiple antibodies. Serologic findings common to many autoimmune diseases will be discussed first, followed by findings in specific autoimmune diseases.

Serologic Findings Common to Many Autoimmune Diseases

Antinuclear Antibodies

Antibodies to nuclear antigens (ANA) are antibodies directed against components of the cell nucleus, such as nucleoproteins and nucleic acids. ANA are associated with many systemic diseases, including systemic lupus erythematosus (SLE), mixed connective tissue disease (MCTD), and rheumatoid arthritis (RA). ANA can be used as a diagnostic indicator, as a prognostic indicator, or as a means of monitoring the effectiveness of therapy.

The first recognition of an antinuclear factor was made by Hargraves when he described the lupus erythematosus (LE) cell in patients with SLE.[8] The LE cell, seen primarily *in vitro*, requires heparinized blood to be incubated with glass beads to damage the cells releasing nuclear material. The nuclei can then be recognized by a factor called the LE factor and, in the presence of complement, will alter the chromatin. When the altered chromatin is phagocytosed by an intact neutrophil, the altered chromatin appears ho-

Table 29-2: Spectrum of Autoimmune Disease

Organ Specific	Intermediate	Non–Organ Specific
Hashimoto's thyroiditis	1° biliary cirrhosis	SLE
Graves' disease	Sjögren's syndrome	Rheumatoid arthritis
Pernicious anemia	Myasthenia gravis	PSS
Juvenile insulin-dependent diabetes	Goodpasture's syndrome	MCTD
	Chronic active hepatitis	

SLE = systemic lupus erythematosus
PSS = progressive systemic sclerosis
MCTD = mixed connective tissue disease

mogeneous and is called a hematoxylin body. The LE factor is now known to be an antinuclear antibody directed against deoxyribonucleoprotein; it is found predominantly in individuals with systemic lupus erythematosus but is also detected in other systemic rheumatic diseases.

The development of the immunofluorescence technique and its application to detect antinuclear antibodies provided greater sensitivity and specificity, allowed semiquantitation, and was easier to perform than the LE cell preparation. Indirect immunofluorescence is the method of choice to screen for ANA. A representative protocol follows: Fixed substrate containing nuclei (mouse liver or tissue culture cells) is incubated with patient or control serum. After washing, the tissue is incubated with anti–human immunoglobulin conjugated with fluorescein; following a second wash, the slide is viewed with a fluorescence microscope. The pattern and titer are recorded.

Several patterns of nuclear fluorescence can be described and are shown in Figure 29-3. Using mouse liver cells, the patterns are diffuse, peripheral, speckled, and nucleolar. The diffuse, or homogeneous, pattern evenly stains the nuclei and is associated with deoxyribonucleoprotein; the peripheral, or rim, pattern appears as bright fluorescence near the edge of the nuclei and is associated with native DNA; the speckled pattern appears as numerous evenly distributed speckles of fluorescence within the nuclei and is associated with many saline extractable nuclear antigens; and the nucleolar pattern appears as two or three large, nearly round fluorescent areas within the nucleus and is associated with nucleolar RNA. If a human epithelial tissue culture cell line, such as HEp-2 or KB cells, is used as the substrate, the antigens present are those in the mouse liver cells plus the SSA/Ro antigen and the centromere antigen. The centromere antigen is present in cells that are actively replicating and produces a characteristic discrete speckled pattern when the centromere fluoresces. A summary of the immunofluorescence patterns and nuclear antigens is presented in Table 29-3.[9]

Thus, from the indirect immunofluorescence procedure, not only can the presence and titer of an ANA be demonstrated, but the pattern of fluorescence can also be described. Positive ANA are seen in a variety of diseases. The pattern, though not a diagnostic marker for any specific disease, may suggest the specificity of the antibody or antibodies present. Multiple ANA can be present in a patient specimen, and further testing can confirm the antibody specificity.

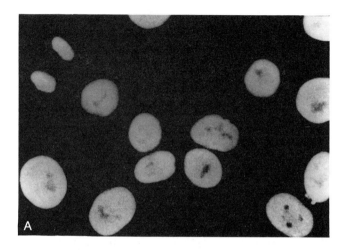

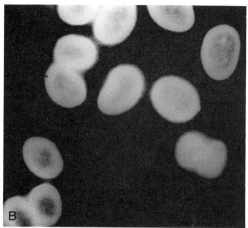

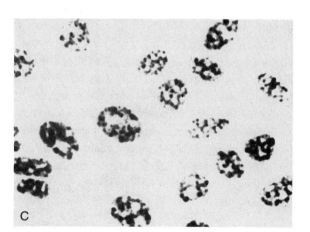

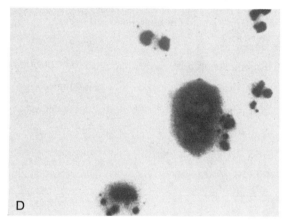

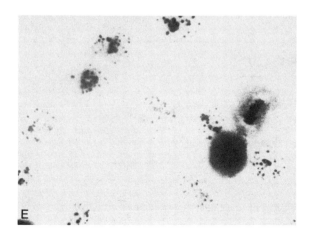

FIGURE 29-3. Patterns of ANA. The indirect immunofluorescence technique uses HEp2 tissue culture cells as the substrate. The magnification is 400×. (*A*) Homogeneous pattern with positive chromosome staining. (*B*) Peripheral pattern with positive chromosome staining. (*C*) Speckled pattern with negative chromosome staining. (*D*) Nuclear pattern with negative chromosome staining. (*E*) Centromere (discrete speckled) pattern with positive chromosome staining. (Reproduced with permission from Kallestad Diagnostics, Austin, TX.)

Table 29-3: Nuclear Antigens and Associated Immunofluorescence Pattern

Nuclear Antigen	Pattern
Double-stranded DNA	Peripheral and/or homogeneous
Single-stranded DNA	Negative
Native DNA	Peripheral and/or homogeneous
Deoxynucleoprotein	Peripheral and/or homogeneous
Histone	Homogeneous
Soluble extractable nonhistones	Speckled
Sm	Speckled
Ribonucleoprotein	Coarse speckled
SSA (Ro)	Fine speckled
SSB (La)	Fine speckled
Scl-70	Fine speckled
4S-6S RNA	Nucleolar
Centromere	Discrete speckled

The antibodies specifically associated with the diagnosis of systemic rheumatic diseases are marker antibodies (Table 29-4).[9,10] The antibody directed against the nonhistone antigen, Sm antigen, is a marker antibody found in 30% to 40% of patients with systemic lupus erythematosus. Some SLE patients also have an antibody that reacts only with double-stranded DNA; this antibody indicates active systemic lupus erythematosus and is rarely seen in other diseases. A second marker antibody is directed against the nonhistone antigen Scl-70 and is present in 15% to 20% of patients with progressive systemic sclerosis (scleroderma). The centromere antibody is a marker antibody found in a subset of progressive systemic sclerosis, CREST, with a frequency of 70% to 90%.

The frequency and association of other defined antigens are presented in Table 29-5. Note the considerable overlap of the presence of an antibody with several diseases; for diagnostic purposes, a panel of antibodies is useful. Principal methodologies to characterize the ANA specificity include double diffusion, passive hemagglutination, enzyme immunoassay, radioimmunoassay, and indirect immunofluorescence.

Native DNA (n-DNA) antibodies can be detected by radioimmunoassay (RIA) or indirect immunofluo-

Table 29-4: ANA: Marker Antibodies

IIF Pattern	Antigen	Disease (frequency)
Speckled	Sm	SLE (30% to 40%)
Peripheral	double-stranded DNA	SLE, active disease (60% to 70%)
Speckled	Scl-70	scleroderma (15% to 20%)
Centromere	centromere	CREST variant of PSS (70% to 90%)

IIF = indirect immunofluorescence
CREST = syndrome of calcinosis, Raynaud's phenomenon, esophageal dysmotility, sclerodactyly, and telangiectases
PSS = progressive systemic sclerosis

Table 29-5: ANA Profiles

	RNP	nDNA	histone	Sm	SSB	SSA	Scl-70	centro-mere	nucle-olar	JO-1	PM-1
MCTD	+[1]	+(L)									
SLE	+	+	+	+[3]	+	+			+		
PSS	+	+(L)					+[4]	+[5]	+		+
DM/PM		+(L)								+	+
SS	+	+(L)			+	+			+		
RA	+	+(L)	+								
DRUG INDUCED LE			+[2]								

RNP =	ribonucleoprotein		(L)	low titer
MCTD =	mixed connective tissue disease		1	high titers of only anti-RNP antibodies is suggestive of MCTD
SLE =	systemic lupus erythematosus		2	high titers of only anti-histone antibodies is suggestive of drug-induced LE
PSS =	progressive systemic sclerosis		3	marker antibody for SLE
DM/PM =	dermatomyositis/polymyositis		4	marker antibody for PSS
SS =	Sjögren's syndrome		5	marker antibody for CREST variant of PSS
RA =	rheumatoid arthritis			
LE =	lupus erythematosus			

rescence (IIF) techniques.[9] The RIA method, or Farr technique, uses radiolabeled DNA to capture the n-DNA antibody; the complex is then precipitated with saturated ammonium sulfate. Following centrifugation, the radioactivity in the precipitate is measured and is directly related to the amount of n-DNA antibody present. The IIF method uses *Crithidea luciliae* as the substrate, since the hemoflagellate possesses n-DNA in its kinetoplast. After incubating the substrate with patient serum, washing, incubat-

ing with fluorescent labeled anti–human globulin, and final washing, the slide is viewed with a fluorescence microscope. As seen in Figure 29-4, specific fluorescence of the kinetoplast indicates the presence of n-DNA antibodies.

Double diffusion is used to detect antibodies against the saline extractable nuclear antigens, such as Sm, SSA, SSB, Jo-1, Scl-70, and ribonucleoprotein (RNP). An extract of calf or rabbit thymus is the source of antigen and is placed in the center well; the

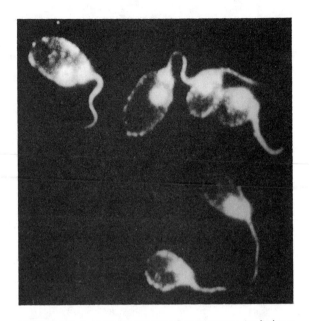

FIGURE 29-4. Indirect immunofluorescence technique demonstrating anti–native-DNA antibody. The substrate is *Crithidia luciliae* and the magnification is 1000×. (Reproduced with permission from Kallestad Diagnostics, Austin, TX.)

prototype (known positive) serum, known negative serum, and unknown patient serum are placed in the surrounding wells. During incubation, the antigen and antibody diffuse toward each other and form a precipitin line when the reactants meet. Comparing the positive serum control reaction with the patient serum reaction can define the specific antibody. In Figure 29-5, a line of identity confirms the presence of anti-Sm antibody in patient A and anti-RNP antibody in patient B. Reference sera containing antibodies of known specificity can be obtained from the Centers for Disease Control.

Rheumatoid Factor

Rheumatoid factor (RF) is an immunoglobulin that reacts with the Fc portion of an IgG molecule; therefore, RF is an anti-antibody. *In vivo*, RF can be of the

IgA, IgE, IgG, or IgM class; however, only RF of the IgM class is serologically detectable. This antibody will react with human IgG as well as IgG of other species.

Two agglutination methods are commercially available to measure RF: latex agglutination (or latex fixation) and hemagglutination.[11] The latex agglutination method described by Singer and Plotz[12] utilizes a latex particle coated with Cohn fraction II of human IgG. When patient serum is heat inactivated and mixed with the antibody-coated latex particle, macroscopic agglutination occurs when RF is present. Using a tube method, semiquantitation of positive sera results in the titer; weakly positive sera have a titer from 20 to 40, whereas a titer greater than 80 is considered a positive reaction, suggesting rheumatoid arthritis. Though this test is easy to perform, there are some disadvantages associated with

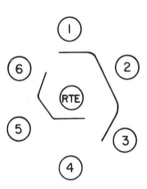

FIGURE 29-5. Immunodiffusion to identify Sm and RNP antibodies

Well 1: anti-Sm prototype serum.
Wells 2 and 3: patient A serum.
Well 4: anti-U1-RNP prototype serum.
Wells 5 and 6: patient B serum.

The center well contains the antigens from rabbit thymus extract. Note the precipitin reaction of identity with wells 1 and 2 (patient A serum contains the Sm antibody); note the precipitin reaction of identity with wells 4 and 5 (patient B serum contains the U1-RNP antibody).

it. Individuals without disease can exhibit low titers of RF, the frequency of which increases with age. False positive reactions can occur when excess lipids, microbial contamination, or C1q are present in the serum.

The other commercially available method, the Rose-Waaler test,[13,14] uses sheep red blood cells coated with hemolysin (an anti–sheep erythrocyte IgG antibody produced in rabbits). Sera containing RF will react with the antibody coating the sheep red blood cells and cause macroscopic agglutination. Antibody-coated sheep red blood cells exhibit fewer false positive reactions with serum from normal individuals than antibody-coated latex particles and exhibit more specificity for those RF associated with rheumatoid arthritis. Since this assay uses cells from another species, heterophile antibodies may interfere, causing a false positive reaction.

Cryoglobulins

Cryoglobulins are proteins that reversibly precipitate or gel at 0 to 4°C. They are classified as follows.[15] Type I cryoglobulins are monoclonal immunoglobulins. Type II represent mixed cryoglobulins in which a monoclonal immunoglobulin is directed against a polyclonal immunoglobulin. Type III cryoglobulins are polyclonal and consist of one or more immunoglobulins, none of which are homogeneous. Types I and II cryoglobulins are associated with monoclonal gammopathies, a group of diseases in which a monoclonal protein is produced by neoplastic plasma cells or lymphocytes. Types II and III cryoglobulins are circulating immune complexes produced in response to a variety of antigens, including viral, bacterial, and autologous antigens.

Symptoms resulting from cryoglobulinemia are related to the tendency of the protein to precipitate at low temperatures and to occlude blood vessels; symptoms include Raynaud's phenomenon, vascular purpura, bleeding tendencies, cold-induced urticaria, pain, and cyanosis. The concentration of the cryoglobulin, the temperature at which the protein precipitates out of solution, and the ability of the cryoglobulin to bind complement determine the extent of symptomatology. Essential mixed cryoglobulinemia is an idiopathic disease with arthralgia, purpura, weakness, and frequently lymphadenopathy, hepatosplenomegaly, and renal failure. This disease can be progressive and may result in death.[16]

Cryoglobulins can be detected and characterized in the clinical laboratory. Blood should be collected, allowed to clot, and centrifuged; the serum should be separated at 37°C to ensure that the cryoglobulins will remain in the serum. If the serum is then refrigerated, cryoglobulin will appear as a white precipitate or gel. Warming the serum to 37°C will reverse the precipitation. The cryoglobulin is quantitated by filling a hematocrit tube with serum, incubating at 1°C, centrifuging at 1°C at 750 g for 30 minutes, and reading the cryocrit. To characterize the cryoprotein, remove the supernatant and wash the precipitate three times using cold normal saline. Redissolve the cryoprecipitate by adding saline and then warming the suspension to 37°C for 30 minutes. Immunoelectrophoresis of the protein solution will identify the immunoglobulin class or classes present.[17]

Cryoglobulins can interfere in a number of laboratory tests. Complement activation and consumption can occur when C1q binds to immune complexes. Spurious elevation of leukocyte counts can occur because of their interaction with cryoglobulins and fibrinogen.[17]

Immune Complexes

When an antigen combines with an antibody and this complex circulates in the blood, it is called a circulating immune complex (CIC). It is a nonspecific indicator of immune activation and is commonly found in autoimmune disease. When immune complexes become lodged in tissue, damage often results.

The methods for quantitating CIC are based on

physical properties of CIC, and some are shown in Figure 29-6. Some methods rely on the ability of immune complexes to bind C1q: solid-phase or liquid-phase immunoassays are available.[18] In the solid-phase immunoassay, C1q is bound to the solid phase; incubation with patient serum captures immune complexes that bind to the C1q. The bound immune complexes can be detected by radio- or enzyme-labeled anti–human immunoglobulin and quantitated by measuring the label. In liquid-phase immunoassay the sample is incubated with radiolabeled C1q, the complexes are precipitated, and the label is quantitated. Assays using C1q most avidly bind larger, potentially pathologic, immune complexes (19–27S) and will detect only those immune complexes containing IgG1, IgG2, IgG3, or IgM.

A second general strategy to measure CIC involves the interaction of the immunoglobulin portion of the immune complex with rheumatoid factors.[18] Monoclonal RF obtained from the sera of patients with macroglobulinemia or mixed cryoglobulinemia is used to quantitate CIC. A competitive inhibition radioimmunoassay procedure allows radiolabeled monoclonal RF to bind to sample CIC competing with IgG-bound sepharose. The greater the CIC concentration in the sample, the less binding of monoclonal RF will occur with the IgG-sepharose. RF reacts with an Fc component of IgG which is different from

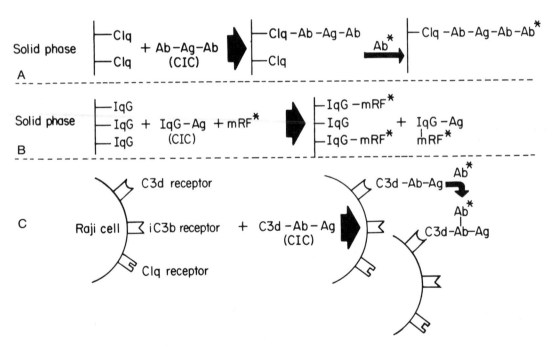

FIGURE 29-6. Methods to detect circulating immune complexes. (A) Solid-phase immunometric assay. Circulating immune complexes (CIC) bind to solid-phase C1q. The labeled immunoglobulin (Ab*) is quantitated and is directly related to the bound CIC. (B) Competitive inhibition radioimmunoassay. Unlabeled rheumatoid factor competes for binding sites on immobilized IgG and on the CIC. The labeled rheumatoid factor (mRF*) is quantitated and is inversely related to the bound CIC. (C) Raji cell assay. CIC bind to the cell surface receptors of the lymphoblastoid cell line, Raji cell. The labeled immunoglobulin (Ab*) is quantitated and is directly related to the bound CIC.

the binding site of C1q; RF does not bind to IgM. RF preferentially recognizes smaller CIC, as small as 8S.

Raji cells can also bind circulating immune complexes.[19] This cultured human lymphoblastoid cell line is derived from Burkitt's lymphoma and has receptors on its surface for C3d, iC3b, and C1q. When serum containing circulating immune complexes is incubated with Raji cells, the complexes will bind to the cell surface receptors; the bound complexes can then be quantitated using radiolabeled anti–human globulin.

The clinical utility of quantitating circulating immune complexes has been questioned because of the lack of reliable assays. Although the various methods available can detect different characteristics of immune complexes, lack of a stable, reproducible calibrator has hampered standardization of quantitative assays. Interfering substances also prevent standardization. For instance, antilymphocyte antibodies can react with Raji cells. Circulating immune complexes represent a diverse group of substances containing antigen and antibody; some methods may preferentially measure one type of complex over another.[20] The dynamics of the presence of CIC, degree of disease activity, and immune complex deposition in tissue require further investigation to assess clinical usefulness.

Non–Organ-Specific Autoimmune Diseases

Systemic Lupus Erythematosus

Systemic lupus erythematosus (SLE) is a chronic noninfectious, inflammatory disease that may involve many organs. Episodes of exacerbation alternate with remissions. The onset of the disease can be insidious or acute, and the course of the disease is variable. Women are four times more likely to develop SLE, particularly during the childbearing years; however, the diagnosis has been made in patients aged 2 to 97 years.[16] There is a higher incidence of SLE in blacks, compared with whites.[21]

SLE is an immune complex disease. Tissue injury is mediated by immune complexes that, when deposited in tissue, can initiate an inflammatory response. Where do the immune complexes come from? Most evidence suggests that depressed suppressor T-cell function allows the overproduction or inappropriate production of autoantibodies; these autoantibodies combine with common autoantigens and form immune complexes.[22] Most important is the production of DNA–anti-DNA complexes.

The cause of SLE is unknown, but the expression of the autoimmune reaction is influenced genetically. In identical twins, if one twin has SLE, 50% to 60% of the other twins will also have the disease,[23] and in first-degree relatives of patients with SLE, the incidence of SLE is more than 200 times greater than that in the general population.[21] There is an association between SLE and the presence of HLA-DR3.[4] Recent evidence suggests that asymptomatic first-degree relatives of patients with SLE have impaired suppressor T-cell function.[24] The increased frequency of SLE in women of childbearing age suggests that hormones influence the disease; the production of anti-DNA antibodies appears to be enhanced by estrogens.[25]

The severity of the disease varies from one individual to another; there is no single, common clinical pattern. Preliminary criteria for the classification of systemic lupus erythematosus were prepared by the American Rheumatism Association in 1971 and revised in 1982. These criteria were developed to identify patients to be included in clinical studies; the presence of 4 of 11 criteria was sufficient for inclusion. The patient history and symptoms are often insufficient; when serologic and immunopathologic tests are included in the criteria, there is greater chance to establish a diagnosis.[21]

Clinical manifestations may include signs and symptoms related to any organ system. General manifestations include fever, weight loss, malaise, and weakness. Arthritis is the most common manifestation of SLE and may precede multisystem involvement. Joint involvement in SLE is symmetrical, is rarely deforming, and can involve almost any joint.

Skin lesions and photosensitivity are the next most common findings in SLE. Usually the rash is erythematous and primarily involves areas exposed to ultraviolet radiation. The classic butterfly rash (malar rash) found in a minority of patients is diagnostically useful. The direct immunofluorescence test performed on a lesional skin biopsy to demonstrate immunoglobulin (usually IgG or IgM) and complement at the epidermal–dermal junction is the lupus band test. Immune complexes can also be demonstrated in the involved skin in discoid lupus erythematosus, a skin disease that may exist independent of or in conjunction with SLE.

The systemic nature of SLE is apparent from the presence of immune complexes in skin biopsies from areas without an active rash and in non-sun-exposed skin. The presence and nature of the lupus band test has been used to predict the presence of renal disease, a serious manifestation of SLE: A negative lupus band test or one with IgM only is associated with low incidence of lupus nephritis, whereas the presence of IgG, with or without other immunoglobulins, is associated with a greater incidence of renal disease. Active immune complex disease process in SLE is associated with hypocomplementemia and the presence of anti-DNA antibodies.[21,26]

Renal involvement occurs in the majority of patients with SLE. According to the World Health Organization's Classification of Lupus Nephropathy, five classes of glomerulonephritis are associated with SLE.[27]

Class I   Normal—No changes are seen when a kidney biopsy is evaluated by light microscopy, electron microscopy, and immunofluorescence microscopy.

Class II   Mesangial changes—Immune complexes in the mesangium are seen by electron microscopy and direct immunofluorescence; hypercellularity of the mesangial region may be present when evaluated by light microscopy.

Class III   Focal and segmental proliferative, necrotizing, or sclerosing glomerulonephritis—Hypercellularity of the mesangial region and focal and segmental proliferation of intracapillary and extracapillary cells are seen in less than 50% of the glomeruli or less than 50% of the glomerular surface when evaluated by light microscopy. Subendothelial and mesangial deposits are seen by electron microscopy and immunofluorescence microscopy.

Class IV   Diffuse proliferative glomerulonephritis—The light microscopy findings are the same as in class III, except that greater than 50% of the glomeruli or greater than 50% of the glomerular surface is involved. Abundant subendothelial deposits are present.

Class V   Membranous glomerulonephritis—A diffuse uniform thickening of the glomerular capillary walls is present owing to intramembranous immune deposits.

In class I the renal function is normal and the urine sediment may be normal or a minimal amount of protein may be excreted. Class II changes are associated with slightly abnormal renal function and hematuria, pyuria, and slight proteinuria. Class III changes have increased abnormal renal function, nearly all show proteinuria, and some have nephrotic syndrome. Class IV changes are the most severe; azotemia, hematuria, pyuria, and proteinuria are present in nearly all patients, and two thirds have nephrotic syndrome. Renal failure may occur. All patients with class V changes have proteinuria; most have nephrotic syndrome; and some have azotemia, hematuria, and pyuria.

Almost any organ system can be involved in SLE. Clinical features may include pleurisy, pericarditis, seizures, psychosis, ocular changes, pancreatitis, and small-vessel vasculitis.

Hematologic findings are normochromic, normocytic anemia, leukopenia, thrombocytopenia, and deficiency in the function of suppressor T cells.[21] Although the LE factor can be demonstrated in most patients with SLE and is shown by a high titer of an IgG antibody directed against deoxyribonucleoprotein, the insensitivity and the labor-intensive nature of the test has made it impractical; the ANA test is preferred.

Virtually all patients with SLE have a high titer of ANA ($\geq$160). Although the IF pattern may be diffuse, peripheral, or speckled, sera may contain multiple ANA evidenced by detecting more than one pattern. One pattern (*e.g.*, speckled) may be masked by another (*e.g.*, diffuse). Multiple antibodies may be present in different concentrations, so the pattern may change as the titer changes. Specific characterization of the ANA can be useful in making a diagnosis of SLE. Antibodies to double-stranded DNA (DS-DNA) and to the Sm antigen are nearly specific for SLE. In patients with active disease, approximately 60% to 75% have anti–DS–DNA antibodies, and 25% have Sm antibodies.[10,21,28] DS–DNA antibodies are strongly associated with SLE, especially at high levels. Some evidence also suggests that this antibody is associated with renal disease. Sm antibodies represent a marker for SLE: They are present only in SLE and not in other rheumatic diseases. Sm antibodies can be detected by immunodiffusion, counterimmunoelectrophoresis, and hemagglutination.[9]

The immunologic nature of SLE is supported by the presence of numerous serum antibodies. Red blood cell antibodies are detected by the direct Coombs test and may cause hemolytic anemia. Anti-lymphocyte antibodies are associated with lymphocytopenia. Antiplatelet antibodies occur in 75% to 80% of patients with SLE and are believed to be responsible for thrombocytopenia. The lupus anticoagulant is an antibody directed against phospholipid and prolongs the partial thromboplastin and prothrombin times. The biological false positive test for syphilis, caused by an autoantibody to the phospholipid cardiolipin, occurs in about 15% of the patients with SLE. Commonly, both phospholipid antibodies occur simultaneously. Rheumatoid factor, another autoantibody, is present in low titer in nearly 30% of patients with SLE.[21]

During the active phase of the disease, complement is decreased. The immune complexes activate the complement cascade, thereby decreasing the serum complement components C3 and C4 and also decreasing the functional activity when serum CH_{50} is measured. Cryoglobulins and circulating immune complexes may be detected in serum. The erythrocyte sedimentation rate also increases, indicating an inflammatory response. Acute-phase reactants, such as C-reactive protein, are also elevated.[29]

Rheumatoid Arthritis

Rheumatoid arthritis (RA) is a chronic noninfectious systemic inflammatory disease of unknown etiology that primarily affects the joints. Women are affected two to three times more often than men. The frequency of the disease increases with age, and the peak incidence occurs in women between 30 and 50 years of age.[21]

Pathogenetically, RA is believed to begin with the production of IgG by lymphocytes in the synovium, because of an unknown stimulus. The IgG is recognized as foreign, stimulating the production of rheumatoid factors (RF). Most RF are of the IgG and IgM (both monomeric and pentameric forms) classes, both of which can recognize the Fc portion of the IgG molecule. Immune complexes are formed, either IgG aggregates or IgM–IgG complexes, and the classical pathway of complement is activated and amplified by the alternative pathway of complement. The inflammatory response proceeds via the bioactive complement fragments, and inflammatory cells enter the synovial space and release intracellular products (*e.g.*, the lysosomal content, prostaglandins, and leukotrienes) that damage the synovium. T cells contribute to the inflammatory process.[24,30] A consequence of the inflammatory response in the joint is the production of a pannus, an abnormal growth of synovial cells following enzymatic destruction of the cartilage.

Clinical manifestations of RA include nonspecific findings of fatigue, weight loss, weakness, mild fever, and anorexia. Morning stiffness and joint pain that improve during the day are present in all patients with RA. The inflammatory joint changes, most often in the small joints, may result in loss of function and permanent deformity. Extra-articular manifestations, most common in patients with high titers of RF, include vasculitis, rheumatoid nodules, and Sjögren's syndrome. Rheumatoid nodules, found in approximately 20% to 25% of patients with RA, especially the more severe forms, are round or oval firm masses located in the subcutaneous tissue near joints. They are areas of collagen necrosis surrounded by a granulomatous inflammation with histiocytes, lymphocytes, and plasma cells. Sjögren's syndrome is an inflammation of salivary and lacrimal glands causing decreased secretion from these glands and results in dryness of the mouth and eyes. It is present in approximately 30% of patients with RA. The association of splenomegaly, neutropenia, and rheumatoid arthritis is referred to as Felty's syndrome.[21]

Laboratory findings in RA include a normochromic, normocytic anemia and thrombocytosis. The erythrocyte sedimentation rate is commonly elevated, as is the concentration of C-reactive protein. RF are detected serologically in about 70% of patients with RA. The hemagglutination method is more specific for RA than the latex agglutination test, because it is more likely to be negative in conditions other than RA, such as hypergammaglobulinemia, syphilis, and old age. In seronegative RA, RF cannot be detected by conventional serologic methods; this is possibly due to the presence of RF that are IgG, monomeric IgM, or RF complexed to IgG.[25] Cryoglobulins may also be present, but serum complement levels are usually normal. Low titers of ANA are present in 20% to 70% of patients.[21]

During active disease, the synovial fluid has the characteristics of an inflammatory exudate; it is cloudy, with a cell count usually between 5000 and 20,000/μL, most of which are neutrophils. The protein concentration is elevated; depolymerization of hyaluronate reduces the viscosity of the fluid and causes a poor mucin clot. Complement is often decreased, and RF may be detected.[25]

Sjögren's Syndrome

Sjögren's syndrome can occur alone (primary Sjögren's syndrome) or in conjunction with other diseases (such as rheumatoid arthritis). Serologic findings that may be observed are polyclonal hypergammaglobulinemia (50% of patients); rheumatoid factor (90%); ANA (70%), usually a speckled or diffuse pattern; and autoantibodies directed against the salivary duct. Specific ANA include SS-B (in primary Sjögren's syndrome), SS-A (associated with SLE), and rheumatoid arthritis nuclear antigen (associated with rheumatoid arthritis).[9,21]

Progressive Systemic Sclerosis (Scleroderma)

Progressive systemic sclerosis (PSS) is a systemic disease in which fibrosis and degenerative changes occur in skin, synovium, and some internal organs. PSS may be associated with Sjögren's syndrome and thyroiditis. The disease may be severe, with generalized skin and internal organ involvement, or more benign, restricted to the skin. CREST syndrome is the milder form of scleroderma manifested by *c*alcinosis, *R*aynaud's phenomenon, *e*sophageal dysmotility, *s*clerodactyly, and *t*elangiectases. Raynaud's phenomenon, pain in the extremities when exposed to cold temperatures, is the most common symptom of the disease (>90% of patients). Laboratory findings include polyclonal hypergammaglobulinemia and ANA (70% of patients) with speckled or nucleolar pattern.[25] Scl-70 antibody is a marker ANA detected in 15% to 20% of patients with PSS, whereas centromere antibody is a marker antibody for the CREST variant with a frequency of 70% to 90%.[9]

Polymyositis–Dermatomyositis

This group of diseases shows acute or chronic inflammatory changes in muscle and skin. Laboratory findings include polyclonal hypergammaglobulinemia, rheumatoid factor, antinuclear antibody, myoglobinemia, increased erythrocyte sedimentation rate, elevated creatine kinase from striated muscle, and increased urine creatine.[25] Specific ANA are PM-1, associated with polymyositis–progressive systemic sclerosis overlap syndrome, and Jo-1, which is the serum antibody most often detected in patients with polymyositis.[9]

Organ-Specific Autoimmune Diseases

Autoimmune Thyroiditis

The two common autoimmune diseases of the thyroid gland are chronic lymphocytic thyroiditis and Graves' disease. Chronic lymphocytic thyroiditis or Hashimoto's thyroiditis most often appears in women between 30 and 60 years of age, with a 5:1 female-to-male ratio.[31] Both humoral and cellular immunity are active in Hashimoto's thyroiditis, as demonstrated by serum antibodies to multiple thyroid antigens and a prominent lymphocytic infiltrate. Destruction of normal thyroid tissue leads to hypothyroidism, loss of thyroid function and low levels of circulating thyroid hormones. The inflammatory response in the thyroid gland is probably initiated by antibody-dependent cell-mediated lymphocytotoxicity.[31]

The thyroid autoantibodies detectable in the serum are directed against three thyroid antigens: thyroglobulin in the follicle, the microsomal antigen in the cytoplasm of the epithelial cells, and the second colloid antigen (CA-2) in the follicle. Approximately 75% of patients with Hashimoto's thyroiditis demonstrate antithyroglobulin antibodies; 70%, antimicrosomal antibodies; and 40%, anti-CA-2.[8] Nearly all (97%) patients with Hashimoto's thyroiditis have at least one of these three antibodies, often in very high titers.[31] The best screening test for thyroid autoantibodies is the indirect immunofluorescence method using primate thyroid sections as the substrate. Using sections fixed in methanol, the presence of thyroglobulin antibodies will cause the follicle to appear flocculent and CA-2 antibodies to appear diffuse; unfixed sections are used to detect microsomal antibodies in which the cytoplasmic staining of the epithelial cells is granular. Most commonly used to detect thyroglobulin and microsomal antibodies is the tanned red cell agglutination method. The need for pure antigen in this test and heterophile antibody interference are disadvantages, but its ease of performance and greater sensitivity are advantages when compared with the indirect immunofluorescence method.[8]

In Graves' disease the thyroid gland is overstimulated, causing diffuse hyperplasia of the gland and the development of a goiter. The continuous stimulation results in hyperthyroidism with elevated serum concentrations of thyroid hormones. Exophthalmos and infiltrative dermopathy also are common findings in Graves' disease.

In normal thyroid function, the gland is stimulated by thyroid stimulating hormone (TSH) to release thyroid hormones. When a sufficient serum level of thyroid hormone is achieved, TSH is no longer secreted by the anterior pituitary; consequently, the thyroid no longer is stimulated. In Graves' disease an autoantibody mimics thyroid stimulating hormone and reacts with the TSH receptor on thyroid cells. Some of these autoantibodies stimulate the thyroid and have been called long-acting thyroid stimulator (LATS) and thyroid-stimulating antibodies (TSab); other antibodies inhibit the action of TSH and have been called thyrotropin binding–inhibiting immunoglobulin (TBII). To clarify the terminology for antibodies that react with the TSH receptor, the American Thyroid Association recently recommended the term *TSH receptor antibody* (TRAb) be used to describe all antibodies reacting with the TSH receptor.[32]

Two different methods have evolved to measure TRAb. One measures the ability of the antibody to stimulate the thyroid gland, and the other measures the ability of the antibody to compete with TSH for receptor binding. The ability of some TRAb to stimulate the thyroid gland while others do not suggests that different epitopes on the TSH receptor are recognized. TRAb directed against the glycoprotein portion of the TSH receptor fails to stimulate the gland, whereas antibodies against the ganglioside portion of the receptor are stimulatory for the thyroid.[33,34]

Other thyroid autoantibodies may also be present in a significant number of patients with Graves' disease: thyroglobulin antibodies in 40%, microsomal antibodies in 50%, and CA-2 antibodies in 5% to 10%.[8]

Idiopathic Adrenal Failure

The idiopathic form of Addison's disease (adrenocortical failure) is associated with the production of antibodies directed against the microsomal component of the adrenal cortical cells in approximately 50% of patients.[35] These antibodies are detected by the indirect immunofluorescence method. Adrenal insufficiency is often accompanied by other autoimmune disorders, such as Hashimoto's thyroiditis, Graves' disease, pernicious anemia, diabetes mellitus, or hypoparathyroidism.[8]

Diabetes Mellitus

Insulin-dependent or type I diabetes mellitus is associated with islet cell antibodies early in the disease. By indirect immunofluorescence, approximately 60% to 85% of patients with insulin-dependent diabetes mellitus have cytoplasmic staining of the β cells of the pancreas.[35]

Chronic Atrophic Gastritis With Pernicious Anemia

Atrophy of the stomach mucosa results in decreased pepsinogen secretion by the chief cells and decreased secretion of hydrochloric acid and intrinsic factor by the parietal cells. Pepsinogens are hydrolytic enzymes necessary to digest protein; hydrochloric acid reduces the pH in the stomach, and intrinsic factor is necessary for vitamin B_{12} absorption. There are two binding sites on intrinsic factor: One can bind to dietary vitamin B_{12} and the other to receptors of the ileum. Thus, the absorption of vitamin B_{12} is achieved. Absence of functional intrinsic factor, therefore, leads to decreased vitamin B_{12} absorption, resulting in pernicious anemia.[36]

In pernicious anemia an inflammatory cell infiltrate destroys the gastric mucosa. Three types of humoral antibodies are frequently associated with pernicious anemia: parietal cell antibodies and two antibodies reactive with intrinsic factor. Parietal cell antibodies, detected by indirect immunofluorescence, appear as a granular, cytoplasmic staining pattern of parietal cells. This granular appearance mimics the staining pattern of mitochondrial antibodies but can be distinguished from it by comparing the reactivity on two tissue substrates, gastric mucosal and renal epithelial cells. Parietal cell antibody will react with the lipoprotein antigen of the parietal cell but not with the mitochondria of epithelial cells of the renal tubules, whereas the mitochondrial antibody will react with mitochondria in both parietal cells and renal tubular epithelial cells.[36]

There are two intrinsic factor antibodies: a blocking antibody (type I) that prevents vitamin B_{12} from binding to intrinsic factor and a binding antibody (type II) that reacts with intrinsic factor or intrinsic factor–vitamin B_{12} complex. The blocking antibody occurs twice as frequently as the binding antibody. In patients with pernicious anemia, approximately 90% have parietal cell antibodies, and 60% to 70% have intrinsic factor antibodies.[36] Parietal cell antibodies are detected in other diseases, such as atrophic gastritis without hematologic changes (60%), chronic thyroiditis (30%), thyrotoxicosis (25%), and diabetes mellitus (21%).[8,36] Intrinsic factor antibodies, however, are found nearly exclusively in pernicious anemia. Low levels of thyroid antibodies may also be present in patients with pernicious anemia.

Autoimmune Chronic Active Hepatitis

Of the many forms of chronic active hepatitis, evidence for autoimmune factors is prominent in one type, classic autoimmune chronic active hepatitis. Histologic changes include intraportal and periportal infiltration of lymphocytes and plasma cells. Diminished number and function of suppressor T cells explain the polyclonal increase in serum immunoglobulin (especially IgG) and the presence of autoantibodies to different organs. Antinuclear antibodies are commonly present; hence, this disease is sometimes called lupoid chronic active hepatitis. Smooth muscle antibodies are present, usually in high titer.[36]

Primary Biliary Cirrhosis

Primary biliary cirrhosis, an autoimmune disease, affects the small bile ducts in the liver and eventually leads to liver failure. Nearly all patients (99%) with primary biliary cirrhosis have high titer mitochondrial antibody, though this antibody may be found less frequently and in lower titers in other liver diseases. The mitochondrial antigen is a lipoprotein located on the inner mitochondrial membrane. Detection of the mitochondrial antibody is most often accomplished by indirect immunofluorescence on rat kidney substrate in which the tubular epithelial cells serve as the source rich in mitochondria. Extrahepatic manifestations of the disease—arthritis, arteritis, and glomerulonephritis—are probably related to the circulating immune complexes. Reduction in number and function of suppressor T cells leads to the overproduction of monomeric IgM and the failure to switch from IgM to IgG production. Patients with primary biliary cirrhosis are severely anergic.[36,37]

Myasthenia Gravis

Myasthenia gravis is a neuromuscular disease in which the innervation of muscles is impaired. Muscle weakness results, especially after sustained exercise, when acetylcholine is prevented from stimulating muscle to contract. Antibodies to acetylcholine receptors, present in approximately 90% of patients with myasthenia gravis, are believed to bind to the acetylcholine receptors, causing endocytosis of the receptors; thus, acetylcholine cannot bind or stimulate the muscle. Other findings contribute to the immunologic basis of the disease, thymic hyperplasia with an increased number of germinal centers and increased B cells (70%), thymoma (a tumor of epithelial cells in the thymus gland; 10%), anti-smooth muscle antibodies, and a greater than expected association with other autoimmune disorders.[38] Experimentally, an anti–acetylcholine receptor antibody, an anti-idiotype antibody, can produce a myasthenialike syndrome in rabbits and mice,[39,40] which has led to the speculation that in human myasthenia gravis the increased number of B cells of the germinal centers in the thymus produce an auto-anti–acetylcholine receptor antibody that is responsible for the impaired neuromuscular transmission.[41] Following thymectomy, two thirds of patients with myasthenia gravis improve, further supporting the role of the thymus in the production of acetylcholine receptor antibodies and the pathogenesis of myasthenia gravis.[38]

Multiple Sclerosis

Multiple sclerosis, a chronic progressive inflammatory disease, is associated with demyelination of the white matter of the central nervous system. Affecting primarily young adults, there is a familial association and a geographic distribution of the disease. The etiology of this disease is unknown; however, an immunologic mechanism is suggested by the presence of lymphocytes in early lesions and plasma cells, lymphocytes, and macrophages in older lesions. Increased γ globulin concentration in cerebrospinal fluid (CSF) is detected in 60% to 80% of multiple sclerosis patients. Faulty T-cell immunoregulation is present in multiple sclerosis; decreased suppressor T-cell function during active disease episodes can explain the increased CSF concentration of IgG.[38] The active lesions of multiple sclerosis, also called plaques, contain suppressor T cells, helper T cells, and macrophages that actively break down myelin. Demyelination results in the release of myelin basic protein into CSF; a concentration greater than 4 ng/mL is associated with multiple sclerosis and other demyelinating diseases.[42]

Increased immunoglobulin concentration in CSF is present in the majority of patients with multiple sclerosis. The two methods for evaluation of central nervous system production of immunoglobulins are the IgG index and CSF protein electrophoresis. With the IgG index one can determine if an increase in CSF IgG is caused by local IgG production or by a change in the permeability of the blood–brain barrier.

$$\text{IgG index} = \frac{\text{CSF IgG/serum IgG}}{\text{CSF albumin/serum albumin}}$$

The normal range for the IgG index is 0.4 to 0.53. An index greater than 0.7 is considered elevated and an indication that IgG production occurs within the central nervous system. The second method to evaluate the production of immunoglobulin in the central nervous system is high-resolution agarose gel electrophoresis of CSF to demonstrate oligoclonal banding in the γ globulin region. Oligoclonal banding is seen as several discrete protein bands in the γ-globulin region and represents immunoglobulins produced by several clones of lymphocytes. Ninety percent of multiple sclerosis patients have oligoclonal banding; however, it is not specific for multiple sclerosis, since it can also be demonstrated in viral meningitis, neurosyphilis, SLE with central nervous system involvement, and other immunologic diseases of the central nervous system.[43]

Autoimmune Bullous Skin Diseases

Pemphigus, bullous pemphigoid, and dermatitis herpetiformis are blistering autoimmune skin diseases.[44] Pemphigus vulgaris is characterized by intraepidermal blisters caused by damage to the intercellular bridges of the cells in the epidermis. Using the direct immunofluorescence technique on a biopsy of perilesional skin, the intercellular space consistently demonstrates the presence of IgG. Circulating serum autoantibodies directed against the intercellular substance can be demonstrated by indirect immunofluorescence using monkey esophagus as the substrate. These autoantibodies are of the IgG class and are present in approximately 90% of patients with pemphigus vulgaris. There is a close association between pemphigus and HLA-DR4.

Bullous pemphigoid is a subepidermal blistering disease in which IgG and C3 can be demonstrated by direct immunofluorescence in biopsies of perilesional skin. The staining pattern is linear, indicated by smooth, continuous fluorescence. By immunoelectronmicroscopy the immune complexes are located in the lamina lucida of the basement membrane. Serum autoantibodies directed against the basement membrane are found in approximately 80% of patients with bullous pemphigoid. These autoantibodies are detected by indirect immunofluorescence and are of the IgG class.[44]

Dermatitis herpetiformis is a chronic bullous disease in which a granular pattern of IgA deposition in perilesional skin can be demonstrated by direct immunofluorescence. Circulating IgA autoantibodies are absent. Dermatitis herpetiformis is nearly always associated with gluten-sensitive enteropathy. A current pathogenetic hypothesis suggests that gluten, or another dietary substance, damages the small intestine and stimulates antibody production. The antibody combines with its antigen and forms circulating immune complexes that lodge in the skin. The alternative pathway of complement is activated, and the resulting production of inflammatory mediators is responsible for the blister formation. Restriction of dietary gluten improves the skin disease.[44] There is a strong association between dermatitis herpetiformis and HLA-DR3 and HLA-B8.[4]

Goodpasture's Syndrome

In Goodpasture's syndrome, circulating antibodies directed against basement membranes combine with the alveolar basement membrane of the lung and the glomerular basement membrane of the kidney. Following complement activation, tissue damage results

in pulmonary hemorrhage and progressive glomerulonephritis. Complement components and anti–basement membrane antibodies can be demonstrated by direct immunofluorescence. The fluorescence pattern is linear and appears smooth, in contrast to the granular pattern associated with immune complex glomerulonephritis. Circulating anti–glomerular basement membrane antibodies of the IgG class can be demonstrated in approximately 89% of patients with Goodpasture's syndrome by indirect immunofluorescence,[45] but enzyme immunoassay is the preferred test because of its greater sensitivity and specificity.

Conclusion

Autoimmunity is an immune process involving recognition of host antigens. This may be beneficial when initiating and regulating an immune response or harmful when damaging host tissue. The spectrum of harmful autoimmunity is great, ranging from organ-specific involvement to non-organ-specific involvement. Both humoral immunity and cell-mediated immunity may contribute to host damage. Evidence of an autoimmune process may be documented by identifying circulating or tissue-lodged immune complexes, circulating autoantibodies, complement consumption or activation, or histologic changes.

References

1. Jerne NK: Towards a network theory of the immune system. Ann Immunol (Paris) 125C:373, 1974
2. Silverstein AM: The history of immunology. In Paul WE (ed): Fundamental Immunology, p 23. New York, Raven Press, 1984
3. Bellanti JA, Calabro JJ, Gelfand MC: Immunologically mediated disease involving autologous antigens. In Bellanti JA (ed): Immunology III, p 409. Philadelphia, WB Saunders, 1985

4. Theofilopoulos AN: Autoimmunity. In Stites DP, Stobo JD, Wells JV (eds): Basic and Clinical Immunology, 6th ed, p 128. East Norwalk, Appleton and Lange, 1987

5. Shoenfeld Y, Schwartz RS: Immunologic and genetic factors in autoimmune diseases. N Engl J Med 311:16, 1984

6. Burdette S, Schwartz RS: Idiotypes and idiotypic networks. N Engl J Med 317:219, 1987

7. Kennedy RC: Anti-idiotype antibodies: prospects in clinical and laboratory medicine. Lab Management 8:33, 1987

8. Zweiman B, Lisak RP: Autoantibodies: Autoimmunity and immune complexes. In Henry JB (ed): Clinical Diagnosis and Management by Laboratory Methods, 17th ed, p 924. Philadelphia, WB Saunders, 1984

9. Nakamura RM, Peebles CL, Molden DP, et al: Autoantibodies to Nuclear Antigens, 2nd ed. Chicago, American Society of Clinical Pathologists Press, 1985

10. Isenberg DA, Maddison PJ: Detection of antibodies to double stranded DNA and extractable nuclear antigen. (Broadsheet 117) J Clin Pathol 40:1374, 1987

11. Linker JB III, Williams RC Jr.: Tests for detection of rheumatoid factors. In Rose NR, Friedman H, and Fahey JL (eds.): Manual of Clinical Laboratory Immunology, 3rd ed, p 759. Washington, DC, American Society for Microbiology, 1986

12. Singer JM, Plotz CM: The latex fixation test. I. Application to the serologic diagnosis of rheumatoid arthritis. Am J Med 21:888, 1956

13. Waaler E: On the occurrence of a factor in human serum activating the specific agglutination of sheep blood corpuscles. Acta Pathol Microbiol Scand 17:172, 1940

14. Rose HM, Ragan C, Pearce E, et al: Differential agglutination of normal and sensitized sheep erythrocytes by sera of patients with rheumatoid arthritis. Proc Soc Exp Biol Med 68:1, 1948

15. Stites DP, Rodgers RPC: Clinical laboratory methods for detection of antigens and antibodies. In Stites DP, Stobo JD, Wells JV (eds): Basic and Clinical Immunology, 6th ed, p 241. East Norwalk, Appleton and Lange, 1987

16. Peacock JE, Tomar RH: Manual of Laboratory Immunology, p 125. Philadelphia, Lea and Febiger, 1980

17. Kyle RA: Classification and diagnosis of monoclonal gammopathies. In Rose NR, Friedman H, Fahey JL (eds): Manual of Clinical Laboratory Immunology, 3rd ed,

p 204. Washington, DC, American Society for Microbiology, 1986

18. Toth CA, Pohl D, Agnello V: Methods for detection of immune complexes by utilizing C1q or rheumatoid factors. In Rose NR, Friedman H, Fahey JL (eds): Manual of Clinical Laboratory Immunology, 3rd ed. Washington, DC, American Society for Microbiology, 1986

19. Theofilopoulos AN, Aguado MT: Assays for detection of complement-fixing immune complexes: Raji cell, conglutinin, and anti-C3 assays. In Rose NR, Friedman H, Fahey JL (eds): Manual of Clinical Laboratory Immunology, 3rd ed, p 197. Washington, DC, American Society for Microbiology, 1986

20. Levinson SS, Goldman J, Nathan LE: Routine immune complex assays for the clinical laboratory: Present status and worth. J Clin Immunoassay 7:328, 1984

21. Rodnan GP, Schumacher HR: Primer on the rheumatic diseases, 8th ed. Atlanta, Arthritis Foundation, 1983

22. Miller KB, Schwartz RS: Autoimmunity and suppressor T lymphocytes. Adv Intern Med 27:281, 1982

23. Winchester RJ, Nunez-Roldman A: Some genetic aspects of systemic lupus erythematosus. Arthritis Rheum 25:833, 1982

24. Miller KB, Schwartz RS: Familial abnormalities of suppressor-cell function in systemic lupus erythematosus. N Engl J Med 301:803, 1979

25. Fye KH, Sack KE: Rheumatic diseases. In Stites DP, Stobo JD, Wells JV (eds): Basic and Clinical Immunology, 6th ed, p 356. East Norwalk, Appleton and Lange, 1987

26. Diaz LA, Provost TT: Dermatologic diseases. In Stites DP, Stobo JD, Wells JV (eds): Basic and Clinical Immunology, 6th ed, p 516. East Norwalk, Appleton and Lange, 1987

27. Silva FG: The nephropathies of systemic lupus erythematosus. In Rosen S (ed): Pathology of Glomerular Disease, p 79. New York, Churchill Livingstone, 1983

28. Ginsberg B, Keiser H: A Millipore filter assay for antibodies to native DNA in sera of patients with systemic lupus erythematosus. Arthritis Rheum 16:199, 1973

29. Tucker ES, Nakamura RM: Laboratory studies for the evaluation of systemic lupus erythematosus and related disorders. Laboratory Medicine 11:717, 1980

30. Roitt I: Essential Immunology, 6th ed. Oxford, Blackwell Scientific Publications, 1988

31. Rose NR, Lorenzi M, Lewis M: Endocrine diseases.

In Stites DP, Stobo JD, Wells JV (eds): Basic and Clinical Immunology, 6th ed, p 582. East Norwalk, Appleton and Lange, 1987

32. Larsen PR, Alexander NM, Chopra IJ, et al: Revised nomenclature for tests of thyroid hormones and thyroid-related proteins in serum. J Clin Endocrinol Metab 46:1089, 1987

33. Valente WA, Vitti P, Rotella CM, et al: Antibodies that promote thyroid growth: A distinct population of thyroid-stimulating autoantibodies. N Engl J Med 309:1028, 1983

34. Yavin E, Yavin Z, Schneider MD, et al: Monoclonal antibodies to the thyrotropin receptor: Implications for receptor structure and the action of autoantibodies in Graves' disease. Proc Natl Acad Sci USA 78:3180, 1981

35. Bigazzi PE, Burek CL, Rose NR: Antibodies to tissue-specific endocrine, gastrointestinal, and neurological antigens. In Rose NR, Friedman H, Fahey JL (eds): Manual of Clinical Laboratory Immunology, 3rd ed, p 762. Washington, DC, American Society for Microbiology, 1986

36. Taylor KB, Thomas HC: Gastrointestinal and liver diseases. In Stites DP, Stobo JD, Wells JV (eds): Basic and Clinical Immunology, 6th ed, p 457. East Norwalk, Appleton and Lange, 1987

37. McMillan SA, Alderdice JM, McKee CM, et al: Diversity of autoantibodies in patients with antimitochondrial antibody and their diagnostic value. J Clin Pathol 40:232, 1987

38. Hoffman PM, Panitch HS: Neurologic diseases. In Stites DP, Stobo JD, Wells JV (eds): Basic and Clinical Immunology, 6th ed, p 598. East Norwalk, Appleton and Lange, 1987

39. Wasserman NH, Penn AS, Freimuth PI, et al: Anti-idiotypic route to anti-acetylcholine receptor antibodies and experimental myasthenia gravis. Proc Natl Acad Sci USA 79:4810, 1982

40. Cleveland WL, Wassermann NH, Sarangarajan R, et al: Monoclonal antibodies to the acetylcholine receptor by a normally functioning auto-anti-idiotypic mechanism. Nature 305:56, 1983

41. Vincent A, Scadding GK, Thomas HC, et al: In vitro synthesis of anti-acetylcholine-receptor antibody by thymic lymphocytes in myasthenia gravis. Lancet 1:305, 1978

42. Gerson BS, Cohen R, Gerson IM, et al: Myelin basic protein, oligoclonal bands, and IgG in cerebrospinal fluid as indicators of multiple sclerosis. Clin Chem 27:1974, 1981

43. Mehl VS, Penn GM: Electrophoretic and immunochemical characterization of immunoglobulins. In Rose NR, Friedman H, Fahey JL (eds): Manual of Clinical Laboratory Immunology, 3rd ed, p 126. Washington, DC, American Society for Microbiology, 1986

44. Dahl MV: Clinical immunodermatology. Chicago, Year Book Medical Publishers, 1981

45. Wilson CB, Yamamoto T, Ward DM: Renal diseases. In Stites DP, Stobo JD, Wells JV (eds): Basic and Clinical Immunology, 6th ed, p 495. East Norwalk, Appleton and Lange, 1987

Glossary

Acquired agammaglobulinemia: Immunodeficiency characterized by a severe decrease or absence of immunoglobulins and occurring in adults with a previously healthy immune system.

Active immunity: The immune response produced by an immunocompetent individual following exposure to a foreign challenge.

Acute glomerulonephritis: A nonsuppurative sequel to group A streptococcal infection characterized by proteinuria, hematuria, hypertension, and general impaired renal function.

Acute lymphoblastic leukemia (ALL): A malignant disease characterized by increased blast cells of lymphoid origin present in the bone marrow and frequently seen in the peripheral blood.

Acute phase proteins: Plasma proteins whose concentration increases or decreases during inflammation.

Adaptive immunity: Immunity that is acquired or learned by an individual only after a challenge is encountered.

Adjuvants: Agents that potentiate or enhance an immune response.

Adoptive immunity: The transfer of immunocompetent cells from one individual to a second individual to establish immunocompetence in the second individual.

Adsorption: In ligand assays, a technique that uses particles to trap free ligand.

Affinity: The tendency for one epitope to unite with one antigen combining site of an antibody molecule.

Affinity maturation: A phenomenon in which antibodies produced later in the secondary immune response have a higher affinity for the antigen than those produced earlier.

Agammaglobulinemia: A humoral deficiency marked by the decrease or absence of serum immunoglobulins.

Agglutination: The cross-linking of a particulate or insoluble antigen by the corresponding antibody.

Agglutination inhibition: A serologic technique in which soluble antigen in the patient's sample reacts with known antibody reagent to form an invisible complex; the antibody reagent is then unavailable to react with the particulate antigen reagent; in this procedure no agglutination yields a positive result.

Agglutinin: Antibody that participates in agglutination reactions.

Agglutinogens: Antigens that participate in agglutination reactions.

AIDS: Acquired immunodeficiency syndrome, caused by the human immunodeficiency virus.

Allergens: Exogenous antigens that elicit an overproduction of IgE.

Allergy: A harmful reaction experienced by some people to commonly encountered environmental antigens, usually caused by the overproduction of IgE.

Allogeneic: Belonging to the same species yet genetically different.

Allograft: Transplanted tissue from a donor to a genetically different recipient of the same species.

Allotype: Genetic variation within a species of the constant region of the heavy or light chain of an immunoglobulin molecule.

α **heavy chain disease:** The most common heavy chain disease characterized by an infiltration of lymphoid and plasma cells into the small intestines; the disease is common in the Middle East.

α_1**-antitrypsin:** An acute phase protein that is a serine protease inhibitor.

α_2**-macroglobulin:** An acute phase protein that is a protease inhibitor.

Alpha-feto protein (AFP): An oncofetal protein normally produced by fetal liver; in adults, elevated serum levels may indicate a hepatoma, testicular teratoblastomas, or other inflammatory diseases.

Amboceptor: Anti–sheep red blood cell antibody that causes hemolysis of sheep red cells in the presence of complement.

Amplification: The generation of C3b in the complement pathway, by either the classical or alternative pathway, to provide a feedback loop to increase the activation of C3 through C9 components.

Anamnestic response: The secondary immune response in which the immune system remembers previous antigenic exposure.

Anaphylatoxin: Biologically active peptides that mediate inflammation by inducing the release of histamine, contracting smooth muscles, and increasing vascular permeability.

Anaphylaxis: Systemic immediate hypersensitivity that occurs when mast cell mediators affect more than one organ.

Anti–deoxyribonuclease B test: A neutralization test in which antibodies in patient serum will prevent the enzyme DNAse B from depolymerizing DNA.

Anti–human globulin: An antibody preparation that contains antibody to a range of globulins (polyspecific) or to a single globulin (monospecific, such as anti-C3b) used to detect sensitized particles.

Anti–hyaluronidase test: A neutralization assay in which antibodies inactivate hyaluronidase and prevent subsequent enzymatic breakdown of the substrate by hyaluronidase.

Antilymphocyte globulin: A form of immune suppression in which serum contains antibodies directed against lymphocytes.

Antinuclear antibody: An autoimmune antibody directed against a component of the nucleus, commonly found in systemic lupus erythematosus.

Antibody-dependent cell-mediated cytolysis (ADCC): An effector mechanism in which cells coated with antibody react with the Fc receptors on lymphocytes to cause target cell damage.

Antigen–antibody complex: The union of an antibody with a homologous antigen.

Antigen-presenting cells (APCs): Accessory cells that present antigen to lymphocytes in conjunction with MHC class II molecules; APCs are required in the initial step of an immune response.

Antigen valency: The number of antigenic determinants present on an antigen.

Antigenic determinant (epitope): The portion of the immunogen molecule that can bind with antibody.

Antigenicity: The ability of a substance to react with immune products.

ARC (AIDS Related Complex): Following HIV exposure, the intermediate clinical state between an asymptomatic infection and AIDS.

Arthus reaction: A type III hypersensitivity reaction, induced experimentally by the intradermal injection of the sensitizing antigen, that allows preexisting antibody to combine with the antigen and causes localized destructive inflammation at the site of immune complex formation.

ASO neutralization test: An enzyme inhibition reaction in which streptolysin O antibodies neutralize the streptolysin O reagent, thus preventing hemolysis of human group O red blood cells by the streptolysin O reagent.

Ataxia telangiectasia: An autosomal recessive immunodeficiency characterized by variable humoral and cellular immune defects, as well as sinopulmonary infection and ataxia.

Atopy: A genetically determined hypersensitivity usually referring to allergic patients who produce an abnormally large amount of specific IgE when exposed to small concentrations of antigen.

Atypical (reactive) lymphocytes: In infectious mononucleosis, suppressor and cytotoxic T lymphocytes capable of recognizing and killing B lymphocytes infected with the Epstein-Barr virus.

Autofluorescence: The natural fluorescence of a tissue or substrate.

Autograft: Tissue transplanted back to the original donor.

Autoimmunity: An immune response directed against self.

Avidity: The tendency for multiple antibodies and multivalent antigens to combine; the cumulative binding strength of all antibody–epitope pairs.

Azathioprine: An immunosuppressive drug that inhibits purine metabolism and DNA proliferation so that cell division is prevented.

AZT (azidothymidine): Used to treat HIV infection, this purine analog inhibits reverse transcriptase, thus preventing viral RNA from being converted to DNA.

Becquerel (Bq): A standardized unit of radioactivity that equals one disintegration per second.

Bence Jones protein: Free light chains.

β particles: Particles emitted from radioisotopes that can be negatively charged electrons (negatrons) or positively charged particles (positrons).

Bruton's X-linked agammaglobulinemia: A congenital X-linked defect in which B cells fail to mature and secrete immunoglobulin.

Burkitt's lymphoma: A malignant neoplasm of B lymphocytes associated with Epstein-Barr virus infection and found primarily among children in a restricted area of Africa and in New Guinea.

C-reactive protein: An acute phase protein produced by the liver in early inflammatory response, capable of precipitating the C-polysaccharide extract of pneumococcus.

Cachectin: Identical to tumor necrosis factor, this monokine mediates inflammation.

CALLA (common acute lymphoblastic leukemia antigen): A 100-kd glycoprotein (CD10) that serves as a useful marker, since it is present in 75% of non-T, non-B acute lymphoblastic leukemia and 40% of lymphoblastic lymphoma.

Carcinoembryonic antigen (CEA): A glycoprotein normally synthesized, secreted, and excreted by the gastrointestinal tract; however, it can be detected in serum in disorders of the gastrointestinal tract. For tumors that secrete CEA, CEA measurements are used to monitor the efficacy of therapy and the recurrence of disease.

Carrier: A molecule that when coupled to a hapten renders the hapten immunogenic.

Cell-mediated immunity: A form of adaptive immunity in which T lymphocytes recognize and react with a challenge through direct cell-to-cell interaction or through lymphokines.

Ceruloplasmin: An acute phase protein that is the principal copper-transporting protein in human plasma.

CH$_{50}$ assay: A hemolytic assay used to assess the function of the classical pathway of complement. Sheep red blood cells coated with rabbit anti–sheep red blood cell antibody are incubated with patient sample. If there is sufficient concentration and function of complement in the patient sample, the classical pathway is activated and hemolysis results.

CH$_{100}$ assay: A diffusion assay used to assess the function of the classical pathway of complement. This test is based on the principle of mixing sensitized sheep red blood cells with agar and placing serum in wells. As diffusion occurs, complement in the serum hemolyzes the cells, producing a measurable clear zone that is proportional in size to the complement activity.

Chancre: A firm, eroded, painless papule with raised margins found in the early stages of syphilis that usually progresses to a clean-based, nonbleeding, painless ulcer.

Chemotactic factor: A substance that directs the migration of neutrophils and monocytes into an area of inflammation.

Chemotaxis: The directed movement of phagocytic cells either toward or away from particles in the environment.

Chessboard titration: Used in indirect immunofluorescence, a serial dilution of conjugated antiserum is reacted with a serial dilution of positive control serum to determine the optimal dilution of conjugated antiserum.

Chiasmata: The crossing-over of genetic information (specifically, genes coding for an MHC antigen) from one chromosome to the sister chromosome.

Chimeras: The exchange of tissue between fraternal twins during fetal life so that each twin recognizes the other's tissue antigens as ''self'' and tolerates the antigens.

Chronic lymphocytic leukemia (CLL): Most often, a B-cell malignancy characterized by an elevated white blood cell count in the peripheral blood and the bone marrow; malignant B cells are morphologically similar to small resting lymphocytes.

Class I antigen: A dimer present on nucleated cell surfaces that is composed of β_2 microglobulin noncovalently bonded to the major histocompatability complex product, a single glycoprotein chain composed of 338 amino acids with a molecular weight of 44,000 d.

Class II antigen: A heterodimer major histocompatibility product composed of two glycoprotein chains, an α and a β chain, which are not covalently bound to each other but are located next to each other on the cell membrane.

Clonal abortion: One proposed mechanism of immune tolerance in which an immature B cell exposed to a low concentration of antigen arrests its maturation process so that it cannot respond to subsequent antigen exposure.

Clone: A population of genetically identical cells derived from a single parent cell.

Cluster of differentiation (CD): Leukocyte surface glycoproteins that are characteristic of specific leukocytes and their stage of maturation or activation; most often detected by monoclonal antibodies.

Cold agglutinins: Autoantibodies of the IgM class that agglutinate human erythrocytes at temperatures less than 37°C and that may be found following *Mycoplasma pneumoniae* infection and other diseases.

Competitive binding assay: A heterogeneous ligand assay in which labeled and unlabeled ligand compete for a limited number of binding sites on the binding reagent.

Competitive radioimmunosorbent test (RIST): A competitive RIA to detect total IgE based on the simultaneous incubation of radiolabeled IgE and unknown IgE with anti-IgE bound to a solid phase.

Complement: A humoral mechanism of nonspecific immune response consisting of at least 14 components that proceed in a cascading sequence of activation, which results in cell lysis.

Complement fixation: A serologic technique in which the test system and indicator system compete for the binding of complement. If complement binds to the specific test antigen–antibody complex, complement will be unavailable to react with the visible indicator system of sensitized sheep red blood cells.

Concanavalin A (Con A): A mitogen derived from the jack bean and used to stimulate T-cell mitosis.

Congenital rubella syndrome: During pregnancy, maternal infection with the rubella virus may result in the virus crossing the placenta and infecting the fetus; detrimental effects of rubella syndrome include congenital heart disease, cataracts, and neurosensory deafness.

Congenital syphilis: The transfer of *Treponema pallidum* across the placenta, which can result in late abortion, stillbirth, neonatal disease, or latent infection; transferral of the organisms can occur at any stage of syphilis.

Contact sensitivity: Systemic sensitization caused by direct skin contact in which a second encounter with the same antigen results in epidermal inflammation.

Countercurrent immunoelectrophoresis: A gel precipitation reaction in which one column of wells contains antibody and a second column of wells contains the antigen. When placed in an electric field, each migrates toward the other until precipitation occurs at the zone of equivalence. It is commonly used to detect autoantibodies, microbial antigens, and antibodies to infectious agents.

CREST: A mild form of scleroderma manifested by *c*alcinosis, *R*aynaud's phenomenon, *e*sophageal dysmotility, *s*clerodactyly, and *t*elangiectases.

Cromolyn (disodium cromoglycate): A therapeutic drug that protects asthmatic patients by stabilizing the lysosomes and preventing the release of mediators from mast cells.

Crystal scintillation: Used to measure γ radioactivity, this technique detects the energy released during decay by exciting a fluor that releases a photon of visible light.

Curies (Ci): The traditional unit of radioactivity; it equals 3.7×10^{10} Bq.

Cutaneous lymphoma: Also referred to as mycosis fungoides, this malignant disease is characterized by malignant T lymphocytes in the skin; malignant T cells in the blood are called Sezary cells.

Cyclosporin: An immunosuppressive drug used in transplantation that inhibits interleukin-2 production and secretion, suppresses helper T-cell activity, and reduces cellular and humoral immunity.

Cyroglobulins: Serum proteins that reversibly precipitate or gel between 0 and 4°C.

Cytokines: Protein molecules secreted by leukocytes that transmit messages to regulate cell growth and differentiation.

Cytotoxicity: Cell destruction; cytotoxicity techniques are commonly used to detect HLA antigens in transplantation.

Cytotoxic T cells (T_c): A subpopulation of T lymphocytes that destroys cells by direct cell-to-cell interaction without the presence of antibody.

Cytotropic: Having a specificity for; IgE is cytotropic for basophils and mast cells.

Dane particle: A complete hepatitis B virion.

Davidsohn differential: A hemagglutination test in which the characteristics of the heterophile antibody are defined by their absorption by guinea pig and beef cell antigens. The heterophile antibodies associated with infectious mononucleosis are absorbed by beef erythrocytes but not by guinea pig antigen.

Delayed hypersensitivity (cell-mediated immune reaction): Type IV hypersensitivity mediated by lymphokines released from sensitized T lymphocytes.

Density gradient centrifugation: The most common procedure for the separation of mononuclear cells in which diluted blood is added to a tube containing a density gradient preparation and centrifuged. Four layers can be identified from top to bottom of the tube: plasma, mononuclear cells, density gradient, and finally red cells and granulocytes.

Diapedesis: The emigration of cells through a blood vessel wall to enter the adjacent tissue.

DiGeorge Syndrome (thymic hypoplasia): An immunodeficiency disease characterized by the failure of parathyroid and thymus glands to develop during fetal life; decreased or absent T lymphocytes and hypocalcemic tetany become apparent shortly after birth.

Direct agglutination: An agglutination reaction in which the antigen is found naturally on the surface of cells (such as red blood cells or bacteria).

Direct anti–human globulin test: An agglutination procedure to detect *in vivo* sensitized red blood cells using anti–human globulin reagent.

Direct immunofluorescence: An immunofluorescence technique in which an antibody labeled with a fluorochrome reacts with a tissue, cell, or microbial test antigen.

Disseminated intravascular coagulation: A secondary pathophysiologic state in which coagulation proteins and platelets are consumed in the microcirculation causing bleeding tendencies; the activated coagulation enzymes also catabolize C3 resulting in decreased serum concentration of C3.

Electrophoresis: A procedure to separate molecules in an electrical field based on differences in migration related to the charge of the particles.

Electrostatic force: The attraction of a positively charged portion of a molecule for a negatively charged portion of a molecule.

Endodermal: Pertaining to the inner layer of a tissue.

Enzyme immunoassay: A ligand assay in which the label is an enzyme and the binding reagent is an antibody.

Eosinophil chemotactic factor of anaphylaxis (ECF-A): A preformed mediator released during mast cell degranulation that stimulates eosinophils to migrate to the site of antigen–antibody reaction.

Eosinophilia: The increased number of eosinophils in the peripheral blood, usually associated with allergic reactions or parasitic infections.

Eosinophilic chemotactic factor (ECF): A preformed mediator released from the mast cell during an allergic response that is responsible for attracting eosinophils to the site of activated mast cells.

Epi-illumination fluorescence microscope: A fluorescence microscope in which excitation light travels from the light source through the excitation filter and is reflected by the dichroic mirror at a 45° angle to the specimen. Light emitted from the specimen travels through the objective, dichroic mirror, and barrier filter before it is viewed.

Epitope (antigenic determinant): The portion of the immunogen molecule that can bind with antibody.

Epstein-Barr virus: A double-stranded enveloped virus belonging to the Herpetoviridae family capable of transforming B lymphocytes, which then become self-perpetuating.

Equivalence: The relative concentration of soluble antibody and soluble antigen that produces maximal antigen–antibody complex formation.

F(ab')₂: The fragment of immunoglobulin molecule generated by pepsin cleavage consisting of the two antigen combining sites joined by disulfide bonds.

Fab: The fragment of an immunoglobulin molecule generated by papain cleavage that binds to one antigen binding site.

Fc: The fragment of immunoglobulin molecule generated by papain cleavage that cannot bind to antigen. The Fc portion of rabbit IgG crystallizes; hence, this is the crystallizable fragment.

Febrile agglutinins: Antibodies produced in response to bacterial infections in which fever is a prominent feature.

Flow cytometry: A method in which a large number of cells pass through an aperture, where they are exposed to light or electric current to generate a signal that is measured. Cell surface markers, cell size, and cell volume are detected by this technique.

Fluid phase diffusion: One of the earliest precipitation reactions to detect unknown antigen or antibody, in which soluble antigen is layered on top of soluble antibody in a capillary tube and each diffuses toward the other until antibody–antigen complex and precipitate at the interface.

Fluorescence: A form of luminescence in which a molecule absorbs light energy of one wavelength and emits light energy of a longer wavelength in less than 10^{-4} seconds.

Fluorescent microscopy: A modified darkfield microscope that uses special components to separate excitation wavelengths from emission wavelengths.

Fluorescent treponemal antibody absorption test (FTA-ABS): An indirect fluorescent antibody test that uses dried Nichols strain *Treponema pallidum* as the antigen. Absorbed patient serum is added to the antigen and fluorescein isothiocyanate labeled anti–human gamma globulin is added to visualize the patient antibody.

Fluorochrome: An organic compound that fluoresces when exposed to short wavelengths of light and that is used to label an antibody so that it can be visualized.

Forbidden-clone theory: A theory of autoimmunity that states that during fetal development those lymphocyte clones that are capable of reacting to self are eliminated.

Fulminant: Occurring with great rapidity.

Functional deletion: One proposed mechanism of immune tolerance in which helper T cells are absent and cannot help to produce an immune response to T-dependent antigens; this occurs with high concentrations of the antigen.

γ emission: A portion of the electromagnetic radiation spectrum that consists of very short wavelengths originating from an unstable nucleus.

γ heavy chain disease: A heavy chain disease characterized by fever, recurrent infection, lymphadenopathy, and progressive proliferation of plasma cells.

Graft versus host disease (GVHD): The clinical and pathologic sequelae that occur when immunocompetent T cells in the graft recognize and attack antigens of the immunoincompetent host.

Granulocytic macrophage colony stimulating factor: A lymphokine that induces the growth of hematopoietic cells that are committed to become granulocytes or macrophages.

Granulomatous hypersensitivity: Cellular reaction resulting when microorganisms persist within macrophages.

Graves' disease: An autoimmune disease of the thyroid in which an antibody to the thyrotropin receptor (thyroid stimulating hormone receptor) stimulates the thyroid.

Gummas: Lesions commonly seen in tertiary syphilis that are believed to be the result of delayed hypersensitivity; lesions may occur in the skin, bones, mucosa, and muscles.

Hairy cell leukemia (leukemic reticuloendotheliosis): A disease characterized by infiltration of irregular "hairy" malignant cells with cytoplasmic projections into the bone marrow and spleen but without peripheral lymphadenopathy.

Half-life: The time needed for 50% of the radionuclide to decay and to become more stable.

Haplotype: A sequence of closely linked alleles on a chromosome that are inherited as a unit.

Hapten: A substance that is antigenic (can bind to an immune product) but not immunogenic (cannot stimulate an immune response).

Haptoglobin: An acute phase protein that binds irreversibly to free hemoglobin, thus forming a complex that is rapidly cleared.

Hashimoto's thyroiditis: An autoimmune thyroid disease characterized by a chronic lymphocytic infiltrate.

Heavy chain: The portion of the immunoglobulin molecule consisting of about 440 amino acids and arranged in one variable domain and three or four constant domains.

Heavy chain disease: Rare lymphoproliferative disorder characterized by the presence of fragments of free heavy chains without light chains.

Helper T cells (T$_H$): A subpopulation of circulating T lymphocytes that function to help other antigen-specific T or B cells to proliferate and differentiate into functional effector cells.

Hemagglutination: Agglutination that occurs when red blood cells are the particles.

Hemolysin (amboceptor): Anti–sheep red blood cell antibody that causes hemolysis of sheep red cells in the presence of complement.

Hemolytic disease of the newborn (HDNB): Present at birth, this disease is caused by maternal–fetal red cell incompatibility. Most commonly, an RhD-negative mother becomes sensitized to the D antigen present on fetal red blood cells; the maternal antibody crosses the placenta and increases the destruction of fetal red blood cells.

Hepatomegaly: Enlargement of the liver.

Heterodimer: A molecule composed of two unrelated units.

Heterogeneous ligand assay: A test procedure that requires the separation of the free label from the bound label in order to quantitate the bound label.

Heterophile antibody: An antibody that is produced in response to one antigen and that reacts with a second, genetically unrelated antigen.

Heterozygous: Having a different allele at the locus on each of the paired chromosomes.

Histamine: A bioactive amine and preformed mediator released from mast cells during allergic responses that is responsible for the immediate effects of bronchoconstriction, increased mucous production, pruritus, increased vasopermeability, and vasodilation in allergic reactions.

Histiocytes: Macrophages that are fixed in various tissues and that are actively involved in phagocytosis.

HIV: Human immunodeficiency virus; the etiologic agent of AIDS.

Hodgkin's disease: A lymphoma characterized by binucleated Reed–Sternberg cells.

Homogeneous ligand assay: A test procedure that does not require a separation step prior to quantitating the label because the bound label selectively separates from the free label or is active only when it is free.

Homology: The degree of sameness; usually used to compare the similarity between genomes (such as HIV-1 and HIV-2) or amino acid sequences (such as IgG1 and IgG2).

Homozygous: Having the same alleles at the locus on both chromosomes.

Humoral immunity: A form of adaptive immunity in which B lymphocytes and plasma cells produce specific antibodies that recognize and react to a challenge.

Hyaluronidase: An enzyme produced by group A β-hemolytic streptococci.

Hydrogen bonding: The attraction of two negatively charged atoms for the positively charged hydrogen ion to create a weak bond.

Hydrophobic force: The attraction between nonpolar groups in an aqueous environment.

Hyperemia: An increased flow of blood into the affected area following injury.

Hypergammaglobulinemia: Increased production of immunoglobulins.

Hypersensitive pneumonitis (extrinsic allergic alveolitis): A type III hypersensitivity reaction in which inhaled antigens combine with preexisting antibody to initiate inflammation.

Hypersensitivity: An exaggerated immune response that causes tissue damage to the host.

Icteric: Pertaining to jaundice.

Identity: In gel precipitation reactions, a smooth continuous line formed when one antigen, identical to the second antigen, reacts with antiserum.

Idiotopes: Antigenic determinants within the variable region of an immunoglobulin molecule.

Idiotype: Genetic variation within the variable domain of an immunoglobulin molecule.

Idiotype network: The interaction between one product of the immune system (such as an antibody) and another product of the immune system (such as a second antibody); the result is the regulation of the production of immune molecules.

IgA: The second most abundant immunoglobulin in serum and the predominant immunoglobulin in secretions.

IgD: The immunoglobulin that is the least abundant in serum and most abundant on the surface of B lymphocytes.

IgE (reagin antibody): The homocytotropic antibody that binds to mast cells and is responsible for allergic responses.

IgG: The most abundant immunoglobulin in serum; prominent in immunity against viruses and bacteria. It is the only immunoglobulin class that crosses the placenta.

IgG index: The comparison of the ratio between cerebrospinal fluid and serum IgG compared to cerebrospinal fluid and serum albumin. An index greater than 0.7 suggests IgG production in the central nervous system.

IgM: The third most abundant immunoglobulin in serum, consisting of a pentameric macromolecule that functions as the first antibody produced in response to an antigen.

Immediate hypersensitivity: An exaggerated immune reaction that occurs within minutes following exposure to the antigen or allergen.

Immune adherence: The covalent bonding between the cleaved form of C3 (C3b) as part of an immune complex and cell surfaces that promotes their removal by the reticuloendothelial system.

Immune complex disorder: The pathophysiology associated with clinical features secondary to immune complex formation and deposition.

Immune status: The measurement of specific antibody to determine whether an individual is resistant or susceptible to an infection.

Immune surveillance theory: The immune response of normal individuals that regularly eliminates malignant or potentially malignant cells, thereby preventing tumor growth.

Immune tolerance: The state of unresponsiveness to an immunogen.

Immunoelectrophoresis (IEP): An immunologic method in gel in which a mixture of proteins is separated by electrophoresis. Antiserum is placed in troughs and diffuses toward the separated proteins until precipitin arcs appear at equivalence. Used to characterize monoclonal proteins in serum or urine.

Immunofluorescence: A histochemical or cytochemical technique to detect an antigen associated with tissue, serum, microorganisms, or cells using an antibody labeled with a fluorochrome.

Immunogen: A substance that causes a detectable immune response.

Immunogenicity: The ability of an antigen to produce an immune response.

Immunologic deficiency theory: A theory of autoimmunity that states that a defect in immune regulation is responsible for autoimmunity.

Immunology: The study of the mechanisms that protect an individual from injury.

Immunometric assay: A ligand assay in which the amount of antigen in the test sample is directly proportional to the measured bound labeled antibody.

Immunosuppression: Reduced activity of T and B lymphocytes and macrophages, including decreased antibody and cytokine production.

Immunotherapy: Therapy to manipulate the immune system against disease and malignancy.

Indirect anti–human globulin test: An agglutination procedure to detect *in vitro* antibody–antigen reactions using anti–human globulin reagent. It is commonly used to detect red cell compatibility.

Indirect immunofluorescence: An immunofluorescence technique used to detect circulating patient antibody after it reacts with a source of known antigen. The bound patient antibody is detected by its reaction with fluorochrome-labeled antibody.

Inducer cells: A T-cell subset that causes the maturation of active T-cell subpopulations.

Innate immunity: Immunity that is present from birth in all individuals and that is activated in the same manner each time the individual is exposed to a challenge.

Innocent bystander cells: Cells in the vicinity of an immune event, most often activated complement, that may be destroyed even though the immune event is directed against different cells.

Interleukin-1 (IL-1): A soluble mediator that promotes proliferation and differentiation of effector cells, specifically antigen-sensitized lymphocytes, including helper T cells.

Interleukin-2 (IL-2): A lymphokine produced and secreted by antigen-sensitized helper T lymphocytes that promotes growth of other activated T cells.

Interleukin-3 (IL-3): A lymphokine that stimulates proliferation of cells in the bone marrow.

Interleukin-4 (IL-4): Also known as B-cell growth factor, this lymphokine stimulates proliferation of antigen-activated B cells and induces differentiation of proliferating B cells into antibody-secreting plasma cells.

Isograft: Transplanted tissue between genetically identical individuals.

Isotype: Different heavy and light chains found in all healthy members of a species as defined by the constant domains of the immunoglobulin molecule.

J chain: A small glycoprotein with a molecular weight of 15,000 d believed to initiate polymerization in IgM and secretory IgA.

Jaundice: The symptom characterized by a yellow coloration of the skin and sclera; it is associated with bilirubinemia and may be seen in hepatitis.

Kinin activation: The interaction of C2b with plasmin to produce polypeptides that promote smooth muscle contraction, mucous gland secretion, vascular permeability, and pain.

Kupffer cells: The most active phagocytic cells of the reticuloendothelial system lining the sinusoids of the liver.

Latency: The stage of acquired or congenital syphilis characterized by the absence of signs and symptoms, yet nontreponemal and treponemal antibody tests are positive.

Leukemia: Malignant proliferation of white blood cells originating in the bone marrow with a peripheral blood phase.

Leukocyte adherence inhibition technique: A one-step technique in which activated lymphocytes are added to a test tube; if the lymphokine is produced, it will inhibit the migration of leukocytes. The cells that do not adhere to the test tube are counted.

Leukotriene: A mediator synthesized from arachidonic acid after initial mast cell stimulation that constricts bronchial smooth muscle and stimulates mucus production and secretion.

Ligand: A molecule that combines with specific complementary configurations of the binding reagent (such as receptors, proteins, or antibody).

Light chain: The portion of the immunoglobulin molecule consisting of approximately 220 amino acids and arranged in one variable domain and one constant domain.

Luminescence: The property of a molecule to emit a photon of light as it reverts to the stable ground state.

Lymph node: An encapsulated collection of lymphocytes and antigen-presenting cells that is a site of antigen interaction, lymphocyte recirculation, and lymphocyte proliferation.

Lymphadenopathy: Enlarged lymph nodes.

Lymphocytosis: An increase in the number of lymphocytes present in peripheral blood.

Lymphokine-activated killer cell (LAK): Cells that respond to IL-2, share many cell surface antigens with NK, cells and can lyse target cells.

Lymphoma: Malignant tumor of lymphoid tissue.

Lymphoplasmapheresis: A method to remove lymphocytes and immunoglobulin from the blood of a transplant recipient.

Lymphoproliferative diseases: The clonal expansion of the cells of the immune system that undergo malignant transformation at a particular maturational or activation stage.

Lysozyme: An enzyme found in secretions that disrupts the cell wall of bacteria, thus killing the organism.

M antigens: Proteins in the cell wall of group A streptococci that determine the serotype and allow the bacterium to adhere to the host cell.

Maturational arrest: The phenomenon that results in the accumulation of malignant lymphocytes with a similar degree of maturation.

Mediator cells: Cells that participate in immunologic reactions by releasing biochemical substances.

Mesodermal: Pertaining to the middle layer of a tissue between the endoderm and the ectoderm.

MHC restriction: The phenomenon that occurs when a lymphocyte population is activated only in the presence of an antigen and a specific class of MHC molecule.

Micro-indirect immunofluorescence test (IFA): The reference assay for rickettsial infections, in which twofold dilutions of patient serum react with multiple rickettsial antigens; the patient antibody is detected using fluorescein-conjugated anti–human IgM or IgG.

Migration inhibition assay: A one-step procedure used to detect the presence of macrophage inhibitory factor (MIF) by incubating lymphocytes, mononuclear cells, and an antigen to activate the lymphocytes. Once activated, the lymphocytes will produce MIF, which inhibits the migration of monocytes/macrophages *in vitro*.

Mitogenic factor: A substance produced by thymic macrophages that induces T-cell development.

Mitogens: Substances that induce cell division. For T and/or B cells these substances serve as the stimulus in lymphocyte transformation.

Mixed lymphocyte culture (MLC): A laboratory technique in which lymphocytes are transformed when exposed to genetically dissimilar lymphocytes; commonly used to detect MHC Class II molecules.

Monoclonal antibody: The transformation of one clone of B cells to produce one class of immunoglobulin with one specificity.

μ heavy chain disease: A rare heavy chain disease that mimics chronic lymphocytic leukemia because vacuolated lymphocytoid plasma cells frequently appear in the peripheral blood.

Multiple myeloma: A neoplasm of single clone of plasma cells that results in an excess of homogeneous immunoglobulin.

Mycoplasma: A genus of organisms lacking a cell wall; the species *Mycoplasma pneumoniae* is the etiologic agent in most cases of atypical pneumonia and can cause upper respiratory tract infections.

Nasopharyngeal carcinoma: A rare form of squamous cell carcinoma associated with Epstein-Barr virus infection.

Natural immunity: Immune reaction that is present spontaneously in normal individuals, does not depend on previous exposure to an antigen, and occurs in the same manner each time an antigen is encountered.

Natural killer cells (NK): A group of lymphocytes that contain cytoplasmic granules and are capable of destroying virus-infected, neoplastic, or allogeneic cells without previous sensitization.

Neoantigens: New antigens expressed by tumor cells.

Neoplasm: An abnormal growth of tissue.

Nephelometric endpoint: In an immunoprecipitation reaction, maximal light scatter due to immune complex formation.

Nephelometric inhibition immunoassay: A nephelometric assay in which haptens form soluble complexes with the antihapten antiserum and prevent detectable complexes from forming between haptens bound to carrier proteins and hapten antiserum.

Nephelometry: A direct measurement of light scattered by particles suspended in solution.

Nezelof's syndrome: A cellular immune deficiency syndrome that is marked by T-cell dysfunction and abnormal immunoglobulin synthesis.

Non-Hodgkin's lymphoma: A heterogeneous group of lymphoid cell cancers that are not Hodgkin's disease.

Nonicteric: Lacking jaundice.

Nonidentity: In gel precipitation reactions, a crossed precipitin line formed when two different antigens react with antiserum.

Nonimmune precipitation: In ligand assays, precipitation of protein-bound ligand by altering its solubility without using antibody.

Nonspecific staining: A nonimmunologic interaction of the conjugated antibody with an antigen; it may be due to the presence of free fluorochrome, interference from serum protein other than immunoglobulin, or mishandled specimens.

Nucleocapsid: A virion without a capsule.

Oncology: The study and treatment of tumors or neoplasms.

Opsonins: Substances that enhance phagocytosis by increasing the rate and quality uptake of a particle.

Opsonization: The process of coating an antigen with antibody to provide more effective phagocytosis.

Partial identity: In gel precipitation reactions, a single precipitin line with a spur formed when one antigen shares common elements with the second antigen and both antigens react with the antiserum.

Passive agglutination (indirect): An agglutination reaction in which an inert carrier particle is coated with a specific antigen.

Passive immunity: The transient protection acquired when preformed immune products, such as antibodies, sensitized lymphocytes, and lymphokines are administered to an individual.

Pathogenicity: The ability to cause disease.

Paul Bunnell test: A screening test to detect heterophile antibodies by reacting dilutions of heat-inactivated patient serum with a standard concentration of sheep erythrocytes and observing agglutination.

Phagocytosis: In nonspecific immune response, the process of engulfment and uptake of particles from the environment by polymorphonuclear neutrophils.

Phosphorescence: A type of luminescence in which the length of time between excitation and emission of light is long (greater than 10^{-4} seconds).

Phytohemagglutinin (PHA): A mitogen derived from kidney bean plant that transforms T cells predominantly.

Platelet-activating factor: A phosphorylcholine derivative that is chemotactic for neutrophils and aggregates platelets.

Pluripotent stem cell: A precursor cell that can differentiate into many different cell types; cells of the immune system originate from primordial cells in the embryonic yolk sac and later in the bone marrow.

Pokeweed mitogen (PWM): A mitogen that stimulates predominantly B cells to divide.

Polyclonal antibody: The increased production of different classes of immunoglobulins due to the transformation of many clones of B cells.

Polyethylene glycol: Commonly used in nephelometric assays to promote antigen–antibody complex formation.

Polymorphism: Multiple alleles at a single locus.

Postcapillary high endothelial venule: Specialized endothelial cells of postcapillary venules in the lymph node to which T and B cells adhere when entering a lymph node and which allows lymphocytes to leave the bloodstream and enter the interstitial fluid of the lymph node.

Postzone: Relative antigen excess compared to the antibody concentration that results in diminished or absent detectable antigen–antibody complex.

Precipitation reaction: The formation of an insoluble complex composed of soluble antigen and soluble antibody.

Primary amyloidosis: A rare disorder characterized by the accumulation of a complex, extracellular, proteinaceous substance dominated by a fibrillar component.

Primary immune response: The cellular and humoral events that occur the first time an antigen is encountered by an individual.

Primary syphilis: The first stage of *Treponema pallidum* infection characterized by the appearance of a chancre.

Primed: Immune cells that have been previously exposed to an antigen.

Properdin (P): A protein of the alternative complement pathway that stabilizes the C3bBb complex to prolong the activity of C3 and C5 convertase.

Prostaglandin D$_2$: An arachidonic acid derivative produced in mast cells that is responsible for a wheal and flare reaction in immediate hypersensitivity.

Prozone: Relative antibody excess compared to the antigen concentration that results in diminished or absent detectable antigen–antibody complex.

Purified protein derivative (PPD): Antigenic material derived from a filtrate of *Mycobacterium tuberculosis* culture used in the skin test to determine exposure to *M. tuberculosis*.

Radial immunodiffusion (RID): Gel precipitation reaction in which monospecific antiserum is incorporated into the gel and soluble antigen is placed in the wells. Antigen diffuses in all directions, combines with the antibody, and forms a precipitin ring surrounding the well.

Radioallergosorbent test (RAST): A sandwich immunoassay to quantitate IgE antibodies directed against specific allergens.

Radioisotope: An atom with an unstable nucleus that spontaneously emits radiation as it decays to a stable nucleus.

Rapid plasma reagin card test (RPR): A rapid macroscopic flocculation test performed on a disposable cardboard slide that uses the VDRL antigen with charcoal particles added to allow macroscopic visualization of the flocculation.

Raynaud's phenomenon: Pain in the extremities when exposed to cold temperatures.

Reagin screen test (RST): A macroscopic flocculation test based on the use of modified VDRL antigen with added Sudan black B for visualization of flocculation. The test can be read qualitatively and quantitatively for the screening and diagnosis of syphilis.

Reaginic antibody: Immunoglobulin E.

Relative risk: The degree of association between a particular HLA antigen and a disease.

Reticuloendothelial system (RES): Mononuclear phagocytes located primarily in the reticular connective tissue framework of the spleen, liver, and lymphoid tissue.

Retrogenetic antigens (oncofetal antigens): Antigens that are normally expressed by fetal tissue and that can be expressed in transformed adult tissue.

Retrovirus: An RNA virus that contains reverse transcriptase, which enables the virus to make DNA from viral RNA.

Reverse passive agglutination: A passive agglutination reaction in which the carrier particle is coated with antibody.

Rheumatic fever: Following untreated streptococcal pharyngitis, this immune-mediated acute inflammatory disease is characterized by carditis, chorea, and erythema marginatum.

Rheumatoid factor: An antibody directed against the Fc portion of an IgG molecule; only those of the IgM class are serologically detectable.

Rocky Mountain spotted fever (tick-borne typhus): A febrile disease marked by skin rash, fever, headache, and myalgia; caused by *Rickettsiae rickettsii*.

Rosetting: A technique to identify T cells that express receptors for sheep red blood cell (E-rosette receptor) or CD3; when SRBCs are incubated with purified lymphocytes, the SRBC will bind to the E-rosette receptor, thus identifying T cells.

Rubella (German measles): A mild contagious illness caused by the rubella virus and characterized by an erythematous maculopapular rash occurring primarily in children 5–14 years old and in young adults.

Sandwich assay (antigen capture assay): A ligand test in which the binding reagent (usually antibody) is immobilized to an inert surface; unlabeled antigen binds to the immobilized antibody and is quantitated after labeled antibody is added.

Secondary immune response: The cellular and humoral events that occur when an antigen is encountered after the first time; this immune response is shorter, faster, and wider than the primary immune response due to immunologic memory.

Secondary syphilis: The disseminated stage of *Treponema pallidum* infection that is marked by skin rashes, low-grade fever, malaise, and the presence of large numbers of treponemes throughout the body; all serologic tests are positive during this stage of the disease.

Secretory component (SC): A glycoprotein added to secretory IgA and secretory IgM and believed to add resistance to proteolytic enzyme digestion.

Self-tolerance: The ability of the body not to respond to autologous antigens.

Sensitization: (1) The induction of an immune response; (2) the attachment of antibody to an antigen-coated particle without agglutination.

Sequela: A disease caused by a previous disease.

Sequestered antigen theory: A theory of autoimmunity that states that some self antigens are hidden from cells of the immune system.

Seroconversion: The detection of specific antibody in the serum of an individual in whom this antibody was previously undetectable.

Serum sickness: An immune complex disorder frequently found in patients who received heterologous serum during immunotherapy and produced antibodies to the serum proteins.

Severe combined immunodeficiency (SCID): The most severe of the immunodeficiencies, characterized by the decrease or absence of both T and B lymphocytes.

Slow-reacting substances of anaphylaxis (SRS-A): Allergic metabolites of arachadonic acid (leukotrienes B_4, C_4, and D_4) that sustain smooth muscle contraction, vasodilatation, and increased vasopermeability.

Specific staining: Fluorescence that results from an immunologic reaction between the conjugated antibody and the antigen.

Splenomegaly: Enlargement of the spleen.

Staphylococcal protein A (SpA): A cell wall protein that interacts with the Fc receptor on B cells and is mitogenic for some lymphocytes.

Stasis: The complete cession of blood flow during severe injury.

Streptococcus pyogenes: Group A, gram-positive, β-hemolytic bacteria that cause oropharyngitis, pyoderma, scarlet fever, and rheumatic fever.

Streptozyme: A rapid, passive hemagglutination slide test to detect antibodies to any of the 5 streptococcal extracellular enzymes produced by group A β-hemolytic streptococci; patient serum and sheep erythrocytes coated with streptococcal enzymes are mixed together and observed for agglutination.

Sucrose density gradient ultracentrifugation: A technique used to separate IgM antibodies physically from IgG antibodies; the antibody-rich fraction can then be tested for the presence of a specific antibody.

Surface immunoglobulin (sIg): The unique surface marker on B cells that is synthesized by the B cell, is expressed on its surface, and serves as the antigen receptor.

Surrogate testing: One test that is performed to indicate indirectly a second infectious or chemical antigen.

Swiss-type agammaglobulinemia: An autosomal recessive immunodeficiency that occurs in infants and is characterized by nonfunctional T and B cells.

Syngeneic: Members of the same species that are genetically identical.

Systemic lupus erythematosus: A chronic inflammatory, multisystem, autoimmune disease characterized by periods of remission and exacerbation.

T-dependent antigens: Antigens that require helper T cells to generate an antibody response.

T-independent antigens: Substances capable of activating B cells without help from T cells.

Terminal deoxynucleotidyl transferase (TdT): An enzyme needed for DNA replication found predominantly in immature T cells.

Tertiary syphilis (gummatous syphilis): A slow, progressive, inflammatory disease that can produce clinical illness 2–40 years after initial infection and that results in neurologic and cardiovascular damage.

Theophylline: A methylxanthine that relaxes bronchial smooth muscle.

Thymocyte: Lymphoid cells of the thymus that mature and differentiate into T lymphocytes before being released into the peripheral circulation.

Thymoma: An epithelial cell tumor of the thymus.

Thymosin: A thymic hormone that promotes T-cell differentiation.

Thymus: Derived from the embryonic pharyngeal pouches, this organ provides a microenvironment in which T cells mature.

Transformation: Lymphocytes proliferate in response to a stimulus and become immunoblasts with increased cell size, nuclear size, and DNA content; the ability of lymphocytes to respond is useful to assess and monitor congenital defects, immunosuppressive therapy, and lymphokine production.

Transmitted light microscope: A fluorescent microscope in which light travels from the light source through the excitation filter, darkfield condenser, specimen, and barrier filter before it is viewed.

Treponema pallidum: An aerobic bacterium belonging to the order Spirochaetales that causes syphilis.

***Treponema pallidum* immobilization test (TPI):** A confirmatory test for syphilis based on measuring the ability of antibody and complement to immobilize a suspension of live treponemes.

Tumor: Swelling; neoplasm.

Tumor necrosis factor (TNF): A monokine that has direct cytolytic activity against tumor cells.

Turbidimetry: The measurement of light transmitted through a suspension of particles.

Unheated serum reagin test (USR): A nontreponemal, microscopic flocculation screening test that uses the choline chloride–EDTA modified VDRL antigen and that is primarily used to monitor the efficacy of syphilis treatment.

Van der Waals force: A weak attractive force between the electron cloud of one atom and the nucleus of another atom.

Vasculitis: A group of syndromes that have common clinicopathologic features associated with an inflammatory reaction in vessel walls.

Venereal Disease Research Laboratory slide test (VDRL): A standard nontreponemal screening test based on the principle of microscopic examination of patient heat-treated serum (source of reagin antibodies) for its ability to flocculate with VDRL antigen containing 0.03% cardiolipin, 0.9% cholesterol, and 0.21% lecithin.

Viral hemagglutination: A natural phenomenon that occurs when a virus agglutinates red blood cells by binding to receptors on the surface of the red blood cells.

Virion: A virus particle.

Waldenström's macroglobulinemia: A rare disorder characterized by an uncontrolled proliferation of a single clone of plasma cells that synthesize homogeneous IgM.

Weil–Felix test: An assay to detect rickettsial antibodies by observing agglutination with certain strains of *Proteus vulgaris.*

Wiscott–Aldrich syndrome: An X-linked recessive disorder that involves multiple immune defects, the presence of eczema, thrombocytopenic purpura, increased susceptibility to infection, and increased IgA and IgE levels.

Xenogeneic: Denoting members of different species with a different genetic background.

Xenograft: Transplanted tissue from a donor to a recipient of different species.

Zidovudine (3′azido-3′deoxythymidine): Used to treat HIV infection, this purine analog inhibits reverse transcriptase, thus preventing viral RNA from being converted to DNA.

Index

Entries followed by *f* indicate figures; those followed by *t* indicate tabular material; those followed by *g* indicate glossary entries. Drugs are listed under their generic names. When a drug trade name is listed, the reader is referred to the generic drug name.

Goodpasture's syndrome (*continued*)
glomerulonephritis in, 77
HLA antigens in, 16t
Gout, complement levels increased in, 147t
gp41, of HIV, 242, 244
gp120, of HIV, 242, 244
gp160, of HIV, 244
Grafts. *See also* Transplantation
types of, 12t
Graft versus host disease, 15, 346g
immune deficiency and, 316
Granulocyte-monocyte colony stimulating factor, 40t
Granulocytes
degranulation of in phagocytosis, 46
polymorphonuclear, 23–24
Granulocytic macrophage colony stimulating factor, 42, 346g
Granulocytopenia, and complement-mediated cell lysis in type II hypersensitivity reactions, 74
Granulomatous disease, chronic, 46–47
Granulomatous hypersensitivity, 79, 347g
Graves' disease, 333, 347g
and antibody-mediated tissue damage in type II hypersensitivity reaction, 73
anti-idiotypes in, 320–321
HLA antigens in, 16t
Gummas, 208, 347g
GVHD. *See* Graft versus host disease

H
Hairy cell leukemia, 295, 347g
Half-life, 347g
Haplotype, 8, 347g
Haptens, 31–32, 108–109, 347g
antibody affinity and, 118–119
Haptoglobin, in acute phase response, 60–61, 347g
Hashimoto's thyroiditis (Hashimoto's disease), 333, 347g
HLA antigens in, 16t
Hassall's corpuscles, 25f, 26
HAV. *See* Hepatitis A virus
HBcAg. *See* Hepatitis B core antigen
HBeAg. *See* Hepatitis B e antigen
HBsAg. *See* Hepatitis B surface antigen
HBIG. *See* High-titer anti-HBs HBV immune serum globulin
HBV. *See* Hepatitis B virus
hCG. *See* Human chorionic gonadotropin
HCG-B combi RIA, 174t
HCV. *See* Hepatitis C virus
HDV. *See* Hepatitis delta virus

HDV-antigen, 265
Heart-lung transplantation, HLA typing and, 11t
Heart transplantation, HLA typing and, 11t, 14
Heavy-chain diseases, 288, 347g
Heavy chains, 93–94, 95f, 97, 347g. *See also specific type*
Helper-inducer T cells
CD markers and, 21
differentiation of, 22
Helper-suppressor (CD4/CD8) cell ratio, in AIDS, 247
Helper T cells, 347g. *See also* Helper-inducer T cells
HIV affecting, 246, 247t
measurement of, 194
MHC restriction and, 17
Hemagglutination, 347g
inhibition test in rubella, 219–220
interpretation of, 220
principle of, 219
procedure for, 219–220
for rheumatoid factor identification, 327
in syphilis, 212–213
treponemal test, 212
viral, 138–139, 356g
Hematopoietic hypoplasia, SCID with, 313
Hemoglobinuria
paroxysmal cold, decreased CH50 levels in, 148t
paroxysmal nocturnal, C3 and C4 levels in, 149t
Hemolysin (amboceptor), 347g
Hemolytic anemia, and antibody-mediated tissue damage in type II hypersensitivity reaction, 73
Hemolytic disease of the newborn, 347g
and complement-mediated cell lysis in type II hypersensitivity reactions, 73
Heparin, in mast cells, 48
Hepatitis A, 259–260
antigen and antibody response in, 260f
clinical manifestations of, 259–260
epidemiology of, 259
laboratory diagnosis of, 260
Hepatitis A virus, 259
detection of, 258
Hepatitis B, 260–263
acute, antigen and antibody response in, 263f
chronic, antigen and antibody response in, 263f
clinical manifestations of, 262

epidemiology of, 261–262
laboratory diagnosis of, 262–263
Hepatitis B core antigen, 261
antibodies to, 261
Hepatitis B e antigen, 261
antibodies to, 261
and laboratory diagnosis of HBV infections, 262–263
Hepatitis B surface antigen, 260, 261
antibodies to, 261
blood screened for, 262
chronic carriers and, 262
and laboratory diagnosis of HBV infections, 262–263
Hepatitis B vaccine, 262
Hepatitis B virus, 260–261
detection of, 258
Hepatitis C virus, 264
Hepatitis delta virus, 164. *See also* Delta hepatitis
Hepatitis (viral), 257–266. *See also specific type*
active chronic, HLA antigens in, 16t
acute, complement levels increased in, 147t
autoimmune chronic active, 335
delta, 264–265
enzyme-linked immunosorbent assay in diagnosis of, 258–259
infective, with arthritis, decreased CH50 levels in, 148t
non-A/non-B, 263–264
radioimmunoassay in diagnosis of, 258
serum, 261
testing for, 257–259
general principles of, 257–258
type A, 259–260
type B, 260–263
Hepatomegaly, 347t
mononuclear phagocyte system activity and, 50
Hereditary angioedema
C1INH deficiency and, 56–57, 148
C4 levels in, 149
decreased CH50 levels in, 148t
Heterodimer, 347t
Heterogeneous ligand assay, 347t
Heterophile antibody, 120–121
in EBV infections, 228
test for, 140t
Heterozygous, 347g
Hexose monophosphate, in chronic granulomatous disease, 46
HI. *See* Hemagglutination, inhibition test
High-grade lymphoma, 294–295
High-titer anti-HBs HBV immune serum globulin, in hepatitis B exposure, 262

LPS. *See* Lipopolysaccharide
LTC₄, 48
LTD₄, 48
LTE₄, 48
LTR. *See* Long terminal repeats
Luminescence, 350*g*
Luminescent labels, in ligand assays, 172
Lupus erythematosus
  drug-induced, ANA profile in, 325*t*
  systemic. *See* Systemic lupus erythematosus
Lymphadenopathy, 350*g*
  mononuclear phagocyte system activity and, 49
Lymphadenopathy-associated virus. *See* Human immunodeficiency virus
Lymph nodes, 26–27, 350*g*
  macrophages of, 49
  structure of, 26*f*
Lymphocyte activation products, lymphocyte function assessed by, 199–200
Lymphocyte cytotoxicity procedure, in HLA antigen detection, 6
Lymphocyte markers, 290–292
Lymphocytes, 19–23. *See also* B lymphocytes; T lymphocytes
  atypical (reactive), 227–228, 231, 342*g*
  circulation of, 28–29
  enumeration of subsets of, 191–194
  in immunodeficiency diseases, 308*t*
  large granular, 23
  separation of, 191*f*
  transformation of, 356*g*
    lymphocyte function assessed by, 197–198, 203*t*
Lymphocytic thyroiditis, 333
Lymphocytosis, 350*g*
  in infectious mononucleosis, 231–232
Lymphoid malignancy, 290–297. *See also* Leukemia; Lymphoma
  lymphocyte marker analysis in diagnosis of, 290–292
Lymphoid organs
  primary, 25–26
  secondary, 26–28
Lymphokine-activated killer cells, 85, 350*g*
Lymphokines, 42
  lymphocyte function assessed by, 199–200
  in tumor immunity, 82
Lympholysis, cell-mediated, 202, 203*t*
Lymphoma, 292–295, 350*g*
  Burkitt's, 342*g*
    Epstein Barr virus associated with, 227

CALLA expressed in, 291
CD markers in study of, 195
cutaneous T-cell, 295
diffuse
  large cells, 293–294
  mixed small and large cells, 293
  small cleaved cells, 293, 294*f*
follicular
  mixed small cleaved and large cells, 293
  predominantly large cells, 293
  predominantly small cleaved cells, 293
high-grade, 294–295
Hodgkin's, 292, 348*g*
  radiotherapy in, 90
intermediate-grade, 293–294
large cell, immunoblastic, 294
low-grade, 292–293
lymphoblastic, 294
non-Hodgkin's, 292–295, 352*g*
small lymphocytic cell, 292–293
small noncleaved cell, 294–295
Lymphoplasmapheresis, 14, 350*g*
Lymphoproliferative diseases, 290–297, 350*g*. *See also* Leukemia; Lymphoma
  lymphocyte marker analysis in diagnosis of, 290–292
Lysis, complement-mediated
  in nonspecific immune response, 54
  in type II hypersensitivity reactions, 73–74
Lysozyme, 350*g*

M

MAb. *See* Monoclonal antibodies
MAC. *See* Membrane attack complex
MAC inactivator. *See* Membrane attack complex inactivator
α₂-Macroglobulin, 60*t*, 62, 341*g*
Macroglobulinemia, Waldenström's, 287–288, 356*g*
  clinical findings in, 287
  laboratory findings in, 287
Macrophage activation factor, 40*t*, 41
  in tumor immunity, 82
Macrophage colony stimulating factor, granulocytic, 42, 346*g*
Macrophage-mediated cytotoxicity, in tumor immunity, 84
Macrophage migration inhibitory factor (migration inhibitory factor), 40*t*, 41
  lymphocyte function assessed by, 199, 200*f*, 203*t*
  macrophage response to, 50
  in tumor immunity, 82
Macrophages, 23, 41, 49

MAF. *See* Macrophage activation factor
Major histocompatibility antigens, 4–10
  class I, 4–5
  class II, 5–6
  class III, 6
  cytotoxicity test in identification, of, 200–201
  mixed-lymphocyte culture in identification of, 198–199
Major histocompatibility complex, 4–18
  HLA regions in, 4
  in immune response regulation, 15–17
  location of, 4
  restriction by, 15–17, 38, 351*g*
Malaria
  C3 and C4 levels in, 149*t*
  P. falciparum, CD4 and CD8 T cells affected by, 195*t*
Malignancy. *See* Cancer
Malignant lymphoma
  diffuse
    large cells, 293–294
    mixed small and large cells, 293
    small cleaved cells, 293, 294*f*
  follicular
    mixed small cleaved and large cells, 293
    predominantly large cells, 293
    predominantly small cleaved cells, 293
  large-cell, immunoblastic, 294
  lymphoblastic, 294
  small lymphocytic cell, 292–293
  small noncleaved cell, 294–295
MALT. *See* Mucosal-associated lymphoid tissues
M antigens, 234, 234*f*, 351*g*
Marek's disease, immunoprophylaxis of, 90
Marker antibodies, 324
  in CREST syndrome, 324, 324*t*, 333
  in progressive systemic sclerosis, 324, 324*t*, 333
  in systemic lupus erythematosus, 324, 324*t*, 331
Mast cells, 24, 48
  sensitization of, 68–69
  in type I hypersensitivity reaction, 69–71
Maturational arrest, 290, 351*g*
Mediator cells, 48–49, 351*g*
  biologic activities of, 48*f*
Mediators
  of nonspecific immune response, 48–49
  of type I hypersensitivity reaction, 71–72

Polymorphonuclear neutrophils
  (*continued*)
  dysfunctions of, 46–47
  emigration of in inflammation,
    63–64
  locomotion of, 45
  phagocytosis and, 45–46
Polymyositis/dermatomyositis, 333
  antinuclear antibodies in, 325*t*, 333
Postcapillary high endothelial venule,
    27, 353*g*
Poststreptococcal glomerulonephritis,
    acute, 236
  reliability of tests for, 236*t*
Postzone, 353*g*
PPD. *See* Purified protein derivative
Precipitation curve, 124*f*
  nephelometry and, 181*f*
Precipitation reaction, 123–134, 353*g*
  agglutination reactions compared
    with, 136*t*
  capillary tube, advantages and dis-
    advantages of, 133*t*
  countercurrent immu-
    noelectrophoresis, 125*t*,
    129–131
    advantages and disadvantages of,
      133*t*
  fluid phase, 124–125
    kinetics of in nephelometry,
      180–182
  in gel, 125–134
  immune, for separation in ligand as-
    says, 169*t*, 170
  immunoelectrophoresis, 125*t*, 130*f*,
    131*f*, 132–133
    advantages and disadvantages of,
      133*t*
  immunofixation electrophoresis,
    125*t*, 131*f*, 133–134
    advantages and disadvantages of,
      133*t*
  nonimmune, for separation in ligand
    assays, 169–170, 352*g*
  Ouchterlony double diffusion,
    125–127
    advantages and disadvantages of,
      133*t*
  radial immunodiffusion, 125*t*, 126*f*,
    127–129
    advantages and disadvantages of,
      133*t*
  rocket technique, 125*t*, 132*f*, 134
    advantages and disadvantages of,
      133*t*
  techniques for
    advantages and disadvantages of,
      133*t*
    types of, 125*t*
  test procedures using, 132*t*

time course of, nephelometry and,
    181*f*
Pregnancy
  complement levels increased in, 147*t*
  hCG tests for, 174*t*, 176–177
  tests for, 140*t*
Pregnosis, 174*t*
Primary amyloidosis, 288–289, 353*g*
Primary immune response, 34–35,
    353*g*
Primed, 353*g*
Progressive systemic sclerosis,
    332–333
  ANA profile in, 325*t*
Proliferation, in inflammation, 65
Properdin, 58, 353*g*
  functional assay of, 146
  reference range for, 146*t*
Prostaglandin D₂, in immediate (type
    I) hypersensitivity reaction,
    72, 299, 353*g*
Protein electrophoresis, serum, in hy-
    pergammaglobulinemia,
    278–280
Protein(s)
  acute phase, 60*t*, 340*g*. *See also*
    Acute phase response;ep C-
    reactive, 59–60, 342*g*
  receptor for, in tumor immunol-
    ogy, 83*t*
  structure of, 60, 61*f*
  test for, 140*t*
  H, 57
    in amplification loop, 57*f*
    disease associated with deficiency
      of, 55*t*, 57
  I, 57
    in amplification loop, 57*f*
    disease associated with deficiency
      of, 55*t*, 57
Proteus vulgaris, in rickettsial dis-
    ease, 121, 270
  agglutination reaction and, 138
Prozone, 353*g*
Psoriasis, HLA antigens in, 16*t*
PSS. *See* Progressive systemic scle-
    rosis
Pulmonary macrophages, in pha-
    gocytosis, 49
Purified protein derivative, 78, 353*g*
Purine analogs, as immunosuppressive
    agents, 113
Purpura, idiopathic thrombocytopenic,
    and complement-mediated
    cell lysis in type II hypersen-
    sitivity reactions, 73–74
PWM. *See* Pokeweed mitogen

Q
Q fever, 267, 268

R
Rabbit syphilis, 205
Radial immunodiffusion, 126*f*,
    127–129, 353*g*
  advantages and disadvantages of,
    133*t*
  complement components measured
    by, 146–147
  immunoglobulins measured by, 279
Radiation, as immunosuppressive
    agent, 113
Radioactive labels, in ligand assays,
    171
Radioallergosorbent test, 302–303,
    353*g*
Radioimmunoassay
  complement components measured
    by, 147
  in delayed hypersensitivity, 300,
    301
  in hepatitis, 257, 258
  for HIV, 253
Radioimmunoprecipitation assay, for
    HIV, 253
Radioimmunosorbent test
  competitive, 344*g*
  in delayed hypersensitivity, 300,
    301
Radioisotope, 353*g*
Radiotherapy, for cancer, 90
Raji cells, 329
R antigens, 235
Rapid plasma reagin test, 140*t*, 211,
    353*g*
  percentage of patients reactive in,
    209*t*
  time needed for, 137
Rapid tests for infectious mono-
    nucleosis, 230
  interpretation of, 230
  principle of, 230
  procedure for, 230
  results of, 230
RAST. *See* Radioallergosorbent test
Rayleigh-Debye light scattering, 180
Rayleigh light scattering, 180
Raynaud's phenomenon, 327, 353*g*
Reaction Rate Analyzer, 184*t*
Reactive lymphocytes, 227–228, 231,
    342*g*
Reagin, 104. *See also* IgE
Reaginic antibody, 353*g*. *See also* IgE
Reagin screen test, 211, 353*g*
Receptors, sheep red blood cell
  in ALL typing, 296*t*
  on T cells, 21